'Shibley Rahman's last book in ~~his trilogy~~ ... its a comprehensive and thought-provoking tour de force through the subject matter – great reading for any health and social care professional, academic and interested lay person. Here is a perspective from an author who in himself integrates academic qualifications in medicine, law and management with a lived experience of disability. A unique read!'
– *Reinhard Guss, Chair, Faculty of the Psychology of Older People*

'Practitioners, family carers and people with dementia looking for a comprehensive resource about dementia need look no further. Few books combine detailed explanations about clinical aspects of dementia with policy analysis and yet remain so centred on people's individual experiences. This is an important resource for anyone who wants to understand more about providing better dementia support.'
– *Jo Moriarty, Senior Research Fellow, King's College London*

'An absolute gem of a book. Through his career, Shibley Raman has been sequentially academic neurologist, service user, family carer and blogging activist. His learning and wisdom have been distilled into a highly readable, comprehensively referenced and bang up-to-date companion for anyone who needs to learn and understand about people with dementia and what can be done to help them, their families and professional carers to get the very best out of life.'
– *Robert Howard, Professor of Old Age Psychiatry, University College London*

'The third of Rahman's books on issues relating to dementia. Another must-read text that discusses the many and varied elements of what is required to enhance the lives and wellbeing of people with dementia. I particularly like his style of telling us what we can expect to learn from each section and suggestions for further reading. This, as well as the first two books from the author, is an essential read for all health and social care students in gaining an overview of caring in dementia.'
– *Dr Karen Harrison Dening, Head of Research & Evaluation, Dementia UK*

'There can be no doubt that *Enhancing Health and Wellbeing in Dementia* should be essential reading for anyone with an interest in improving the lives, and rights, of people living with dementia. It is an important book which is both comprehensive and practical – no easy matter to achieve! His encyclopaedic span concludes appropriately with the primacy of person-centred approaches, the importance of dignity, quality and leadership – yes, yes, yes!'
– *Des Kelly OBE, Chair, The Centre for Policy on Ageing*

'Shibley's voice has emerged as an important one to take notice of within dementia care. His ability to draw together a huge range of knowledge from many different spheres of research, practice and policy and to use it to light our way rather than confuse us further is unique.'

– Professor Dawn Brooker, Director of the Association for Dementia Studies at the Worcester University

'This important book continues our journey of what it means to see the person beyond their diagnosis of dementia, with a fresh focus on freedom, dignity and human rights. Dr Shibley challenges the idea that nothing can be done to improve dementia care. He brings practical thinking around how we can move towards truly integrated, person-centred ways of working – making a timely and valuable contribution to our collective understanding.'

– Dr Helen Sanderson, author of Person-Centred Thinking with Older People

—— Enhancing Health and Wellbeing in Dementia ——

Enhancing Health and Wellbeing in Dementia

— A Person-Centred Integrated Care Approach —

Dr Shibley Rahman

Forewords by Professor Sube Banerjee
and Lisa Rodrigues

Afterword by Lucy Frost

Jessica Kingsley *Publishers*
London and Philadelphia

Boxes 10.3, 11.2 and 13.1 are reproduced with kind permission of the King's Fund.
Box 11.4 is reproduced by kind permission of the Royal College of Opthalmologists.
Figure 13.1 is reproduced by kind permission of the World Health Organization.

First published in 2017
by Jessica Kingsley Publishers
73 Collier Street
London N1 9BE, UK
and
400 Market Street, Suite 400
Philadelphia, PA 19106, USA

www.jkp.com

Library of Congress Cataloging in Publication Data
Names: Rahman, Shibley, author.
Title: Enhancing health and wellbeing in dementia : a person-centred integrated care approach / Dr Shibley Rahman ; foreword by Professor Sube Banerjee.
Description: London ; Philadelphia : Jessica Kingsley Publishers, 2017. | Includes bibliographical references and index.
Identifiers: LCCN 2016050890 | ISBN 9781785920370 (alk. paper)
Subjects: | MESH: Dementia--therapy | Patient-Centered Care--methods | Delivery of Health Care, Integrated--methods | Quality of Life | Social Environment | Great Britain
Classification: LCC RC521 | NLM WM 220 | DDC 362.1968/3-- dc23 LC record available at https://lccn.loc.gov/2016050890

British Library Cataloguing in Publication Data
A CIP catalogue record for this book is available from the British Library

ISBN 978 1 78592 037 0
eISBN 978 1 78450 291 1

Printed and bound in Great Britain

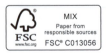

CONTENTS

FOREWORD

Sube Banerjee

Reading the manuscript of this book prompted me to reflect on where we are with dementia. We have come a very long way and very quickly. In less than a decade dementia has gone from being at the very bottom of the pile in terms of health priority to the very top. It is not only on the agenda, but at the top of the agenda, for countries across the world that have developed National Dementia Strategies, from Mexico to South Korea, and from Qatar to Uruguay. Equally, international organisations from the World Health Organization to the G7 have moved dementia from out of the shadows of inactivity into the light of action.

From modest beginnings, fuelled by the experiences of people with dementia and the family members that support them, framed by the sharp and effective advocacy of the voluntary sector Alzheimer's societies and associations worldwide, and informed by research and clinical practice in health and social care, we have crafted a narrative that has caught the imagination of the world. Like all good stories it has developed its own life. It is not now owned by those that first articulated it, it is now part of common discourse, common understanding and common sense.

Simply stated, the story is that dementia is the paramount unsolved health and social care challenge for the 21st century. It is already so common that almost every family is affected and that its cost to society is greater than that of heart disease and cancer combined. In the next generation we know that the numbers will double and the costs will at least triple. We know that there is an immense amount that can already be done to enable people to live well with dementia, but that these opportunities to prevent harms, costs and crises are more often than not missed. The narrative we have is at the point of call for action, of people seeing that dementia is everybody's business and buckling down to grow, develop and deliver the solutions needed. The story has the virtue of being true and it is not over.

It is brilliant and astonishing that we have come so far, so fast. But such rapid progress has consequences. Other health priorities have been built on decades of research and experience, which means that the arguments for assessments and interventions made are strong and well rooted. It means that services are well founded and generally available. In dementia we have not got the deep evidential roots that those working on other conditions, such as heart disease and cancer, have built carefully over the past 50 years. This is understandable when the stakes are so high, the needs are so great and the opportunity is open. However, what this means is that there remain important gaps in the evidence base for the provision of care and services in dementia. For example, we do not have definitive models of how and by whom diagnostic services should be provided and we do not have accepted models and standards for post-diagnostic care. We do not have consensus about what can and should be done in primary care, in secondary care, in social care and by the families and the voluntary sector. Mao Zedong stated, 'The policy of letting a hundred flowers bloom and a hundred schools of thought contend is designed to promote the flourishing of the arts and the progress of science.' In the provision of services for people with dementia we are at the stage of 'a hundred flowers' blooming with as many models of care as there are Clinical Commissioning Groups. While some of the flowers may be wonderful, some are likely to be frankly poisonous and we do not know which is which at the moment. We need to identify where we have needs for more information and secure the data. We need to use those insights to move rapidly to consolidate our service models so that we can generate a clear and simple promise for people with dementia and their families that details what they can expect from services and what they will receive.

This is a complex and difficult journey and Dr Rahman's book is like having an informed, interested, intelligent and profoundly humane friend by your side on the journey through. This book is a friend who is encyclopaedic in knowledge and who is not afraid to have opinions and to express them. We are part-way along the journey; we have come a long way but we have far to go. This book helps us reflect on where we are and the road we have travelled, all the better to plan and travel the road ahead.

Sube Banerjee,
Professor of Dementia,
Brighton and Sussex Medical School

FOREWORD

Lisa Rodrigues

I remember meeting my first patient with a diagnosis of dementia when I was a student nurse. There was a wildness in her eyes that I didn't like; I was frightened by her and what she might do. Slowly I came to recognise that what I saw there was not aggression, but a terror far greater than my own. And which of us would not have been terrified, locked up in a place we didn't recognise, surrounded by strangers and unable to understand what was going on or to articulate how we felt?

I have now reached the stage in life when elderly relatives and the parents of friends are experiencing some of the terror that I saw in that lady's eyes all those years ago. Things are of course better now for people who are diagnosed with one of the causes of dementia than they were in the 1970s. Awareness has increased and the stigma has reduced. And for some, there are treatments that slow the disease process. But things could be a lot better still.

And that is what this meticulously researched, extremely polite but nonetheless challenging book is about. My good friend Dr Shibley Rahman sets out what is best practice in language and attitude as well as care and support. He writes with great authority and humility about what people who have dementia, and their loved ones, face and how we could all do a great deal more to help them.

I can hear Shibley speaking as he reminds us that dementia seldom travels alone, and that it is not in any way true, despite what people are often told, that nothing can be done to help those who experience its effects.

When I was a chief executive running mental health services in Sussex, I also played a number of national roles. I recall being at 10 Downing Street for the launch of the coalition government's Dementia Strategy. There was talk about more and better diagnosis and more money for research. It was an uphill struggle to deliver even a fraction of this, when the money was getting ever tighter and commissioners had no choice but to hope that it could all be dealt with in primary care with no extra resources. But if you had a serious brain disease, you would want a scan and the right diagnosis, wouldn't you? And to be followed up by someone who knew not only the theory about your disease but, given there is currently no cure, also had some practical ways to support you?

I have had a number of conversations recently with friends about the cruelty of dementia. The long lives many people are now living have increased the incidence. And if we are not careful, as Shibley gently but persuasively suggests we should be, it can rob people of their freedom and their dignity. And not just in the loss of privacy around intimate tasks, but also in volition about how to spend one's time. We all need something meaningful to do with which to fill the days. People with dementia become easily bored. But one man's joy at community singing is hell for someone who hates music and wants to go out walking, if only all the doors were not locked.

This is a wonderful book, for students, health professionals, researchers, policy makers, politicians and families, and for people who may be in the early stages of one of the diseases that causes dementia.

This is a book that challenges but also gives hope. Which I think is the greatest gift of all.

Lisa Rodrigues, CBE, writer, coach and mental health
campaigner, www.LisaSaysThis.com

ACKNOWLEDGEMENTS

It is my great pleasure to dedicate this book to two people. First, I am grateful to Prof Martin Rossor. I worked for him in 2002 as a junior at the National Hospital for Neurology and Neurosurgery, Queen Square, London. His contribution to clinical care and research in dementia has been exceptional. Second, I would like to give special thanks to Prof Dawn Brooker. Although I have never worked for Prof Brooker, her contribution to personhood and dementia has been remarkable up against the reality of the NHS, and she has inspired many leaders within the field of international dementia work.

I would like to thank especially Prof Sube Banerjee and Lisa Rodrigues for kindly writing forewords for this book, and Lucy Frost for the afterword. A very special mention of Kate Swaffer and of the contributions from Dementia Alliance International. I hold them both in the highest regard. Finally, tremendous thanks to Chris Roberts for giving me the idea to write this book, my third.

The author and publishers are grateful to the National Institute for Health and Care Excellence (NICE) for help with this text. The author should like to confirm that in no way does inclusion of the NICE material confirm any approval or endorsement of the present text by NICE. Functional hyperlinks to the material, correct at the time of press, are given in the main body of the text. NICE guidance is prepared for the National Health Service in England. All NICE guidance is subject to regular review and may be updated or withdrawn at any time.

PREFACE

More of us living longer will mean more of us developing dementia, as we know the risk of developing it increases with age. There are over a hundred forms of dementia, of which Alzheimer's (more correctly a syndrome) is one. All are common and you're pretty likely, at the very least, to know someone who knows someone with dementia. If current trends continue and no action is taken, the number of people with dementia in the UK is predicted to increase to 1,142,677 by 2025, and to 2,092,945 by 2051, an increase of 40% over the next 12 years or 156% over the next 38 years (Alzheimer's Society, 2014). Disclosing a diagnosis of dementia may sometimes seem as though the 'professional' least wants to talk about it, whereas the patient wants to find out just as much as they can. Dementia is not just a condition of old age, however. At one level, all dementias are conditions of the brain – chronic, progressive conditions which worsen. There are symptomatic treatments, often very limited in time and scope, but sometimes worth a try. Disclosing a diagnosis is never just to one person – or at least it shouldn't. Those close to the patient will often be involved, and they will have hopes, worries and expectations about the future. Reversing the false belief that all people with dementia are in 'advanced stages' has not been easy – and all credit is due to those who have worked towards this.

Nonetheless, there are reasons to be cheerful. We know a lot more about the science of dementia. Many more of us are living beyond young or middle aged. In addition, the political spotlight has recently been shone on dementia, but such scrutiny must be accompanied by responsibility. For some, however, the diagnosis of dementia can come as a devastating shock as society has conditioned us to fear this condition even more than diseases such as cancer, where there has been marked medical progress.

Dementia, perhaps more than any other medical condition, is profoundly human and it is important to see the person beyond the diagnosis. Dementia never travels alone, and it's not uncommon for a patient to be living with multiple conditions, such as lung disease or heart failure. This means that dementia is complex. There are strong reasons why a new national strategy for dementia must be rigorously pursued, as the previous strategy expired in 2014 after five years. We also need to renew our contract not only with the growing number of people with dementia in the UK, but also with the huge army of carers, both paid and unpaid. Without unpaid family carers, the system would implode, so preserving their health and ability to cope is essential. We have reached a tipping point in care where the demand from older people needing care will outstrip family members able to meet that need. This care gap is expected to increase rapidly over the next two decades (Pickard, 2015).

It is essential for us to be able to diagnose the type of dementia accurately and to have the skills to do so no matter the setting. The distinctions between primary and secondary care are becoming increasingly blurred as we progress, albeit at a snail's pace, towards integration. Medical professionals know not to give certain drugs in certain types of dementia to avoid making things worse. But much more importantly, the attitude of 'nothing can be done' must be turned around; if a person has complex visuospatial problems following a dementia such as posterior cortical atrophy, occupational therapists should attend to their needs. Similarly, if a person has complex linguistic problems following a dementia such as primary non-fluent progressive aphasia, that person may need a speech and language therapist. If a person is prone to eating sweet food and drink during progression of dementia, they should have a dietician's input. If a person develops problems in their movement or gait following a dementia, they should see a physiotherapist. The enablement narrative which is emerging puts to full use the skills base of the allied health professionals, and this expertise is much needed in the anticipation of care needs, or care planning, so life can be lived to the full and unnecessary hospital admissions can be avoided.

A national strategy in the UK, where people with dementia and their carers get the right help, in the right place and at the right time, would show that we as a society wish to promote wellbeing as well as quality of care, from diagnosis to beyond death, wherever that may be, for example at home, in hospital and in a care home or hospice. The complexity of living with dementia means that it is no longer reasonable for people to 'blame' people with dementia, writing off those who are distressed due to a combination of pain and communication difficulties as 'challenging' – or people with dementia who talk round a subject as 'confabulating' – or people who are not engaged in environments promoting contentment as 'agitated'. Dementia-friendly care is much more than the décor and colour scheme of buildings – in a nutshell, dementia-friendly care puts personhood first.

A national strategy for dementia would represent an endorsement of a long-term planning commitment by society to valuing people who have contributed much to society. It is said that Ronald Reagan, even with advanced dementia, used to enjoy reminiscing about skills he used at work in his 20s. As dementia 'never travels alone' and comorbidity is a norm rather than an exception, the national infrastructure has to be fit for purpose. Generalists and specialists in the workforce need to build on the great work which has been done in raising awareness, for example by ground-breaking initiatives such as Dementia Friends. There also needs to be a shift in ethos, such as not dosing up people inappropriately in care homes with antipsychotic drugs, a greater readiness for advance care planning, access to key components such as legal advice or appropriate housing, and a willingness to engage with palliative approaches or end-of-life care when that time comes. The infrastructure must also accept some unpalatable truths – we may not be able to provide for the complex needs of residents in care homes when other solutions might be more appropriate, such as community nursing or hospital at home. A more timely diagnosis will mean that there will be more people than ever before living while knowing their diagnosis of dementia. This implies a greater responsibility for signposting knowledge and information beyond 'silos' to encourage, wherever possible, independent living. This ethos – in keeping with the regulatory codes for the NHS and social care – must fulfil essential safeguarding and safety obligations by professionals, ensuring care is not delayed and that health needs are not simply ignored. There needs to be a political, social, economic, legal, technological and financial commitment to this renewed dementia strategy, with integration at its centre.

The narrative has undoubtedly changed in other ways. The link between dementia and disability is much clearer in people's minds, as are the fundamental human rights of people living with dementia (and reciprocal ones from carers) impacting on all aspects, such as diagnosis and care and support, both formal and informal. Thanks to this greater definition, it is hoped there will be greater respect and dignity and a stronger sense of solidarity, reciprocity and citizenship. Research and service provision can no longer be 'done to' people with dementia and their closest ones.

Choice and control can only exist if the necessary resources are in place in the system. We are lucky in the UK in not being a low-income country. Nonetheless, we should be on our guard against inequality, the social determinant of health. Knowledge is power. We know the numbers of people living with dementia are increasing. We know this could need more resources. We know there's a benefit from timely diagnosis. We know there is an obligation for high quality of life and quality of care for all involved.

Above all, a renewed settlement for dementia is needed nationally, with integration at the very heart of it.

The dementia umbrella

I will return to a number of themes in this book to explain what some 'essentials' of good care look like in **integrated, person-centred dementia care**.

The bottom line is that every person with dementia and their carers are entitled to the highest standards in such care.

I would now like to introduce how the key features of integrated person-centred care can be imagined as covering spokes in an umbrella of integrated care.

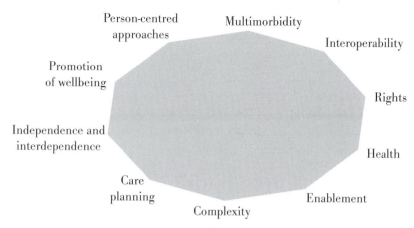

Figure P.1: The dementia 'umbrella'

A description of the key spokes is given in the text: they are multimorbidity, interoperability, rights, health, enablement, complexity, care planning, independence and interdependence, promotion of wellbeing, and person-centred approaches.

These ten spokes are:

Multimorbidity

Dementia rarely travels alone. If diagnosed with dementia, one is likely to be living with several other conditions. It is becoming important to see people beyond the disease. The whole is greater than the sum of its constituent parts. Note that in this book, the terms **comorbidity** and **multiple morbidity** are used interchangeably.

Interoperability

At its most primitive level, this means data can be free flowing between different parts of the system, such as the care home and health and social care. But it probably means more than this: that is, being able to talk the same language of dementia care, whatever the precise operating system is (health care, social care or elsewhere).

Rights

Rights allow one to do something or not to have to do something. Rights are complementary, so it is not possible to talk of the rights of persons with dementia in isolation. They must always be described mutually within the context of someone else's rights (e.g. a carer's precise needs and rights can never be assumed to be exactly the same as those of persons with dementia, and vice versa). Universal human rights are inalienable, and indeed are pervasive in dementia care in a number of guises – for example, the use of video surveillance in care homes or citizenship. However, while legal instruments define some rights, the basis of a 'rights-based consciousness' is much wider and includes moral rights.

Health

Irrespective of care setting, a person with dementia always fundamentally has a right to health. This can be enabled or compromised by health care systems.

Enablement

Like reasonable adjustments for physical disability, enablement conveys the notion that there are ways to help people with dementia with particular difficulties (e.g. memory) by improving quality of life, health and independence. This is a different approach to the biomedical one, which is focused on improvement of symptoms and 'cures'.

Complexity

Dementia is complex. Dementia itself is the umbrella term for more than a hundred conditions, all with distinct presentations, and each individual presenting with a dementia is unique. Catering for any needs of persons with dementia and their nearest needs to acknowledge the complexity of the relationships between different people and organisations. A system is also needed which can make sense out of what might appear at first sight to be chaos.

Care planning

Any journey you make requires you to go from A to B, but planning that journey not only involves some idea of where you might be going but also what you'll need to travel successfully. Care planning is no different, and care pathways must never be so rigid (signposting to non-existent services, for example) as to be useless. Nobody should be left behind in care planning, which means that a minimal requirement might involve participation by the person living with dementia, carers and relevant professionals.

Independence and interdependence

The ideal would be for the person with dementia to 'take control', but suitable tools are needed for this, such as bespoke genomics information, information about care and services, budgets, etc. However, the paradox is that it is impossible to do things alone because of the complexity of the system the principal actors are involved in and their high interdependence.

Promotion of wellbeing

The Care Act (section 1(1)) imposes a statutory duty to 'promote wellbeing', but this may, depending on your perspective, include promoting physical health primarily.

Take, for example, the New Economics Foundation in a discussion of measuring wellbeing (Thompson and Marks, 2008, p.8):

> A cursory glance at the range of policy initiatives referencing wellbeing illustrates what has often been regarded as a difficulty with the concept: namely, its very broad application. In the context of health discourse, for instance, wellbeing is often used as an umbrella term covering a range of positive health behaviours, and is thus understood primarily as a state of good physical health that can be improved by engaging in particular behaviours.

More recently, some psychologists and social scientists have co-opted the term to refer exclusively to subjective aspects of life. (In this view, external factors including physical health and material circumstances may play a role in determining whether a state of wellbeing will emerge, but they are not equivalent to it. Indeed, part of the research agenda has been concerned with attempting to identify just how much of the variability in subjective wellbeing can be attributed to external circumstances relative to factors such as personality, behaviour, attitudes and aspects of the early environment including genetic factors.)

Wellbeing is thus the interplay of a person with their own environment, and this is at the heart of Kitwood's work on the environment. Under such a wide definition, wellbeing can be ameliorated by having one's physical health promoted (though it is worth noting that wellness is not the absence of illness), as well as being involved in certain meaningful activities, such as singing or the theatre.

Person-centred approaches

Personhood is at the heart of this book, and my conclusion (Chapter 14) will attempt to reconcile personhood with other approaches, such as human rights and the biomedical model. Concentrating on a person does not mean, of course, not concentrating on friends, family or other important relationships.

—— How to use this book ——

In addition to using this book as a resource, you are also advised to consult www. evidence.nhs.uk, which offers access to a number of useful sources of clinical evidence. Online medical journals are also an excellent source of peer-reviewed research, such as the *British Medical Journal*, *The Lancet* and *Dementia – The International Journal of Social Research and Practice.* You are also strongly recommended to become familiar with the output of the King's Fund, the Royal Colleges, NHS England and the Care Quality Commission, which have all produced interesting contributions in this field.

You are requested not to take any of this book as professional advice, and you are strongly encouraged to examine the original sources which I have cited. I apologise for any errors I have made in representing my colleagues' arguments. I have tried to represent all published work as accurately as possible to the best of my knowledge.

Also, please take time to listen to the views and opinions of people with dementia and their closest ones, including carers.

—— About this book ——————————————————

This is not a manual on any of the aspects of the provision of care, such as how to 'serve up' activities in a care home. There are very good books for that. Nor is it a book all about care homes, and it is definitely not a book offering any clinical advice. It is, however, I hope, a timely and constructive discussion of some fundamental issues to do with dementia, health and wellbeing.

This book brings different strands in dementia research up to date. It coincides with the publication of the new NICE guidance entitled 'Assessment, Management and Support for People Living with Dementia and Their Carers' to be published in November 2017, as well as publication of the 'Dementia Core Skills Education and Training Framework'. Taking account of relevant Cochrane reviews, it is a comprehensive, evidence-based synthesis of the importance of a person-centred integrated approach, and it discusses how integrated care pathways might facilitate this. It is sometimes forgotten that a fundamental right to health underpins wellbeing across all settings, including care homes, nursing homes, at home and in hospices, but it is also often forgotten that physical health is an important component of wellbeing. This book therefore covers a diverse range of topics including mental health in care homes, meaningful activities in residential settings, the whole health and social care ecosystem (including getting into and out of hospital in a timely manner), as well as enablement through targeted support. Key themes such as dignity in health, care and wellbeing straddle key strands in personhood, human rights and the biomedical approach, and these themes are of critical prominence in service improvement through research, regulation and the nurturing of staff. The book will be of help to people living with dementia, carers, dementia leaders, care home managers, commissioners, policy directors, professionals, practitioners and academics, as well as interested members of the public.

Dr Shibley Rahman
London

—— Essential reading ——————————————

Department of Health. 2015. Dementia Core Skills Education and Training Framework, available at www.skillsforhealth.org.uk/images/projects/dementia/Dementia%20Core%20Skills%20 Education%20and%20Training%20Framework.pdf?s=cw1 (accessed 23 Sept 2016).

Kitwood T. 1997. *Dementia Reconsidered*, Buckingham: Open University Press.

—— References ——————————————————

Alzheimer's Society. 2014. *Dementia 2014*, London: Alzheimer's Society.

Pickard L. 2015. A growing care gap? The supply of unpaid care for older people by their adult children in England to 2032. Ageing and Society, 35(1), 96–123.

Thompson S., Marks N, 2008. *Measuring Wellbeing in Policy: Issues and Applications*. London: New Economics Foundation, available at b.3cdn.net/nefoundation/575659b4f333001669_ohm6iiogp. pdf (accessed 23 Sept 2016).

Chapter 1

PREVENTING AND DIAGNOSING WELL

People are a rich tapestry of needs and preferences, hurts and fears, doubts and insecurities, strengths and weaknesses, likes and dislikes, emotions and habits. (Stokes and Goudie, 2002, p.59)

Learning objectives

At the end of this chapter you should:

» have a general awareness of the economic context of dementia

» be able to define prevalence and incidence

» be able to describe the key features of the common types of dementia

» have been introduced to the concept of the care pathway and integration as a way for persons with dementia and carers to live better after diagnosis

» have some awareness of barriers to integration

» understand some common triggers for crises and 'institutionalisation'

» appreciate some of the current issues concerning diagnosis in primary care

» understand the current reasoning behind the use of cognitive enhancers

» have been introduced to recent developments in policy relevant to service provision in dementia, including new models of care and devolution of powers

» understand the importance of non-communicable diseases, prevention and risk reduction strategies, and be cognisant of the current evidence recommendations

» know how to begin to evaluate critically the notion of quality of life (QoL) with an appreciation of the critical importance of personhood and the uniqueness of individuals

—— Introduction ————————————————

Worldwide, 44 million people live with dementia. This figure is expected to reach 135 million by 2050. Meanwhile, in 2010 the cost of care reached an estimated $604 billion worldwide, equivalent to 1% of global gross domestic product. Costs are expected to exceed $1 trillion annually in the US alone by 2050 (WISH, 2015).

This chapter will evaluate how we got to where we are, against a backdrop of economics and markets. How the initial diagnosis is made, as well as where and when, is of considerable interest not only to England but also to other jurisdictions. The development of care pathways from timely diagnosis to end of life (EoL) can seem curiously ill-defined by English policy.

The main different types of dementia are below (see Box 1.1).

Box 1.1: Common types of dementia

ALZHEIMER'S DISEASE

* This is the most common cause of dementia.

* Its occurrence is likely to be due to a combination of genetic inheritance, environmental effects and overall health (among other factors).

* There are some common symptoms of Alzheimer's disease, but it is important to remember that everyone is unique.

* Clumps of protein, known as *plaques* and *tangles*, gradually form in the brain. They are thought to be responsible for the increasing loss of brain cells.

For most people with Alzheimer's, the earliest symptoms are memory lapses, difficulty remembering recent conversations, forgetting appointments and taking longer to do routine tasks.

These symptoms occur because the early damage in Alzheimer's is usually to a part of the brain called the hippocampus (and the immediately surrounding areas), which has a central role in day-to-day learning and memory.

Alzheimer's disease can be either sporadic or familial:

* Sporadic Alzheimer's disease can affect adults at any age, but usually occurs after age 65 and is the most common form of Alzheimer's disease.

* Familial Alzheimer's disease is a very rare genetic condition, caused by a mutation in one of several genes. The presence of mutated genes means that the person will eventually develop Alzheimer's disease, usually in their 40s or 50s.

MIXED DEMENTIA

An estimated 10% of people with dementia have more than one type at the same time. This is called mixed dementia. The most common combination is Alzheimer's disease with vascular dementia (caused by problems with the blood supply to the brain). The symptoms of this kind of mixed dementia are a mixture of the symptoms of Alzheimer's disease and vascular dementia.

POSTERIOR CORTICAL ATROPHY

Posterior cortical atrophy (PCA) occurs when there is damage to areas at the back and upper-rear of the brain. These are areas that process complex visual information and deal with spatial awareness. This means that the early symptoms of PCA are often problems identifying objects or reading, even if the eyes are healthy. People with this type of dementia are often seen at great length by opticians before a referral is made to cognitive clinic.

FRONTOTEMPORAL DEMENTIA

Typical symptoms include changes in personality and behaviour and difficulty with language.

In an estimated 20% of cases, people who develop frontotemporal dementia (FTD) have inherited a genetic mutation from their parents.

A person with behavioural variant FTD may:

* become disinhibited – behave in socially inappropriate ways and act in an impulsive or rash manner

* lose interest in people and things (apathy) – lose motivation, but (unlike someone with depression) they are not sad.

The following are also common:

* A person with the temporal variant is most likely to have language difficulties.

* In semantic dementia, the ability to assign meaning to words is gradually lost. Reading, spelling, comprehension and expression are usually affected.

* People with progressive non-fluent aphasia (PNFA) have difficulty communicating due to slow and difficult production of words, distortion of speech and a tendency to produce the wrong word.

DEMENTIA WITH LEWY BODIES

Dementia with Lewy bodies (DLB) could account for about 10% of cases of dementia.

Lewy bodies are small, circular lumps of protein that develop inside brain cells. It is not known what causes them. It is also unclear how they damage the brain and cause dementia.

Common symptoms:

* Lewy bodies in the outer layers of the brain are linked to problems with mental abilities (cognitive symptoms), a feature of DLB

* memory loss and attentional difficulties

* sleep disturbances

* well-formed visual hallucinations (seeing things that are not there, e.g. people or animals, and are detailed and convincing to the person with dementia).

Lewy bodies at the base of the brain are closely linked to problems with movement (motor symptoms):

* slowness

* gait imbalance or slow and stiff (rigid) movement with a blank facial expression.

VASCULAR DEMENTIA

This form of dementia is caused specifically by problems with blood supply to the brain, such as suffering a stroke.

Diabetes, heart disease and high cholesterol and blood pressure can also contribute to the onset of vascular dementia.

Multi-infarct dementia is likely to be the most common type of vascular dementia, caused by a number of strokes, often with symptoms that develop progressively over a period of time. The strokes cause damage to the cortex of the brain, the area associated with learning, memory and language. A person with multi-infarct dementia is likely to have better insight in the early stages than people with Alzheimer's disease, and parts of their personality may remain relatively intact for longer.

INVESTIGATIONS

The clinical diagnosis might include:

* a detailed medical history from the person with dementia and someone close

* a thorough physical and neurological examination

* psychiatric assessment

* cognitive neuropsychological tests

* blood and urine tests (blood tests rarely contribute to the diagnosis but are needed to rule out underlying pathology and are necessary for Quality and Outcomes Framework (QOF) reporting (NHS England, 2015a))

* neuroimaging (e.g. MRI, PET, SPECT) (brain scans (CT or MRI) are *not* essential for a clinical diagnosis of dementia. If a scan is justified, detailed clinical information is crucial for the radiologist (NHS England, 2015a))

* lumbar puncture for cerebrospinal fluid tests (often, currently, a research tool)

* EEG (for rarer diagnoses).

RECOMMENDED READING

See NHS England (2015a).

———— Business, economics and markets ————

Tulloch (2005), in referring to Sydenham's philosophy, argues that the role of doctors is to identify and manage people with diseases who present to them. It is expected that the number of people with dementia will rise from 2001 to 2040 by 80–190% in Europe, North America and the developed Western Pacific region, while in Latin America, India, China, North Africa and the Middle Crescent a steep increase of more than 300% is forecast (Hampel et al., 2011).

Statistics vary, but the consequences are important. As Sube Banerjee has stated: 'At a political level, the nature of the problem must become clear at a national level, for the need for policy and action to be recognized' (Banerjee, 2012, p.707). Overall, the increase in life expectancy is to be welcomed, but the risk of developing dementia increases as one gets older. It is thought that 23% of the **global burden of disease** arises in older people. The hypothesised breakdown of this is interesting (nearly half the burden is in high-income countries) (Prince et al., 2015).

The overall costs for health and social care for dementia in the UK are eye-watering (see Figure 1.1).

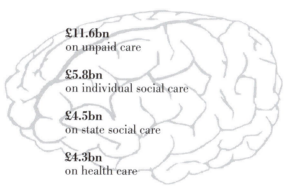

£11.6bn
on unpaid care

£5.8bn
on individual social care

£4.5bn
on state social care

£4.3bn
on health care

£100 million on other costs

Figure 1.1: Costs and care
Source: redrawn from Public Health England (2016).

It is widely known that, despite reassurances of maintained spending in the UK in recent years, the situation for the NHS and social care is precarious. There is of course the additional consideration that more timely diagnosis of dementia might stoke demand for care services (Hampel et al., 2011). Roberts and colleagues (2015), in an influential report entitled 'Filling the Gap: Tax and Fiscal Options for a Sustainable UK Health and Social Care System', comment that there is likely to be a gap between the available health budget and the funding required to maintain the quality and range of services. This gap is estimated to be £2bn by 2020/1, rising to £9bn by 2030/1 (Roberts et al., 2015, p.9). In November 2015, *The Guardian* drew attention to a letter from 15 social care and older people's groups writing about the potential closure of up to half of Britain's care homes unless the funding gap were closed (Campbell, 2015). Unsurprisingly, an urgent debate on how to organise and fund existing and future dementia care services has been called for, in an influential piece in *The Lancet* in March 2015. The piece was entitled 'Dementia: Turning Fine Aspirations into Measurable Progress' (no authors listed, 2015, p.1151).

The discussion about the economics of dementia remains heavily biased towards a narrative of 'costs' and 'burden', rather than value. As a dementia progresses, the cost in health care tends to increase (Caravau and Martin, 2015). Sandra Schaller and colleagues (Schaller et al., 2015) have found that overall the major cost drivers were, rather surprisingly, 'informal costs', including home-based long-term care and nursing home expenditure, rather than direct medical costs (including medication and inpatient and outpatient services). The costs of care in all jurisdictions are important. Epidemiological evidence is crucial for policymakers if we are to arrive at a balanced judgement on the relative resource allocations for cure, care, living well and prevention (for an excellent article on this, see Wu et al., 2016).

Memory services were originally designed to enable a timely intervention in dementia, addressing the issue that only one-third of people had received a formal diagnosis, or had any contact with specialist services during the course of the dementia (Banerjee, 2012). Banerjee and Wittenberg (2009) had previously modelled the impact of the national provision of memory services in preventing admissions to care homes. One of the most striking findings of their modelling was that the memory services for timely diagnosis and intervention for dementia need only achieve a modest increase in average QoL for people with dementia, plus a 10% diversion of people with dementia from residential care, to be held to be cost-effective. The cost-effectiveness of these services continues to be a burning issue more than ever since previous seminal work (e.g. Banerjee et al., 2009).

The overall approach to key questions for decision-makers in the economics of dementia can be summarised as follows (McCrone, 2008).

» What is the overall economic cost of dementia?

» Are interventions to treat dementia cost-saving (i.e. do they save resources now or in the future)?

» Are these interventions cost-effective (i.e. do extra benefits justify any extra costs)?

A fundamental problem is that advances in medicines, biotechnologies and population growth can lead to high-cost services and goods, and this places enormous pressure on the scarce resources of public funds (McHugh et al., 2015). Marmor and Oberlander (2012) stated that the United States not only has the most expensive health care system in the world by a long margin (based on data going up to 2009), but appeared to be also singularly unsuccessful at controlling health care spending. As a way of controlling costs, the overall trend has been for many developed countries to move away from institutional care and towards home care where possible, and this requires the rewiring of the logistics of the supply chain in management (Archer, Bajaj and Zhang, 2008).

Care pathways

As a dementia progresses, a person living with it will have different needs, and require different types of help. But likewise, it would be wrong to offer an unreasonable level of certainty as 'what to expect now' following a diagnosis of dementia.

In a policy paper, entitled 'Dementia: Post-Diagnostic Care and Support', the UK government set out the general gist of their plans (Department of Health, 2016), building on a consensus between some principal stakeholders. Accordingly, for England, once a person with dementia has received a diagnosis, it is essential that they get appropriate post-diagnostic care. This is needed to ensure that people living with the effects of dementia and their families and carers have the right information and support so they can live as fulfilling lives as possible, prepare for the future and that their preferences for EoL are acted upon.

Care pathways, also known as clinical pathways, critical pathways or integrated care pathways, are used all over the world. Patient safety, quality of care and efficiency of health care procedures are international phenomena (Vanhaecht et al., 2010). They originate from industrial processes and were introduced in health care in the early 1980s internationally (Kinsman et al., 2010). In response to this complex challenge, the European Pathway Association adapted the definition as suggested in Vanhaecht, De Witte and Sermeus (2007), and nowadays define a care pathway as: 'A complex intervention for the mutual decision-making and organization of predictable care for a well-defined group of patients during a well-defined period' (Vanhaecht et al., 2010). A good example of the importance of care pathways is the identification of distinguishing features of the approach to care. The integrated cancer care pathways, established in 2009, were based on previously established multidisciplinary guidelines for doctors, nurses and other professionals (Schrijvers, van Hoorn and Huiskes, 2012). Such pathways make the vital relevance of key personnel, such as clinical nursing specialists, crystal clear.

I will provide a final discussion, in light of the subsequent chapters, of the complexity in integrated care pathways in Chapter 14.

There are key defining characteristics of pathways (see Box 1.2).

Box 1.2: Defining characteristics of pathways

* An explicit statement of the goals and key elements of care based on evidence.

* Best practice and patient expectations.

* The facilitation of the communication and coordination of roles, and sequencing the activities of the multidisciplinary care team, patients and their relatives.

* The documentation, monitoring and evaluation of variances and outcomes, and the identification of relevant resources.

SOURCE: BASED ON VANHAECHT ET AL. (2010).

Dementia is particularly complicated because of the dynamics of the people involved in a dementia diagnosis. The disclosure of a diagnosis of dementia has a significant impact on both the individuals with dementia and their families, and spouses have to adjust to increasingly unequal relationships (Bunn et al., 2012). There has been a global push towards the timely diagnosis of dementia, but there is relatively little understanding of the care transitions along the assessment and diagnostic pathway from the perspective of people affected by cognitive impairments, including dementia. In one recent study, feelings of confusion, uncertainty and anxiety about interminable waiting times have dominated (Samsi et al., 2014). There is, notwithstanding, a considerable consensus on the aims of care pathways.

It is acknowledged that care pathways should recognise the individuality and capabilities of each service user and ensure that they are treated with dignity and respect, and help the person with dementia understand and manage their illness and enhance their strengths. The aim of asset-based practice is to promote and strengthen the factors that support good health and wellbeing, protect against poor health and foster communities and networks that sustain health. A health asset is 'any factor or resource which enhances the ability of individuals and communities to maintain and sustain health and wellbeing' (Hopkins and Rippon, 2015, p.3). Care pathways, furthermore, should also have a dual aim of helping all carers, including informal carers, to continue caring for as long as practical, and have a rehabilitative emphasis to help people with dementia have the best QoL possible within the limitations of their illness.

This book has six themes, broadly ranging from 'preventing well' to 'dying well and bereavement' (see Figure 1.2).

Preventing well
Diagnosing well
Living well
Caring well
Supporting well
Dying well and bereavement

Figure 1.2: Six themes

Preventing well

The NICE 'Dementia overview'[1] details a clear pathway which covers supporting people with dementia and their carers in health and social care. It is drawn from a number of other NICE sources (see 'Essential reading'). The section on 'risk factors and prevention' (section 3) provides guidance on risk factors, genetic counselling and prevention.

Diagnosing well

This is considered later in this chapter.

The NICE 'Dementia overview'[2] provides guidance on diagnosing well, in sections on 'early identification', including groups of persons considered to be at high or increased high risk, follow-up for persons identified as having mild cognitive impairment, and 'diagnosis and assessment' (sections 4 and 5).

In the Department of Health's document 'Dementia: A State of the Nation Report on Dementia Care and Support in England' from November 2013 it says: 'Timely diagnosis of dementia really matters. It is the key to helping people with dementia, their families and carers get the support they need, to plan for the future and to make informed choices about how they would like to be cared for' (p.4).

As a starting point, 'Dementia Diagnosis and Management: A Brief Pragmatic Resource for General Practitioners' (NHS England, 2015a) is extremely helpful.

Living well, caring well and supporting well

'The Dementia Guide: Living Well after Diagnosis' from the Alzheimer's Society is an excellent guide for anyone who has been recently told they have dementia.

---

1   Available at https://pathways.nice.org.uk/pathways/dementia (accessed 28 Oct 2016).
2   Available at https://pathways.nice.org.uk/pathways/dementia (accessed 28 Oct 2016).

It includes useful tips about living well, planning ahead, services for people with dementia, support for carers and research.

NICE has published various quality standards relevant to providing support to people with dementia, including the assessment and personalised care plan, reviewing needs and preferences, physical and mental health and wellbeing, and independent advocacy.[3]

Examples of post-diagnosis help and support might include:

» information about available services and sources of support

» a facilitator to provide easy access to appropriate care and advice

» an allied health professional or practitioner to enable and protect patients and carers (e.g. social worker, physiotherapist, occupational therapist) (also for people living with minimal cognitive impairment)

» a clinical nursing specialist for expertise in care (including palliative approaches and end of life) and support enabling continuity of care

» peer support.

Community services are especially important, for example, including help with housing issues, day services/day opportunities, short breaks/respite care, crisis response/rapid response assistance, household aids and adaptations, and assistive technology. The Dementia Roadmap provides high-quality information about the dementia journey alongside local information about services, support groups and care pathways to assist primary care staff to more effectively support people with dementia and cognitive impairment, and their families and carers.[4] Produced in collaboration with the Alzheimer's Society and funded by the Department of Health, the Dementia Roadmap was introduced as a platform to help Clinical Commissioning Groups (CCGs) and other local organisations to bring together information for patients in their area for the first time, so that GPs can refer them to the best care to meet their needs as quickly as possible (Royal College of General Practitioners, 2014).

Coordination of care with integrated care plans as key

The NICE 'Dementia overview'[5] in section 9 (promoting independence and maintaining function) includes recommendations on what care plans should address, including essential components, and makes reference to relevant NICE quality standards.

---

3   Available at pathways.nice.org.uk/pathways/dementia#content=view-info-category%3Aview-quality-standards-menu (accessed 3 Oct 2016).
4   Available at dementiaroadmap.info (accessed 3 Oct 2016).
5   Available at https://pathways.nice.org.uk/pathways/dementia (accessed 28 Oct 2016).

A helpful overview of care and support plans is provided on the NHS Choices webpage.

Dementia-friendly communities are a contribution to this aspect of policy, but also acute clinical services need to interface seamlessly with other areas of the health care ecosystem, including residential homes (care homes and nursing homes) and primary care. The efficacy of getting patients in and out of hospital depends on the state of the social care services.

The House of Care (see Figure 1.3) has been very influential here:

> The House of Care is a coordinated delivery system for personalised care and support planning for people with LTCs [long-term conditions]. The 'house' acts as a checklist to help practices think about how they can adapt their whole system and all its components to enhance the health and wellbeing of people with LTCs. This requires the engagement and commitment of multiple partners and sectors, including NHS providers, social care, and public health and other local government stakeholders. (Taylor, 2015)

The rest of this book is about caring and supporting well, as well as living well, in care homes, hospices, hospitals and at home.

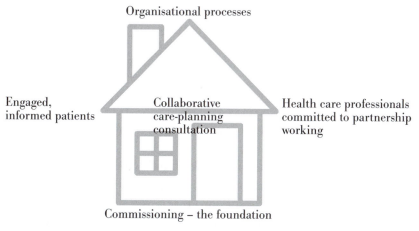

Figure 1.3: House of Care

Source: from Taylor (2015, Fig. 1, p.4).

Dying well and bereavement

It is argued that much of the preparation for bereavement should be as the person with dementia and their closest ones come to grips with the transition from living well with a long-term condition to preparing for a good death. This is discussed in full in Chapter 12.

—— Crises and institutionalisation ——

It has long been of interest what the exact prevalence of people living with dementia living in residential homes is, as national standards pertain to the health and wellbeing of residents (Matthews and Dening, 2002).

At this point, it is worth reviewing the definitions of **prevalence** and **incidence** (see Figure 1.4).

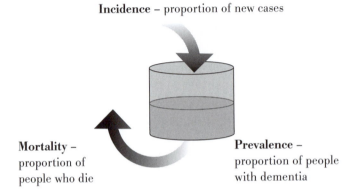

Incidence – proportion of new cases

Mortality – proportion of people who die

Prevalence – proportion of people with dementia

Figure 1.4: Prevalence and incidence

In this model, if we assume that occurrence of new cases (incidence) is comparable to a water stream into a container, and the stream leaking out represents those who die (mortality), the water level would be the prevalence. The flow rate of the water streams (incidence and mortality) therefore affects the water level (prevalence) at different time points.
Source: redrawn from Wu et al. (2016, panel 2, p.119).

Health care policies in many countries aim to enable people with dementia to live in their own homes as long as possible.

Crises in dementia are common, are often multifactorial and frequently result in hospital and care home admissions. A crisis in dementia has been defined as a process where there is a stressor (or stressors) that causes an imbalance requiring an immediate decision (Vroomen et al., 2013). Factors such as living alone, increased dependence and the severity of dementia, high levels of carer burden and poor social support networks contribute to the risk of people with dementia being institutionalised (Ledgerd et al., 2016). It appears that most people want to live in their own homes for as long as possible, if their health permits them to do so (Böckerman, Johansson and Saarni, 2012). Darton, Netten and Forder (2003) suggest that the underlying relationship in England between the needs of individuals and the costs of caring for them is confounded by a number of factors.

Many factors influence the decision that an older person should enter residential care. This book uses the shorthand term **institutionalisation**, reflecting the current published peer-reviewed literature – *but this is not ideal*.

The way that the care for older people with and without dementia is organised may have differed over the years and has certainly been influenced by local and national cultures and political priorities, including financial support for public care services (Helvik et al., 2015). And care in the community may not be necessarily more inexpensive. König and colleagues (2014) found that care for persons with dementia living in the community tends to cost more than care in nursing homes when functional impairment is controlled for. (Chapter 11 resumes this discussion.)

Reasons for nursing home placement are complex, involving patient and carer characteristics, and the cultural and social environment. Variation in the organisation of dementia care and cultural aspects, or the relationship between the informal carer and person with dementia, may be factors influencing the reasons (Aneshensel et al., 1995). A higher carer burden has been associated with an increased risk of patient hospitalisation and a faster time to patient institutionalisation (Brodaty and Donkin, 2009).

In relation to carer-related outcomes, female carers have been shown to experience higher levels of burden than male ones (Yee and Schultz, 2000). Studies have identified a positive relationship between carer burden and the number of hours of care provided (Pinquart and Sorensen, 2003) and an unmet need for emotional support (Hughes et al., 2014). It is widely assumed that placement will alleviate the burden of care, and past research has largely focused on predictors of placement rather than on how carers experience the transition (see review by Dunkin and Anderson-Hanley, 1998). Placement, however, does not end the caring role. Instead, carers often renegotiate their role within the context of the institutional setting (Gaugler, 2005).

The ability to perform activities of daily living (ADLs) deteriorates to a greater extent during the later stages of dementia (Takechi et al., 2012). Indeed, Wübker and colleagues have found that the association between ADLs, independence and cost was on average about three times higher than the association between cognition and total costs (Wübker et al., 2015). Minimising the disruption of disability might also impact on carer burden and the potential to delay or prevent institutionalisation. Interdisciplinary team management of ADL disability is arguably ideal for all settings that manage the care of older adults (Ciro, 2014). Knowledge about the performance deterioration in different ADLs has implications for designing interventions to address specific activities at different stages of the disease (Giebel, Sutcliffe and Challis, 2015).

Delirium represents the most frequent complication of hospitalisation for hospitalised older adults (Fong, Tulebaev and Inouye, 2009). In hospitalised older adults, delirium can initiate or otherwise be a key component in a cascade of events that leads to a downward spiral of functional decline, loss of independence, institutionalisation and, ultimately, death (Marcantonio, 2010). Geriatric care and care coordination from daily team meetings can decrease the probability of transition to a nursing home (Yoo, Nakagawa and Kim, 2013). The phrase 'interface geriatrician' has been coined to refer to a geriatrician working in this way, partly in hospital and partly in the community (Gladman et al., 2015). Interviewees from the integrated care teams in the Leeds interface geriatric service have previously reported that patients appreciated the input of the interface geriatrician and that care is now more streamlined around their social and medical needs; patients are no longer obliged to repeat their story to others in the integrated care team and they see members of staff who are well informed about them (King's Fund, 2014).

—— Diagnosis ——————————————————

There has been a drive for harmonisation of **assessment of dementia** in a number of ways.

For example, the requirement for harmonised innovation and assessment of cognitive, behavioural and functional features has been extensively discussed in the field of dementia research.[6]

Nonetheless, there remains a gradient in the realisation of dementia diagnoses in different care settings. It can take a long time between first noticing symptoms and getting a diagnosis of dementia. It is widely acknowledged that the prevalence of dementia is higher at the institutional level than at the community level (Bartfay, Bartfay and Gorey, 2014).

Physicians may unconsciously hesitate to label a patient as such (Downs and Bowers, 2008), and family members may gradually take over social roles from the patient, without necessarily being aware of what they are doing (De Lepeleire, Heyrman and Buntinx, 1998). GPs play an essential role in the recognition and effective ongoing management of dementia, occupying a key position where they can challenge stereotypes and, with support and targeted training about communicating with people living with dementia, can emphasise the ways in which people with dementia can communicate, thereby enhancing their potential to reciprocate (Gove et al., 2016). Individuals might notice a wider range of signs than just memory and cognitive changes; personality changes and general tensions in relationships at work and at home are also reported (Perry-Young et al., 2016).

Timely diagnosis enables persons with dementia and their families to receive help in understanding and adjusting to the diagnosis and allows them to prepare for the future. Although no cure currently exists, timely diagnosis carries significant personal, social and economic benefits which have the potential to improve QoL for patients and reduce carer burden (Banerjee and Wittenberg, 2009; Getsios et al., 2012).

---

6   See, for example, the JPND Working Group on Longitudinal Cohorts document: www. neurodegenerationresearch.eu/wp-content/uploads/2015/10/JPND-Report-Costa.pdf (accessed 3 Oct 2016).

There have been legitimate concerns about the current English policy. 'The policy comprises proactive memory assessment of people in both primary care and acute hospital settings who may not have symptoms; however, there is little evidence that such initiatives, which inevitably lead to increased referrals to specialist services, are cost-effective and whether they are distressing to patients' (Robinson, Tang and Taylor, 2015, p.1). The Prime Minister's Challenge, launched in 2012, set out a plan to ramp up the diagnosis rate so that two-thirds of the estimated 670,000 people living with dementia in England would get a formal diagnosis. Fox and colleagues (2014) reported on a survey of GPs aimed at understanding the **dementia diagnosis gap** in Norfolk and Suffolk. Participating GPs reported concerns about the quality and availability of post-diagnostic support services for people with dementia and their carers.

It is considered by many that a complete clinical neuropsychological assessment (comprehensive cognitive evaluation) remains today *the only way* to make an accurate diagnosis of early cognitive disorder in Alzheimer's disease or other dementia (Kenigsberg et al., 2016). The authors also noted that cognitive testing is included in memory clinics and in research, but not sufficiently in professional practice in nursing homes. The benefits of population screening for dementia will be overestimated if patients who would have been subjected to case-finding are included in screening studies (Mate et al., 2016). The diagnosis of dementia is in effect a shared responsibility between generalist and specialist disciplines.

Much could be done to improve GPs' knowledge of dementia, and the confidence of older GPs could be an educational resource. However, greater experience may create scepticism about timely diagnosis because of the perceived poor quality of specialist services (Ahmad et al., 2010). Diagnosis is usually thought of as a linear process of performing one or more tests in patients with specific signs or symptoms, but in reality the process is replete with complexity and ambiguity. By the time people arrive at the point of being told of their diagnosis, they may have been through an often lengthy and confusing process of assessment and investigation (Robinson, Clare and Evans, 2005).

Factors which can delay a diagnosis have been reviewed by Perry-Young and colleagues (2016), and appear to comprise four distinct sub-concepts:

» discounting, misattributing and deferring

» interpersonal issues

» delays due to different cultural expectations

» delays due to services.

It appears that some people would appreciate a discussion of the possibility of dementia before the diagnosis is 'officially' confirmed, so that the revelation is not perceived as a shock (Derksen et al., 2006). There is still, unfortunately, a relative paucity in empirical research observing the process of diagnostic disclosure in dementia. Studies exploring the views of patients and their families suggest this should be an ongoing process, with the provision of support and information tailored to individual needs (Robinson et al., 2011). Because of their often close and well-established relationship with patients, GPs may be in the ideal position to recognise the initial signs of a possible dementia, and to initiate appropriate assessment and treatment plans (Dodd et al., 2015). Above all, supporting informal carers, monitoring their health and wellbeing, and providing or referring them for additional practical and psychological support is another crucial role for GPs and the community care service (Robinson, Tang and Taylor, 2015).

There are interesting arguments for and against disclosure of the diagnosis, although many intuitively feel that the 'right to a diagnosis' is very real (see Box 1.3).

Box 1.3: Possible reasons for and against disclosure of a diagnosis of dementia

For disclosure:

* the right to know
* confirmation of suspicions and better understanding
* allowing opportunities for future care planning
* facilitating a focus on the abilities rather than disabilities of the person with dementia
* positive adaptations within family and spouse relationships
* access to early treatments, both pharmacological and psychological
* participation in research studies.

Against disclosure:

* would cause emotional upset
* prior distressing experience
* rejection by family and friends, social stigma and embarrassment
* no effective medical care available
* may cause suicide ideation in patients
* not wishing to cause a burden to family.

Distinguishing between the different neurodegenerative causes of dementia is vitally important to allow affected individuals and their families to access appropriate treatment, support and care (Gaugler et al., 2013). Valuable diagnostic information may be missed unless clinicians and radiologists jointly review and discuss brain imaging in cases of frontotemporal dementia (Dewer et al., 2016). In one study, 60% of patients assigned a single diagnosis of behavioural variant FTD (bvFTD) by community clinicians did not have bvFTD according to specialists (Shinagawa et al., 2016). These results revealed a widespread lack of familiarity with core diagnostic symptoms among non-specialists and suggest that community clinicians require specialised diagnostic support before providing a definitive diagnosis of bvFTD.

In the UK, the Gnosall model of primary care memory clinics was launched in 2006. Within this model, specialist services, families and primary care providers worked together to screen patients for cognitive decline, focusing in particular on patients with a vascular history (Greaves and Greaves, 2011). Factors which could increase the risk of developing vascular dementia are often the same as the factors involved in the risk of cardiovascular disease (e.g. smoking). Further advice include medication compliance (use of a dosette box or other concordance aids as necessary), regular monitoring of blood sugar and blood pressure, regular reviews by the GP, and advice about diet and exercise. In this model, **eldercare facilitators**, including nurses, organised assessment, provided further support and linked with specialist services which were provided at a monthly memory clinic in every GP practice provided by a psychiatrist (Greaves et al., 2015). This primary care dementia service reduced the waiting time for a diagnosis of dementia to just four weeks, and reported significant savings to the NHS, while also showing high levels of service users' and professionals' satisfaction (Greening et al., 2009; Clark et al., 2013).

Another model of primary care-led assessment service was trialled in Croydon. This model involved a low-cost, high-throughput, multiagency service which aims to enable early identification and intervention in dementia (Banerjee et al., 2007). Once the diagnosis has taken place, a structured person-centred care plan should be written summarising the issues discussed and who to contact in the event of the patient or carer needing further advice and support. Any follow-up plans should also be written in this care plan.

There are a number of practices which are now considered helpful in delivering person-centred care. For an excellent handy guide to this, please see Sanderson, Bown and Bailey (2015).

It is worth noting that many find the **one-page profile** very useful.

The foundation of delivering person-centred support is a one-page profile. A one-page profile brings together what people appreciate about the person, and reflects what is important to and for them. It is vital that anyone supporting an older person knows what matters to them as an individual and exactly how they want to be supported. (Sanderson et al., 2015, p.27)

An example of a two-page profile is the **This is Me** tool. It is for people with dementia to complete and lets health and social care professionals know about their needs, interests, preferences, likes and dislikes. It is available from the Alzheimer's Society.

Access to memory services facilitates diagnosis and can improve the QoL of people with dementia (Banerjee et al., 2007) and carers (Logiudice et al., 1999). The UK Memory Services National Accreditation Programme is a quality improvement and accreditation programme for memory services with 106 services enrolled. Using survey data from patient and carer feedback questionnaires collected from services as part of the accreditation process, it was recently reported that patients and carers had very good experiences of memory services overall, whether they had standard or excellent accreditation. However, 'excellent' services were consistently better on a number of factors, providing some evidence for the value of the accreditation process for improving the quality of memory services (Hailey et al., 2016).

The pathway from early identification in primary care of symptoms suspicious of dementia to secondary care assessment is crucial to patients receiving a timely diagnosis. Hayhoe, Majeed and Perneczky (2016) have recently proposed that 'A primary care led process, perhaps staffed by practice nurses carrying out assessments according to protocols, may speed up diagnosis while reducing pressure on general practitioners and specialists', adding that 'memory services should consider accepting referrals directly from sources other than primary care, including hospitals, social services, and patients and carers themselves' (p.414).

A number of possible other actors who could be involved at this stage are:

» local authorities and social services

» professionals and practitioners

» telecare

» fire services

» DVLA

» peer support groups

» Alzheimer's Society – helpline, local guides, 'The Dementia Guide'

» Dementia UK and Admiral nurses

» Dementia advisors and dementia support workers.

Ask the person with dementia and the carer if they are interested in any local or national research programmes. Provide appropriate information and signposting guidance to them. Careful consideration should be given to capacity and consent. The Department of Health has funded an initiative called Join Dementia Research, which is supported by the major dementia charities (please note that this initiative encourages people without dementia to participate in research too).

Other aspects include: financial and legal advice, including Lasting Powers of Attorney (LPA), and advance care planning (planning ahead) and EoL care (see Chapter 12).

Indeed, preliminary evidence suggested that providing GP practices with the support of geriatricians improves the management of elderly patients in care homes and reduces health care crises (Anekwe, 2010).

Finally, clear gaps have been identified in addressing the dementia and mental health needs of culturally diverse communities. For example, according to the Policy Research Institute on Ageing and Ethnicity (PRIAE), in collaboration with the International School for Communities, Rights and Inclusion (ISCRI), the barriers faced by minority communities include the following:

» Members of Black Asian and Minority Ethnic (BAME) communities sometimes have little confidence that services will meet cultural, linguistic or religious needs.

» Interpreting services are in short supply, are inadequately advertised and often have limited funding.

(PRIAE in collaboration with ISCRI, 2010)

I explored this serious and important issue in detail in Chapter 3 on culture and diversity in my book *Living Better with Dementia* (Rahman, 2015).

Pharmacological therapies

Acetylcholinesterase inhibitors are hypothesised to work by inhibiting the enzyme acetylcholinesterase (AChE), which breaks down the neurotransmitter acetylcholine (Li et al., 2015).

The NICE (2011) Final Appraisal Determination 'Donepezil, Galantamine, Rivastigmine (Review) and Memantine for the Treatment of Alzheimer's Disease' (TA217)[7] makes key recommendations on certain treatment options.

The corresponding scientific literature is also noteworthy, although not official guidance.

There is little to choose between acetylcholinesterase inhibitors (AChEIs). Price and tolerability are the key deciders. The main side-effects of AChEIs are syncope and gastrointestinal upset, and they are contraindicated in heart block, significant cardiac conduction problems or if the pulse rate is <60 (NHS England, 2015a).

---

7   Available at https://www.nice.org.uk/Guidance/ta217 (accessed 28 Oct 2016).

Acetylcholinesterase inhibitors (such as galantamine and rivastigmine) are used to treat mild-to-moderate Alzheimer's disease. They can also be used to treat dementia with Lewy bodies, and can be particularly effective at treating hallucinations (NHS Choices, 2015). Individual clinical trials have demonstrated the benefits of donepezil in patients with severe Alzheimer's disease. Data were pooled from three randomised, placebo-controlled trials of donepezil for severe Alzheimer's disease to further evaluate treatment effects and overall tolerability/safety. These findings suggest measurable donepezil-mediated symptomatic benefits in cognition, global function and ADLs in patients with severe Alzheimer's disease (Winblad, 2009). Howard and colleagues (2015) concluded that withdrawal of donepezil in patients with moderate-to-severe Alzheimer's disease increased the risk of nursing home placement during 12 months of treatment, but made no difference during the following three years of follow-up.

Memantine is used to treat severe Alzheimer's disease, but can also be given to people with moderate symptoms if they do not respond well to AChEIs (NHS Choices, 2015). The ability of memantine to decrease symptomatic decline and to improve functioning in patients with moderately severe-to-severe Alzheimer's disease was originally demonstrated in two pivotal phase III trials and has subsequently been confirmed in other studies (Winblad and Poritis, 1999; Reisberg et al., 2003).

The following can also be noted (but note the date of publications):

» There are no currently licensed treatments for vascular dementias within the UK, so treatment strategies have largely focused on control of underlying cardiovascular risk factors and treatment of associated symptoms (O'Brien, Burns and BAP Dementia Consensus Group, 2011).

» Randomised controlled trials of cholinesterase inhibitors have demonstrated benefit in cognitive and non-cognitive symptoms in dementia with Lewy bodies (O'Brien et al., 2011).

» The current data on the pharmacological treatments for frontotemporal dementias appear to indicate that certain medications are effective in reducing some behavioural symptoms, but none of these medications had an impact on cognition (Nardell and Tampi, 2014).

» Cholinesterase inhibitors may also lead to clinical improvement for rarer dementias associated with neurological conditions (Li et al., 2015).

» There is some evidence that antipsychotics can cause a range of serious side-effects for people who have dementia with Lewy bodies (NHS Choices, 2015).

» Patient understanding and beliefs about their illness may impact on their likelihood both to seek help for their symptoms and also to adhere to any recommended therapies. A review of qualitative research proposed that three phases of decision-making are important regarding medication adherence in older people: faith in the prescriber's ability to correctly diagnose and select treatment; testing of the effectiveness of the medication on symptom relief and adverse effects; and patients' beliefs about the illness itself (Banning, 2008). Complex medication regimens have also been associated with increased potential adverse drug events and hospital readmission, and inversely associated with adherence and hospital discharge directly home (Lalic et al., 2016).

—— Introduction to integration ——

An **integrated care service** is defined as a coherent and coordinated set of services which are planned, managed and delivered to individual service users across a range of organisations and by a range of cooperating professionals and informal carers (Raak et al., 2003).

Whereas the rationale for integrated care is evident, the developmental process for integrated care is less clear as it is a complex and long-term one. The integration of care can be complicated by different goals, different funding streams and different stakeholders or care providers (Minkman et al., 2013). Integrated working aims to ensure continuity of care, reduce duplication and fragmentation of services, and places the patient as the focus for service delivery, but there is an urgent need to develop and test interventions that promote integrated working and address the persistent divide between health services and independent providers (Davies et al., 2011).

National Voices' (2013) 'A Narrative for Person-Centred Coordinated Care'[8] sets out what person-centred, coordinated care should mean in practice and is a guide to the sort of things that integrated care will achieve, including:

» better planning

» more personal involvement of the person using the services

» free access to good information.

Enablement (sometimes called reablement or re-enablement) is about helping people become more independent and improve their QoL. Integrated care is a term typically used to describe attempts to improve patient experience and achieve greater efficiency and value from health delivery systems by redesigning services in

8   Available at www.nationalvoices.org.uk/publications/our-publications/narrative-person-centred-coordinated-care (accessed 3 Oct 2016).

such a way as to minimise the fragmentation experienced by some groups of service users (Shaw, Rosen and Rumbold, 2011).

Integrated care is both person-centred and coordinated. The ageing population and increased prevalence of chronic diseases require a strong re-orientation away from the current emphasis on acute care towards prevention, self-care, more consistent standards of primary care and care that is well coordinated and integrated. But the narrative of the medicalisation of Alzheimer's disease faces a large problem. This is elegantly articulated by Callahan and colleagues (2009): 'the initial advances in the treatment of Alzheimer's disease and related dementias may improve survival but also increase the length of time that an older adult needs care. This may paradoxically place an even greater burden on those components of the care system charged with providing this care' (p.369).

The King's Fund established the Commission on the Future of Health and Social Care in England in 2013 to explore what a new settlement for health and social care might entail. The commission's interim report set out a compelling case for a new settlement based on the huge pressures facing the NHS and social care at a time of growing demands and constrained resources.

In 2014, Kate Barker wrote:

> The prize of our new settlement is huge: a more integrated service, a simpler path through it, more equal treatment for more equal need, and a far less distressing experience for those trapped in the confusions of today's arrangements. (Commission on the Future of Health and Social Care in England, 2014)

In an excellent article in *The Lancet* entitled 'Multimorbidity – older adults need health care that can count past one' from February 2015, Banerjee indeed celebrated the improvement in life expectancy for citizens of developed countries, but also legitimately warns against increasing specialist, technology-driven care away from integrated general care. This can impact on poor-quality outcomes and poor-quality service response for people with dementia with comorbidities (Banerjee, 2015). Care home residents undoubtedly have complex care needs; for example, between 75% and 80% of residents have memory problems, 57% are affected by urinary incontinence, 42% have faecal incontinence and some 61% require assistance with mobility (Gordon, 2015 on the BGS blog).

But formidable barriers to integration do exist for dementia (see Box 1.4). The distinction between medical care and social care can be an arbitrary one, and yet the funding implications can be colossal. The distinction between universal health care funded through general taxation, and social care which is means-tested and highly rationed, is becoming a bigger obstacle to the true integration of the two services (Humphries, 2015).

Box 1.4: Barriers to integration in health and social care

* Integration is unlikely to deliver immediate financial savings.

* The current organisational structures in acute, primary and social care have been created under different statutory regimes, which is a challenge to bringing organisations together.

* Concerns about the security and privacy of information and data (including under anticipated EU data protection legislation).

* Inappropriate pay incentives (acute care system and hospitals are largely paid-for activities, whereas part of the solution for integrated care may be capitated budgets).

* Financial sustainability of care providers such as care homes in a consolidating sector.

* Lack of adequate stakeholder input from an early stage (ideally pre-procurement).

* Competition or procurement law regulations are seen by many as expensive and time-consuming hindrances to integration.

* Governance arrangements around pooled budgets become the central focus rather than providing better care.

* The legislative framework is quite specific about the requirement for commissioners to put in place an agreement (known as a section 75 agreement).

* Structural and cultural barriers to providing older people with joined-up care.

* The need for multidisciplinary working involves training.

* Silos in central and local government.

* Health and wellbeing boards across the country are currently concerned about their (lack of) decisions, which significantly restricts their ability to drive integration locally.

SOURCE: AFTER DAC BEACHCROFT (2014) AND INDEPENDENT COMMISSION ON WHOLE PERSON CARE FOR THE LABOUR PARTY (2014).

It is hard to escape the fact that, currently, residential settings are incredibly important in the wider system of the health economy. Primary and community services spend significant amounts of time providing care for older people resident in care homes. Gage and colleagues (2012) argue that 'care homes are a hub for a wide range of NHS activity, but this is ad hoc with no recognised way to support working together' (p.1).

Traditional hierarchical and gender roles within health care have generated a prevailing physician-centric paradigm; misaligned perceptions of nurses' roles as collaborators represent a possible barrier to the success of integrated care delivery (Alcusksy et al., 2015). When a patient's needs cannot be covered by one professional or health care provider alone, collaboration between different providers is required (Minkman et al., 2011). In discussing 'place-based systems of care', Alderwick, Ham and Buck (2015) advise against underestimating collaboration. In creating a new legal entity, for example, the organisations involved will be sharing control and therefore surrendering some of their own autonomy (Alderwick et al., 2015).

Gordon (2015) succinctly addresses some of the challenges ahead:

> Meanwhile, the question is: what can individual providers do? The first answer is to recognise that care homes and NHS providers share a common challenge, which is providing care to residents whose physical and mental health is often complex and challenging. The next is to realise that it is only through collaboration and team-work that the best care will be realised. Further, to consider the practical ways in which care can be constructed to be integrated. Who will do the initial assessment? How will action plans from the assessment be case managed? Who will conduct the regular reviews?

The NHS Five Year Forward View and New Models of Care

NHS England's New Models of Care programme, launched in January 2015, focused on the acceleration of the design and implementation of new models of care in the NHS, with a particular emphasis on achieving integration through the development of comprehensive local services. It set out how the health service needs to change, arguing for a more engaged relationship with patients, carers and citizens to promote wellbeing and prevent ill health (Maruthappu, Sood and Keogh, 2014).

The Five Year Forward View supports clinicians to provide better, higher quality and more integrated care (NHS England, 2014). The priorities of the Five Year Forward View are still on patients and what they need most:

» reshape the NHS's urgent and emergency care services so they respond effectively to the increasing demands placed on them

» strengthen primary care as the foundation for personalised NHS care

» ensure elective care continues to meet service standards and remain accessible for patients

» shape specialised services to improve their quality and future affordability.

(NHS England, 2015b)

The core argument made in the Forward View centres around three gaps, shown in Figure 1.5.

Health and wellbeing gap: radical upgrade in prevention

Care and quality gap: new models of care

Funding gap: efficiency and investment

Figure 1.5: New Models of Care and the three gaps

New Models of Care are presented in this visionary contribution, including multispeciality providers, primary and acute care systems, urgent and emergency care networks, viable smaller hospitals, specialised services, modern maternity services and enhanced care homes. The approach of the New Models of Care in plugging the 'care and quality gap' *essentially provides a menu of different care models* for different localities to consider, and investment and flexibility are both required to support implementation as essential components of a complex, adaptive approach.

Multispeciality community care providers

The aim is to break down boundaries between GPs and hospitals, physical and mental health and between health and social care to enable the NHS to work better with local communities and reduce pressure on A&E and avoid unnecessary hospital admissions.

I will consider integrated personal commissioning in Chapter 11.

Primary and acute care systems

These are vertically integrated services combining hospitals and GP surgeries, permitting, in particular, greater investment and expansion of primary care in areas with high health inequalities. Perhaps most important are longstanding cultural differences between GPs and their teams on the one hand, and hospital clinicians on the other (Ham and Murray, 2015).

Urgent and emergency care networks

Drawing on the success of major trauma centres, networks of linked hospitals will be formed, ensuring that patients with the most serious needs get to specialist emergency centres.

Viable smaller hospitals

NHS England will work with smaller hospitals to examine new models of medical staffing and other ways of achieving sustainable cost structures, building on the earlier work of Monitor and the Royal College of Physicians' 'Future Hospitals' initiative.[9]

Specialised services

Where the relationship between quality and case volume is strong, NHS England will work with local partners to drive consolidation through a programme of three-year rolling reviews.

Modern maternity services

The NHS will conduct a review of future models for maternity units, which will make recommendations on how best to sustain and develop maternity units that deliver fewer than 4000 babies a year.

Enhanced health in care homes

In partnership with local authority social services departments, and using the opportunity created by the establishment of the Better Care Fund, NHS England is working with local NHS organisations and the care home sector to develop new shared models of in-reach support, including medical and medication reviews.

In March 2015, NHS England and its national partners announced the first of 29 new care model vanguards. There were six enhanced 'health in care home vanguards' which will offer older people a better, joined-up health, care and rehabilitation service, and these vanguards were selected following a rigorous process, involving workshops and the engagement of key partners and patient representative groups.[10]

As an example, in Airedale, nursing and residential homes are linked by secure video to the hospital, allowing consultations with nurses and consultants – for

---

9   Available at www.rcplondon.ac.uk/projects/future-hospital-programme (accessed 3 Oct 2016).

10   Available at www.england.nhs.uk/ourwork/futurenhs/new-care-models/care-homes-sites (accessed 3 Oct 2016).

everything from cuts and bumps to diabetes management and the onset of confusion (NHS England, 2014). Emergency admissions from these homes have been reduced by 35% and A&E attendances by 53%. I will consider admissions and care homes in Chapter 10 in some detail. An audit comparing nursing and residential care homes in Airedale before and after the implementation of telemedicine showed a 35% reduction in hospital admissions (based on hospital episode statistics for around 2000 residents in 23 local care homes). There is no doubt telemedicine and technology in general will be incredibly influential in future, and I resume this theme in later chapters.

— Other areas

Devolution of powers

Integrated care must be delivered at scale and pace. This requires work across large populations at a city- and county-wide level. There should be flexibility to take forward different approaches in different areas and to evaluate the impact, with the main emphasis being on people with complex needs. A series of think tank reports published in 2014 (e.g. Blond and Morrin, 2014) called for more radical devolution of powers to local areas to help them grow their economies. It is argued that population health management focused on individuals has a place (e.g. through 'making every contact count'), but needs to be underpinned and complemented by interventions designed to tackle the underlying social, economic and environmental determinants of health across populations (Alderwick et al., 2015).

Better Care Fund

The Better Care Fund (BCF) was seen by some as a way of encouraging integration. However, concerns have been raised about the practicalities and the potential for harmful redundancy costs as a result of streamlining services (DAC Beachcroft, 2014).

An example of the use of this fund is for a programme supporting 11 Hertfordshire care homes with multidisciplinary teams of health experts, including dieticians, geriatricians, pharmacists, mental health professionals, doctors and nurses. It provides a 'rapid response' team of clinicians to assist residents in failing health within 60 minutes of a call, and grants GPs access to comprehensive information about each patient during their visits. Each receives £5000 from the Better Care Fund – a joint NHS and local authority programme – and from the national NHS Vanguard scheme to cover the cost of additional staff time, so particular staff who have been trained to identify potentially deteriorating residents ('staff champions') can be released from the daily rota to attend training sessions (Williams, 2016).

Non-communicable diseases

Chronic non-communicable diseases account for most of the global burden of disease; 'leading contributors are cardiovascular diseases, cancer, chronic respiratory diseases, musculoskeletal diseases, and mental and neurological disorders' (Prince et al., 2015, p.549). Specifically, cancer, coronary heart disease, dementia and stroke are leading causes of death and disability, and were calculated to account for 55% of deaths in 2012 (Murray et al., 2012). It is still, sadly, a general perception that while there has undoubtedly been progress by government to increase levels of research funding for dementia and stroke, these areas are still comparatively underfunded when compared with the overall burden of disease (Luengo-Fernandez, Leal and Gray, 2015).

Prevention and risk reduction

The health and wellbeing gap of the NHS Five Year Forward View mandates a radical upgrade in prevention, with a national approach to major health risks and encouraging prevention initiatives, such as for diabetes. There are clearly synergies with the aims of any future national plans for dementia in England here.

The right to health is a fundamental part of our human rights and of our understanding of a life in dignity. The right to the enjoyment of the highest attainable standard of physical and mental health is not new. Internationally, first articulated in the 1946 Constitution of the WHO, the **right to health** comprises many entitlements, including the right to prevention, treatment and control of diseases (Office of the United Nations High Commissioner for Human Rights, 2008).

Preventing well (risk reduction) is a core part of national policy

Given the evidence that there may be a vascular component to many dementias, interventions to address vascular risk factors (such as tobacco, poor diet, physical inactivity and alcohol; and intermediate disease precursors such as raised blood pressure, raised blood cholesterol, obesity and diabetes which arise from behavioural and other factors) should also help reduce the risk, progression and severity of dementia (Public Health England and UK Health Forum, 2015). Protective factors also play a part, and these include education and intellectual and social engagement.

Various layers of prevention are as follows:

» *Primary prevention*

'You don't have the disease and you never get it.'

» *Secondary prevention*

'You have evidence of disease but you don't get symptoms.'

» *Tertiary prevention*

'You have the disease and symptoms but you don't get any worse.'

The identification of risk factors for dementia of the Alzheimer type may lead to risk reduction strategies. Recent randomised controlled trials of multidomain interventions, such as the Finnish Geriatric Intervention Study to Prevent Cognitive Impairment and Disability (FINGER) (a two-year programme including diet, exercise, cognitive training and vascular risk monitoring components), show that such interventions could improve or maintain cognition in at-risk older people in the general population (Chong et al., 2016). It is believed by some that preventive approaches and cognitive monitoring must be integrated in the primary care setting to be able to prevent Alzheimer and other dementias in clinical practice for the future (Vellas and Oustric, 2014).

The Blackfriars Consensus helped to establish that while recognising the necessary timescales and lag in benefit from preventive strategies aimed at current younger populations at future risk, there is a compelling need to take immediate, targeted action on the emerging and known risk factors such as physical inactivity (including upstream policy measures) (Public Health England and UK Health Forum, 2015). The precautionary principle also requires that, even for those risk factors for which the evidence is less robust, we should recommend actions that could reasonably be presumed to reduce the risk of some types of dementia at least, while carrying out scientific evaluations of their effects.

The Blackfriars Consensus highlighted various risk factors, focusing on the options for vascular risk reduction, since this accounts for substantial attributable risk and has a robust evidence base (Orrell and Brayne, 2015). Methodological challenges regarding midlife risk factors for dementia include: the heterogeneity of the condition, the fact that it is often not a primary endpoint, difficulty in measuring lifestyle factors, and there may be a survivorship bias because of adverse effects. There are ethical issues around designing randomised controlled trials concerning modifiable risk factors, for example in alcohol research, which merit further scrutiny (Rooney, 2014). Dementia prevention trials will gain much from the inclusion of individuals at increased risk of dementia. Genetic tests and family history data are readily available sources that inform estimates of risk. It is likely that families affected by dementia will be screened for possible inclusion in dementia prevention trials (Robertson, Brown and Whalley, 2014).

There are some brilliant initiatives worldwide. The European Prevention of Alzheimer's Dementia (EPAD) project[11] aims to develop an infrastructure that efficiently enables the undertaking of adaptive, multi-arm **proof of concept** studies for early and accurate decisions on the ongoing development of drug candidates or

---

11   Available at http://ep-ad.org (accessed 3 Oct 2016).

drug combinations for the prevention of Alzheimer's disease. The drive to 'universalise the best', as Nye Bevan called it, extends to other international jurisdictions. For example, the *Gesundes Kinzigtal* system is one of the few population-based integrated care approaches in Germany (NHS Confederation, 2015). The system was developed around ten years ago through a partnership between a network of local physicians and a management company. This approach puts significant emphasis on prevention and health promotion programmes, with the overall objective of improving population health and QoL. This involves running health literacy and healthy lifestyle programmes for specific groups of the population, with particular emphasis on chronic conditions and specific risk groups.

NHS England and Public Health England's (2013) 'A Call to Action: Commissioning for Prevention' is an excellent introduction to this area.

Quality of life

Quality of life (QoL) is a complex, multidimensional construct, and is defined by the WHO as 'individuals' perceptions of their position in life in the context of the culture and value systems in which they live, and in relation to their goals, expectations, standards and concerns' (WHO, 1995). The precise assessment of QoL across different care settings is a pivotal part of contemporary research (Banerjee and Wittenberg, 2009).

Both objective (e.g. behavioural competence and environment) and subjective components are generally considered to be important domains in the QoL of people with dementia (Lawton, 1994). Although common European policy principles aim to keep people with dementia at home for as long as possible, many of them will be admitted to long-term care facilities as the dementia progresses (Prince, Prina and Guerchet 2013). Predictors of QoL within older people living in care homes include perceived autonomy, frequency of available choices, ability to perform activities of daily living, risk of falling, social economic status, amount of time spent with family and perceived social support from and quality of interactions with care staff (Aspden et al., 2014). Measuring QoL in dementia is challenging, not least because of poor recall, time perception, insight and communication on the part of the person with dementia. These problems mean that there are serious questions concerning the validity of the use of generic measures of health-related quality of life (HRQoL) which are not specifically validated for dementia (Banerjee and Wittenberg, 2009).

QoL is often innocently confused with quality of care, which is the way in which care is delivered and the standards that it meets. Separating QoL from quality of care is difficult, especially as the two are not completely distinct. If care is of a high standard, it can support and promote QoL, but it is not necessarily the key contributor (Help the Aged, 2006). Hoe and colleagues (2009) showed that the relationship between lower QoL and living in a 24-hour care setting may be related to higher levels of dependence and behavioural problems among residents and also to people's preference for living at home.

Carers in care facilities and nursing homes, as well as carers in the home situation, strive to offer the best possible QoL to the residents and clients they assist, care for or nurse. An increasing amount of interventional research is being conducted within care homes. QoL represents an important outcome for assessing the impact and cost-effectiveness of these interventions (Owens et al., 2011). People with dementia can express views about their QoL, even in the later stages of the illness. However, in dementia care, staff are often asked to rate the wellbeing of the residents, rather than asking the residents themselves, perhaps due to reservations about people with dementia's ability to comprehend questions and provide reliable accounts (Spector and Orrell, 2006).

Providing good QoL has been recognised as the main goal of currently available dementia care, and recently much research on the QoL of persons with dementia has been performed (Terada et al., 2013). The relationship between the condition of carers and the QoL of persons with dementia is important; for example, depression and the mental health of carers are reported to be correlated with the QoL of persons with dementia as rated by carers (Schiffczyk et al., 2010). Most people move into a nursing home out of necessity, not desire. Adjusting to nursing home life is often a complex and difficult process for older adults, marked by emotional upheaval, personal losses and feelings of abandonment (Chenitz, 1983; Brooke, 1989).

Person-centred care is correlated with residents' ability to perform activities of daily living. Furthermore, residents in units with higher levels of person-centred care were rated as having higher QoL and a better ability to perform activities of daily living compared with residents in units with lower levels of person-centred care (Sjögren et al., 2013).

—— Essential reading ——

Alzheimer's Society, The Dementia Guide: Living Well after Diagnosis, available at www.alzheimers.org.uk/site/scripts/documents_info.php?documentID=2240 (accessed 6 Oct 2016).

Alzheimer's Society, This is Me Tool, available at www.alzheimers.org.uk/site/scripts/download_info.php?downloadID=399 (accessed 6 Oct 2016).

Sanderson H, Bown L, Bailey G. 2015. *Person-Centred Thinking with Older People: Six Essential Practices*, London: Jessica Kingsley Publishers.

Capacity and advocacy

Rahman S. 2014. *Living Well with Dementia*, London: CRC Press. Chapter 11, Decision-Making, Capacity and Advocacy in Living Well with Dementia, pp.175–196.

Culture and diversity

Rahman S. 2015. *Living Better with Dementia*, London: Jessica Kingsley Publishers. Chapter 3, Culture and Diversity in Living Better with Dementia, pp.63–80.

Dementia-friendly communities

Rahman S. 2014. *Living Well with Dementia*, London: CRC Press. Chapter 17, Dementia-Friendly Communities and Living Well with Dementia, pp.285–300.

The debate about screening

Rahman S. 2014. *Living Well with Dementia*, London: CRC Press. Chapter 5, A Public Health Perspective on Living Well with Dementia, and the Debate over Screening, pp.67–100.

—— References ————————————————————

No authors listed. 2015. Dementia: turning fine aspirations into measurable progress. Lancet, 385(9974), 1151.

Ahmad S, Orrell M, Iliffe S, Gracie A. 2010. GPs' attitudes, awareness, and practice regarding early diagnosis of dementia. Br J Gen Pract, 60(578), e360–365.

Alcusky M, Ferrari L, Rossi G, Liu M, Hojat M, Maio V. 2015. Attitudes toward collaboration among practitioners in newly established medical homes: A survey of nurses, general practitioners, and specialists. Am J Med Qual, pii: 1062860615597744.

Alderwick H, Ham C, Buck D. 2015. Population Health Systems: Going Beyond Integrated Care, available at www.kingsfund.org.uk/sites/files/kf/field/field_publication_file/population-health-systems-kingsfund-feb15.pdf (accessed 3 Oct 2016).

Anekwe L. 2010. GP care home support 'cuts deaths and workload', available at www.pulsetoday.co.uk/gp-care-home-support-cuts-deaths-and-workload/11026817.fullarticle (accessed 29 Nov 2016).

Aneshensel CS, Pearlin LI, Mullan JT, Zarit SH, Whitlatch CJ. 1995. *Profiles in Caregiving: The Unexpected Career*, San Diego, CA: Academic Press.

Archer N, Bajaj H, Zhang H. 2008. Supply management for home healthcare services. INFOR, 46, 2, 137–145.

Aspden T, Bradshaw SA, Playford ED, Riazi A. 2014. Quality-of-life measures for use within care homes: a systematic review of their measurement properties. Age Ageing, 43(5), 596–603.

Banerjee S. 2012. The macroeconomics of dementia – will the world economy get alzheimer's disease? Arch Med Res, 43(8), 705–709.

Banerjee S. 2015. Multimorbidity – older adults need health care that can count past one. Lancet, 385(9968), 587–589.

Banerjee S, Wittenberg R. 2009. Clinical and cost-effectiveness of services for early diagnosis and intervention in dementia. Int J Geriatr Psychiatry, 24(7), 748–754.

Banerjee S, Samsi K, Petrie CD, Alvir J, et al. 2009. What do we know about quality of life in dementia? A review of the emerging evidence on the predictive and explanatory value of disease specific measures of health related quality of life in people with dementia. Int J Geriatr Psychiatry, 24(1), 15–24.

Banerjee S, Smith SC, Lamping DL, Harwood RH, et al. 2006. Quality of life in dementia: more than just cognition. An analysis of associations with quality of life in dementia. J Neurol Neurosurg Psychiatry, 77(2), 146–148.

Banerjee S, Willis R, Matthews D, Contell F, Chan J, Murray J. 2007. Improving the quality of care for mild to moderate dementia: an evaluation of the Croydon Memory Service Model. Int J Geriatr Psychiatry, 22(8), 782–788.

Banning M. 2008. Older people and adherence with medication: a review of the literature. Int J Nurs Stud, 45, 1550–1561.

Bartfay E, Bartfay WJ, Gorey KM. 2014. Association of diagnostic delay with impairment severity among institutional care facility residents diagnosed with dementia in Ontario, Canada. Geriatr Gerontol Int, 14, 918e25.

Blond P, Morrin M. 2014. *Devo Max – Devo Manc: Place-Based Public Services*, London: ResPublica, available at www.respublica.org.uk/our-work/publications/devo-max-devo-manc-place-based-public-services (accessed 3 Oct 2016).

Böckerman P, Johansson E, Saarni SI. 2012. Institutionalisation and subjective wellbeing for old-age individuals: is life really miserable in care homes? Ageing and Society, 32(7), 1176–1192.

Brodaty H, Donkin M. 2009. Family caregivers of people with dementia. Dialogues Clin Neurosci, 11, 217–228.

Brooke V. 1989. How elders adjust: through what phases do newly admitted residents pass? Geriatric Nursing, 10, 66–68.

Bunn F, Goodman C, Sworn K, Rait G, et al. 2012. Psychosocial factors that shape patient and carer experiences of dementia diagnosis and treatment: a systematic review of qualitative studies. PLoS Med, 9(10), e1001331.

Callahan CM, Boustani M, Sachs GA, Hendrie HC. 2009. Integrating care for older adults with cognitive impairment. Curr Alzheimer Res, 6(4), 368–374.

Campbell D. 2015. Half of UK Care Homes Will Close Unless £2.9bn Funding Gap Is Plugged, Charities Warn, *The Guardian*, 21 November 2015, available at www.theguardian.com/society/2015/nov/21/half-uk-care-homes-close-funding-gap-nhs-george-osborne (accessed 3 Oct 2016).

Caravau H, Martín I. 2015. Direct costs of dementia in nursing homes. Front Aging Neurosci, 7, 146.

Chenitz WC. 1983. Entry into a nursing home as status passage: a theory to guide nursing practice. Geriatric Nursing, 4, 92–97.

Chong TW, Loi SM, Lautenschlager NT, Ames D. 2016. Therapeutic advances and risk factor management: our best chance to tackle dementia? Med J Aust, 204(3), 91–92.

Ciro CA. 2014. Maximizing ADL performance to facilitate aging in place for people with dementia. Nurs Clin North Am, 49(2), 157–169.

Clark M, Moreland N, Greaves I, Greaves N, Jolley, D. 2013. Putting personalisation and integration into practice in primary care. Journal of Integrated Care, 21, 105–120.

Commission on the Future of Health and Social Care in England. 2014. *A New Settlement for Health and Social Care*, London: King's Fund, available at www.kingsfund.org.uk/sites/files/kf/field/field_publication_file/Commission%20Final%20%20interactive.pdf (accessed 3 Oct 2016).

DAC Beachcroft. 2014. Health and Social Care Integration: A DAC Beachcroft Analysis, available at www.dacbeachcroft.com/media/305758/health_and_social_care_integration_report_m_and_a.pdf (accessed 3 Sep 2016).

Darton R, Netten A, Forder J. 2003. The cost implications of the changing population and characteristics of care homes. Int J Geriatr Psychiatry, 18(3), 236–243.

Davies SL, Goodman C, Bunn F, Victor C, et al. 2011. A systematic review of integrated working between care homes and health care services. BMC Health Serv Res, 24(11), 320.

De Lepeleire J, Heyrman J, Buntinx F. 1998. The early diagnosis of dementia: triggers, early signs and luxating events. Fam Pract, 15: 431–436.

Department of Health. 2013. Dementia: A State of the Nation Report on Dementia Care and Support in England, available at www.gov.uk/government/uploads/system/uploads/attachment_data/file/262139/Dementia.pdf (accessed 3 Oct 2016).

Department of Health. 2016. Policy Paper. Dementia: Post-Diagnostic Care and Support, available at www.gov.uk/government/publications/dementia-post-diagnostic-care-and-support (accessed 3 Oct 2016).

Derksen E, Vernooij-Dassen M, Gillissen F, Olde Rikkert M, Scheltens P. 2006. Impact of diagnostic disclosure in dementia on patients and carers: qualitative case series analysis. Aging Ment Health, 10(5), 525–531.

Dewer B, Rogers P, Ricketts J, Mukonoweshuro W, Zeman A. 2016. The radiological diagnosis of frontotemporal dementia in everyday practice: an audit of reports, review of diagnostic criteria, and proposal for service improvement. Clin Radiol, 71(1), 40–47.

Dodd E, Cheston R, Cullum S, Jefferies R, Ismail S, Gatting L, Fear T, Gray R. 2015. Primary care led dementia diagnosis services in South Gloucestershire: Themes from people and families living with dementia and health care professionals. Dementia (London), pii: 1471301214566476.

Downs M, Bowers B. 2008. Caring for people with dementia. BMJ, 336, 225–226.

Dunkin JJ, Anderson-Hanley C. 1998. Dementia caregiver burden: a review of the literature and guidelines for assessment and intervention. Neurology, 51(Suppl. 1), S53–S60.

Fong TG, Tulebaev SR, Inouye SK. 2009. Delirium in elderly adults: diagnosis, prevention and treatment. Nat Rev Neurol, 5, 210–220.

Fox M, Fox C, Cruickshank W, Penhale B, Poland F, Steel N. 2014. Understanding the dementia diagnosis gap in Norfolk and Suffolk: a survey of general practitioners. Qual Prim Care, 22(2): 101–107.

Gage H, Dickinson A, Victor C, Williams P, et al. 2012. Integrated working between residential care homes and primary care: a survey of care homes in England. BMC Geriatr, 12, 71.

Gaugler JE. 2005. Family involvement in residential long-term care: a synthesis and critical review. Aging & Mental Health, 9, 105–118.

Gaugler JE, Ascher-Svanum H, Roth DL, Fafowora T, Siderowf A, Beach TG. 2013. Characteristics of patients misdiagnosed with Alzheimer's disease and their medication use: an analysis of the NACC-UDS database. BMC Geriatr, 13, 13.

Getsios D, Blume S, Ishak KJ, Maclaine G, Hernandez L. 2012. An economic evaluation of early assessment for Alzheimer's disease in the United Kingdom. Alzheimer's and Dementia, 8(1), 22–30.

Giebel CM, Sutcliffe C, Challis D. 2015. Activities of daily living and quality of life across different stages of dementia: a UK study. Aging Ment Health, 19(1): 63–71.

Gladman J, Harwood R, Conroy S, Logan P, et al. 2015. Medical crises in older people. Programme Grants Appl Res, 3, 4.

Gordon A. 2015. Care Home Residents Deserve the Best Care: The Best Care Is Integrated, available at britishgeriatricssociety.wordpress.com/2015/11/10/care-home-residents-deserve-the-best-care-the-best-care-is-integrated (accessed 3 Oct 2016).

Gove D, Small N, Downs M, Vernooij-Dassen M. 2016. General practitioners' perceptions of the stigma of dementia and the role of reciprocity. Dementia (London), pii: 1471301215625657.

Greaves I, Greaves N, Walker E, Greening L, Benbow SM, Jolley D. 2015. Gnosall primary care memory clinic: eldercare facilitator role description and development. Dementia (London), 14(4), 389–408.

Greaves N, Greaves I. 2011. The Gnosall project: setting new benchmarks for dementia care. Journal of Care Services Management, 5, 49–52.

Greening L, Greaves I, Greaves N, Jolley D. 2009. Positive thinking on dementia in primary care: Gnosall Memory Clinic. Community Practitioner, 82(5), 20–23.

Hailey E, Hodge S, Burns A, Orrell M. 2016. Patients' and carers' experiences of UK memory services. Int J Geriatr Psychiatry, 31(6), 676–680.

Ham C, Murray R. 2015. Implementing the NHS Five Year Forward View: Aligning Policies with the Plan, available at www.kingsfund.org.uk/sites/files/kf/field/field_publication_file/implementing-the-nhs-five-year-forward-view-kingsfund-feb15.pdf (accessed 3 Oct 2016).

Hampel H, Prvulovic D, Teipel S, Jessen F, et al. 2011. The future of Alzheimer's disease: the next 10 years. Prog Neurobiol, 95(4), 718–728.

Hayhoe B, Majeed A, Perneczky R. 2016. General practitioner referrals to memory clinics: are referral criteria delaying the diagnosis of dementia? J R Soc Med, 109, 410–415.

Help the Aged. 2006. My Home Life: Quality of Life in Care Homes, available at www.scie.org.uk/publications/guides/guide15/files/myhomelife-litreview.pdf?res=true (accessed 3 Oct 2016).

Helvik AS, Engedal K, Benth JŠ, Selbæk G. 2015. Prevalence and severity of dementia in nursing home residents. Dement Geriatr Cogn Disord, 40(3–4), 166–177.

Hoe J, Hancock G, Livingston G, Woods B, Challis D, Orrell M. 2009. Changes in the quality of life of people with dementia living in care homes. Alzheimer Dis Assoc Disord, 23(3), 285–290.

Hopkins T, Rippon S. 2015. Head, Hands and Heart: Asset-Based Approaches in Health Care, available at www.health.org.uk/sites/health/files/HeadHandsAndHeartAssetBasedApproachesIn HealthCare.pdf (accessed 3 Sept 2016).

Howard R, McShane R, Lindesay J, Ritchie C, et al. 2015. Nursing home placement in the donepezil and memantine in moderate to severe Alzheimer's disease (DOMINO-AD) trial: secondary and post-hoc analyses. Lancet Neurol, 14(12), 1171–1181.

Hughes TB, Black BS, Albert M, Gitlin LN, et al. 2014. Correlates of objective and subjective measures of caregiver burden among dementia caregivers: influence of unmet patient and caregiver dementia-related care needs. Int Psychogeriatr, 26(11), 1875–1883.

Humphries R. 2015. Integrated health and social care in England – progress and prospects. Health Policy, 119(7), 856–859.

Independent Commission on Whole Person Care for the Labour Party. 2014. One Person, One Team, One System, available at www.yourbritain.org.uk/uploads/editor/files/One_Person_One_Team_One_System.pdf (accessed 29 Nov 2016).

Kenigsberg PA, Aquino JP, Bérard A, Gzil F, et al. 2016. Dementia beyond 2025: knowledge and uncertainties. Dementia (London), 15(1), 6–21.

King's Fund. 2014. Leeds Interface Geriatrician Service, London: The King's Fund, available at www.kingsfund.org.uk/sites/files/kf/media/leeds-interface-geriatrician-service-kingsfund-oct14.pdf (accessed 3 Oct 2016).

Kinsman L, Rotter T, James E, Snow P, Willis J. 2010. What is a clinical pathway? Development of a definition to inform the debate. BMC Med, 8, 31.

König HH, Leicht H, Brettschneider C, Bachmann C, et al. 2014. The costs of dementia from the societal perspective: is care provided in the community really cheaper than nursing home care? J Am Med Dir Assoc, 15(2), 117–126.

Lalic S, Jamsen KM, Wimmer BC, Tan EC, Hilmer SN, Robson L, Emery T, Bell JS. 2016. Polypharmacy and medication regimen complexity as factors associated with staff informant rated quality of life in residents of aged care facilities: a cross-sectional study. Eur J Clin Pharmacol, 72(9), 1117–1124.

Lawton MP, 1994. Quality of life in Alzheimer disease. Alzheimer Disease and Associated Disorders, 8(3), 138–150.

Ledgerd R, Hoe J, Hoare Z, Devine M, Toot S, Challis D, Orrell M. 2016. Identifying the causes, prevention and management of crises in dementia: An online survey of stakeholders. Int J Geriatr Psychiatry, 31(6), 638–647.

Li Y, Hai S, Zhou Y, Dong BR. 2015. Cholinesterase inhibitors for rarer dementias associated with neurological conditions. Cochrane Database of Systematic Reviews, 3. CD009444.

Logiudice D, Waltrowicz W, Brown K, Burrows C, Ames D, Flicker L. 1999. Do memory clinics improve the quality of life of carers? A randomized pilot trial. Int J Geriatr Psychiatry, 14(8), 626–632.

Luengo-Fernandez R, Leal J, Gray A. 2015. UK research spend in 2008 and 2012: comparing stroke, cancer, coronary heart disease and dementia. BMJ Open, 5(4), e006648.

McCrone P. 2008. The economics of dementia. British Journal of Healthcare Management, 14(10), 437–440.

Marcantonio ER. 2010. Delirium. In JT Pacala, GM Sullivan (eds), Geriatrics Review Syllabus: A Core Curriculum in Geriatric Medicine, 7th edn, New York: The American Geriatrics Society.

Marmor T, Oberlander J. 2012. From HMOs to ACOs: the quest for the Holy Grail in U.S. health policy. J Gen Intern Med, 27(9), 1215–1218.

Maruthappu M, Sood HS, Keogh B. 2014. The NHS five year forward view: implications for clinicians. BMJ, 349, g6518.

Mate KE, Magin PJ, Brodaty H, Stocks NP, Gunn J, Disler PB, Marley JE, Pond CD. 2016. An evaluation of the additional benefit of population screening for dementia beyond a passive case-finding approach. Int J Geriatr Psychiatry, doi: 10.1002/gps.4466.

Matthews FE, Dening T. 2002. UK medical research council cognitive function and ageing study: prevalence of dementia in institutional care. Lancet, 360(9328), 225–226.

McHugh N, Baker RM, Mason H, Williamson L, et al. 2015. Extending life for people with a terminal illness: a moral right and an expensive death? Exploring societal perspectives. BMC Med Ethics, 16, 14.

Minkman MM, Vermeulen RP, Ahaus KT, Huijsman R. 2011. The implementation of integrated care: the empirical validation of the Development Model for Integrated care. BMC Health Serv Res, 11, 177.

Minkman MM, Vermeulen RP, Ahaus KT, Huijsman R. 2013. A survey study to validate a four phases development model for integrated care in the Netherlands. BMC Health Serv Res, 13(13), 214.

Murray CJ, Vos T, Lozano R, Naghavi M, et al. 2012. Disability-adjusted life years (DALYs) for 291 diseases and injuries in 21 regions, 1990–2010: a systematic analysis for the Global Burden of Disease Study 2010. Lancet, 380(9859), 2197–2223.

Nardell M, Tampi RR. 2014. Pharmacological treatments for frontotemporal dementias: a systematic review of randomized controlled trials. Am J Alzheimers Dis Other Demen, 29(2), 123–132.

National Voices. 2013. A Narrative for Person-Centred Coordinated Care, available at www.england.nhs.uk/wp-content/uploads/2013/05/nv-narrative-cc.pdf (accessed 3 Oct 2016).

NHS. 2015. NHS Choices: Care and Support Plans, available at www.nhs.uk/Conditions/social-care-and-support-guide/Pages/care-plans.aspx (accessed 6 Oct 2016).

NHS Choices. 2015. How is Dementia Treated? Available at www.nhs.uk/conditions/dementia-guide/pages/dementia-treatment.aspx (accessed 3 Sept 2016).

NHS Confederation. 2015. Germany's Approach to Integrated Care Is Delivering a Trio of Achievements, Says Elisabetta Zanon, 13 July 2015 (blog), available at www.nhsconfed.org/blog/2015/07/improving-health-integrating-services-and-reducing-costs (accessed 3 Oct 2016).

NHS England. 2014. The Five Year Forward View, available at www.england.nhs.uk/wp-content/uploads/2014/10/5yfv-web.pdf (accessed 3 Sept 2016).

NHS England. 2015a. Dementia Diagnosis and Management: A Brief Pragmatic Resource for General Practitioners, available at www.england.nhs.uk/wp-content/uploads/2015/01/dementia-diag-mng-ab-pt.pdf (accessed 3 Oct 2016).

NHS England. 2015b. Building the NHS of the Five Year Forward View: The NHS England Business Plan 2015–16, available at www.england.nhs.uk/wp-content/uploads/2015/03/business-plan-mar15.pdf (accessed 3 Oct 2016).

NHS England and Public Health England. 2013. A Call to Action: Commissioning for Prevention, available at www.england.nhs.uk/wp-content/uploads/2013/11/call-to-action-com-prev.pdf (accessed 3 Oct 2016).

NICE. 2001. Final Appraisal Determination: Donepezil, Galantamine, Rivastigmine (Review) and Memantine for the Treatment of Alzheimer's Disease, available at www.nice.org.uk/guidance/ta111/documents/alzheimers-disease-donepezil-rivastigmine-galantamine-and-memantine-review-final-appraisal-document2 (accessed 3 Oct 2016).

NICE. 2015. Dementia Overview, available at pathways.nice.org.uk/pathways/dementia (accessed 3 Oct 2016).

O'Brien JT, Burns A, BAP Dementia Consensus Group. 2011. Clinical practice with anti-dementia drugs: a revised (second) consensus statement from the British Association for Psychopharmacology. J Psychopharmacol, 25(8), 997–1019.

Office of the UNHCR. 2008. The Right to Health: Fact Sheet No. 31, available at www.ohchr.org/Documents/Publications/Factsheet31.pdf (accessed 3 Oct 2016).

Orrell M, Brayne C. 2015. INTERDEM (early detection and timely INTERvention in DEMentia); Alzheimer Europe; Alzheimer's Disease International; European Association of Geriatric Psychiatry. Dementia prevention: call to action. Lancet, 386(10004), 1625.

Owens DK, Qaseem A, Chou R, Shekelle P. 2011. High-value, cost-conscious health care: concepts for clinicians to evaluate the benefits, harms, and costs of medical interventions. Ann Intern Med, 154, 174–180.

Perry-Young L, Owen G, Kelly S, Owens C. 2016. How people come to recognise a problem and seek medical help for a person showing early signs of dementia: a systematic review and meta-ethnography. Dementia (London), 1471301215626889 (e-pub ahead of print).

Pinquart M, Sorensen S. 2003. Association of stressors and uplifts of caregiving with caregiver burden and depressive mood: a meta-analysis. J Gerontol B Psychol, 58(2): 112–128.

PRIAE in collaboration with ISCRI. 2010. Mental Health Care for Black and Minority Ethnic Elders, available at www.priae.org/assets/4_PRIAE-ISCRI_Managing_Better_Mental_Health_Care_for_BME_Older_People_2010.pdf (accessed 29 Nov 2016).

Prince MJ, Prina M, Guerchet M. 2013. *World Alzheimer Report 2013: Journey of Caring. An Analysis of Long-Term Care for Dementia*, London: Alzheimer's Disease International.

Prince MJ, Wu F, Guo Y, Gutierrez Robledo LM, et al. 2015. The burden of disease in older people and implications for health policy and practice. Lancet, 385(9967), 549–562.

Public Health England. 2016. Health Matters: Midlife Approaches to Reduce Dementia Risk, available at www.gov.uk/government/publications/health-matters-midlife-approaches-to-reduce-dementia-risk/healthmatters-midlife-approaches-to-reduce-dementia-risk (accessed 12 Oct 2016).

Public Health England and UK Health Forum. 2015. Blackfriars Consensus on Promoting Brain Health: Reducing Risks for Dementia in the Population, available at nhfshare.heartforum.org.uk/RMAssets/Reports/Blackfriars%20consensus%20%20_V18.pdf (accessed 3 Oct 2016).

Raak A, Mur-Veeman I, Hardy B, Steenbergen M, Paulus A. 2003. *Integrated Care in Europe: Description and Comparison of Integrated Care in Six EU Countries*, Maarssen: Elsevier Gezondheidszorg.

Rahman S. 2015. *Living Better with Dementia*, London: Jessica Kingsley Publishers.

Reisberg B, Doody R, Stöffler A, Schmitt F, et al. 2003. Memantine in moderate-to-severe Alzheimer's disease. N Engl J Med, 348(14), 1333–1341.

Roberts A, Thompson S, Charlesworth A, Gershlick B, Stirling A. 2015. Filling the Gap: Tax and Fiscal Options for a Sustainable UK Health and Social Care System, available at _www.health.org.uk/sites/health/files/FillingTheGap_1.pdf (accessed 3 Sept 2016).

Robertson M, Brown E, Whalley L. 2014, Dementia prevention: shared questions for research and clinical management. Maturitas, 77(2), 124–127.

Robinson L, Clare L, Evans K. 2005. Making sense of dementia and adjusting to loss: psychological reactions to a diagnosis of dementia in couples. Ageing and Mental Health, 9, 337–347.

Robinson L, Gemski A, Abley C, Bond J, et al. 2011. The transition to dementia – individual and family experiences of receiving a diagnosis: a review. Int Psychogeriatr, 23(7), 1026–1043.

Robinson L, Tang E, Taylor JP. 2015. Dementia: timely diagnosis and early intervention. BMJ, 350, h3029.

Rooney RF. 2014. Preventing dementia: how lifestyle in midlife affects risk. Curr Opin Psychiatry, 27(2), 149–157.

Royal College of General Practitioners. 2014. A New Route to Dementia Care (blogpost, 22 May), available at www.rcgp.org.uk/news/2014/may/a-new-route-to-good-dementia-care.aspx (accessed 3 Oct 2016).

Samsi K, Abley C, Campbell S, Keady J, et al. 2014. Negotiating a labyrinth: experiences of assessment and diagnostic journey in cognitive impairment and dementia. Int J Geriatr Psychiatry, 29(1), 58–67.

Sanderson H, Bown L, Bailey G. 2015. *Person-Centred Thinking with Older People: Six Essential Practices*, London: Jessica Kingsley Publishers.

Schaller S, Mauskopf J, Kriza C, Wahlster P, Kolominsky-Rabas PL. 2015. The main cost drivers in dementia: a systematic review. Int J Geriatr Psychiatry, 30(2), 111–129.

Schiffczyk C, Romero B, Jonas C, Lahmeyer C, Müller F, Riepe MW. 2010. Generic quality of life assessment in dementia patients: a prospective cohort study. BMC Neurology, 10, 48.

Schrijvers G, van Hoorn A, Huiskes N. 2012. The care pathway: concepts and theories: an introduction. Int J Integr Care, 18, 12(Spec Ed Integrated Care Pathways), e192.

Shaw S, Rosen R, Rumbold B. 2011. *What is Integrated Care?* London: The Nuffield Trust, available at www.nuffieldtrust.org.uk/sites/files/nuffield/publication/what_is_integrated_care_research_report_june11_0.pdf (accessed 3 Oct 2016).

Shinagawa S, Catindig JA, Block NR, Miller BL, Rankin KP. 2016. When a little knowledge can be dangerous: false-positive diagnosis of behavioral variant frontotemporal dementia among community clinicians. Dement Geriatr Cogn Disord, 41(1–2), 99–108.

Sjögren K, Lindkvist M, Sandman PO, Zingmark K, Edvardsson D. 2013. Person-centredness and its association with resident wellbeing in dementia care units. J Adv Nurs, 69(10):2196–2205.

Spector A, Orrell M. 2006. Quality of Life (QoL) in dementia: a comparison of the perceptions of people with dementia and care staff in residential homes. Alzheimer Dis Assoc Disord, 20(3), 160–165.

Stokes G, Goudie F (eds). 2002. *The Essential Dementia Care Handbook*, London: Speechmark Publishing Ltd.

Takechi H, Kokuryu A, Kubota T, Yamada H. 2012. Relative preservation of advanced activities in daily living among patients with mild to moderate dementia in the community and overview of support provided by family caregivers. Int J Alzheimers Dis, 418289.

Taylor A. 2015. *Building the House of Care*, London: Health Foundation, available at personcentredcare.health.org.uk/sites/default/files/resources/buildingthehouseofcare_0.pdf (accessed 3 Oct 2016).

Terada S, Oshima E, Yokota O, Ikeda C, et al. 2013. Person-centred care and quality of life of patients with dementia in long-term care facilities. Psychiatry Res, 205(1–2), 103–108.

Tulloch A. 2005. What do we mean by health? Br J Gen Pract, 55(513), 320–323; discussion, 321–322.

Vanhaecht K, De Witte K, Sermeus W. 2007. *The Impact of Clinical Pathways on the Organisation of Care Processes*, Leuven: ACCO, available at https://lirias.kuleuven.be/bitstream/123456789/252816/1/PhD+Kris+Vanhaecht.pdf (accessed 3 Oct 2016).

Vanhaecht K, Panella M, van Zelm R, Sermeus W. 2010. An overview on the history and concept of care pathways as complex interventions. International Journal of Care Pathways, 14, 117–123.

Vellas B, Oustric S. 2014. Alzheimer's preventive approaches and cognitive monitoring must be integrated into the primary care setting. J Am Med Dir Assoc, 15(11), 783–785.

Vroomen JM, Bosmans JE, van Hout HP, de Rooij SE. 2013. Reviewing the definition of crisis in dementia care. BMC Geriatr, 13(1), 10.

WHO. 1995. The World Health Organization Quality of Life Assessment (WHOQOL): Position paper from the World Health Organization. Soc Sci Med, 41, 1403–1409.

Williams N. 2016. The Care Homes at the Vanguard of Better Health, *The Guardian* (15 March 2016), available at www.theguardian.com/society/2016/mar/15/care-homes-vanguard-better-health (accessed 3 Oct 2016).

Winblad B. 2009. Donepezil in severe Alzheimer's disease. Am J Alzheimers Dis Other Demen, 24(3), 185–192.

Winblad B, Poritis N. 1999. Memantine in severe dementia: results of the 9M-Best Study (benefit and efficacy in severely demented patients during treatment with memantine). Int J Geriatr Psychiatry, 14(2), 135–146.

WISH. 2015. A Call to Action: The Global Response to Dementia through Innovation, available at www.imperial.ac.uk/media/imperial-college/institute-of-global-health-innovation/public/Dementia.pdf (accessed 3 Sept 2016).

Wu YT, Fratiglioni L, Matthews FE, Lobo A, et al. 2016. Dementia in western Europe: epidemiological evidence and implications for policymaking. Lancet Neurol, 15(1), 116–124.

Wübker A, Zwakhalen SM, Challis D, Suhonen R, et al. 2015. Costs of care for people with dementia just before and after nursing home placement: primary data from eight European countries. Eur J Health Econ, 16(7), 689–707.

Yee JL, Schultz R. 2000. Gender differences in psychiatric morbidity among family caregivers. Gerontologist, 40, 147–164.

Yoo JW, Nakagawa S, Kim S. 2013. Delirium and transition to a nursing home of hospitalized older adults: a controlled trial of assessing the interdisciplinary team-based 'geriatric' care and care coordination by non-geriatrics specialist physicians. Geriatr Gerontol Int, 13(2), 342–350.

Chapter 2

CARING WELL:
AN OVERVIEW

If we presume that the majority of people in these settings are genteel old ladies pottering about as if in a television sitcom rather than people with significant disability then we are mistaken and will underestimate what level of care needs to be provided. (Gladman et al., 2007, p.186)

Learning objectives

By the end of this chapter, you will:

» be aware of a relationship between complexity science and innovation

» be introduced to the roles of 'person-centred care', 'relationship-centred care' and 'family-centred care' in producing value in therapeutic relationships and the development of services

» understand the background to 'consumer-directed care'

» understand the philosophy and ethos of 'co-production'

» understand the critical relevance of human-rights-based approaches to citizenship, and how such legislation can provide a framework for service provision including physical restraint and surveillance

» appreciate the importance of 'dementia-friendly environments'

» be introduced to the notion of 'quality of care' and how dementia care is approached in hospitals

» have an appreciation of 'organisational culture'

» be introduced to the social movement of cultural change in residential settings

» be introduced to the critical importance of leadership and staff development

Introduction

It is thought that the top priorities for the NHS and social care include putting services on a financially sustainable footing, redesigning care and getting serious about prevention. Ultimately, all innovations involve a trade-off between risk and return. To minimise risk and unintended consequences, users, companies and policymakers alike need to understand how to make informed choices about new products and services (Merton, 2013).

Complexity theory is the study of complex adaptive systems. The core concept in complexity theory is encompassed by the science of emergence (Samet, 2011), where interacting agents lead to system-level behaviour which is not possible to present by simply summing up the behaviour of the individual agent.

Mainstream innovation studies have been increasingly criticised as being too sequential, linear or phasic in providing an understanding of innovation dynamics. Arguably they pay insufficient attention to the dynamic, uncertain and complex nature of innovation (Zhao, 2014). Although the innovation process can seem linear, it is often in reality non-linear and iterative (Anderson, De Dreu and Nijstad, 2004), due to different actors and contexts involved in the process. Instead, organisations may need to switch to dynamic systems of interconnected associations that are able to change in ways that exceed the complex demands and expectations of today's organisations (Duin and Baer, 2010). Complex adaptive systems are changeable structures with numerous, intersecting hierarchies (Uhl-Bien, Marion and McKelvey 2007). The need for organisational innovation as a means of improving health care quality and containing costs is very widely acknowledged. However, although a growing body of research has improved knowledge of implementation, very little research has considered the challenges involved in sustaining change – especially organisational change led 'bottom-up' by frontline clinicians (Martin et al., 2012). As there appears currently to be profound mistrust of UK politicians and their sudden 'top-down' reform, this is important.

In corporate strategy, the strategic reality for most companies has been that both their business and their environment are complex in real time, whereas the proposed solutions have often been simple, even simplistic. On the other hand, the multiple information channels of flexible management processes allow organisations to capture and analyse external complexity. This is clearly no less relevant to our contemporary NHS and social care.

Centres of care

Essential attributes of **person-centred care** include: knowing and respecting the person as an individual with unique values, needs and preferences; maximising freedom of choice and autonomy; nurturing consistent and trusting relationships;

supporting physical and emotional comfort; and engaging the person's family and friends where appropriate (Cherry et al., 2008). The foundation of non-pharmacological management is to recognise that, for the individual with dementia, it is no longer possible to easily adapt to new conditions; the environment must therefore be adapted to the individual's specific needs (Van Hoof et al., 2010).

Although person-centred care and individualised care have been widely applied and have been included in various government policy directions, recent studies demonstrate that issues relating to quality of care exist in all long-term care settings, but they seem to be especially salient in long-term dementia care (Lillekroken, Hauge and Slettebø, 2015). Efforts to promote person-centred residential dementia care have undoubtedly expanded in the last two decades, following the publication of Kitwood's (1997) seminal work *Dementia Reconsidered*. Kitwood famously described personhood as 'a standing or status that is bestowed upon one human being, by others, in the context of relationship and social being...[implying] recognition, respect, and trust' (p.8). He also identified several styles of interaction that either support or undermine the personhood of individuals with dementia.

This philosophy of person-centred care for persons with cognitive loss reconceptualised dementia as a process dependent on the pathological process and the social psychology of the person affected (Kitwood and Benson, 1995; Murray and Boyd, 2009). That paradigm shift was vital. Person-centred care, as opposed to task-orientated or disease-centred care, takes a holistic approach that emphasises the perspective of the person with dementia and their self-defined experiences and needs (Epp, 2003).

Personhood is critical to integrated care in dementia.

Elements of person-centred care have been extensively described elsewhere, but a working definition is helpful:

> Person-centred care is also a way of viewing health and illness that affects a person's general wellbeing and an attempt to empower the patient by expanding his or her role in their health care. Making the patient more informed, and providing reassurance, support, comfort, acceptance, legitimacy and confidence, are the basic functions of this approach. (Paparella, 2016, p.6)

Brooker and Latham (2016) remind us that for personhood to blossom, people need to feel loved. Kitwood identified five psychological needs that are at risk of being unmet in people living with dementia. If these needs go unmet over a period of time then personhood withers.

Box 2.1: Psychological needs in dementia

INCLUSION

Inclusion is about being in or being brought into the social world either physically or verbally, and making someone feel part of the group. Total acceptance of the person.

ATTACHMENT

Attachment relates to bonding, connection, nurture, trust and security in relationships. Without this, it can be difficult to function well. There is every reason to suppose that the need for attachment remains when a person has dementia.

IDENTITY

Identity relates to the need to know who you are and having a sense of continuity with the past. It is about having a life story that is held and maintained either by the person with dementia or for them by others.

OCCUPATION

Occupation relates to being involved in activity that is personally meaningful; having a sense of agency; and having control to make things happen. In the context of person-centred care, it means for the person to be involved in a significant way in the process of life by using their remaining abilities.

COMFORT

Comfort is about the provision of tenderness, closeness and soothing and is provided through physical touch and/or comfort in words and gestures. Comfort also relates to a need for warmth and compassion to soothe inner anxieties.

SOURCE: ADAPTED FROM BROOKER AND LATHAM (2016).

Although there is no universal consensus on the definition of the concept, person-centred care must include striving to maintain personhood despite declining cognitive ability (Normann, Aspland and Norberg, 1999; Skaalvik, Normann and Henriksen, 2010).

It is also worth collecting and using personal experiences of life and relationships to individualise care and the environment (Normann et al., 1999; Ettema et al., 2007). This approach to the care of the person with dementia takes time to nurture and is usually most easily achieved through consistent, longer term relationships with carers (Clissett et al., 2013). On the other hand, Nolan and colleagues (2002, p.203) have argued that person-centred care fails to 'capture the interdependencies and reciprocalities that underpin caring relationships' and it does not elicit 'mutual appreciation of each other's knowledge, recognition of its equal worth, and its sharing in a symbolic way to enhance and facilitate joint understanding'.

The alternative paradigm of **relationship-centred care** is therefore focused on all the actors in the delivery of health care services and population health management services. It has also become a potent force in thinking about integrated dementia services. The relationship with the patient is the most important role in a way that is fully consistent with the theory and application of patient-centred care. It also includes the whole care team – not only the physician, but also the nurse, the care coordinator, the health coach and other individual providers, as well as the clinic and the entire health care delivery system (Nundy and Oswald, 2014).

My Home Life is a collaborative initiative between Age UK, City University, the Joseph Rowntree Foundation and Dementia UK (Owen and Meyer, 2012). It promotes quality of life in care homes. Positive relationships in care homes can enable staff to listen to older people, gain insights into individual needs and facilitate greater voice, choice and control. Relationship-centred care is at the heart of many examples of best practice. Care home managers play a pivotal role in promoting relationships between older people, staff and relatives. With ongoing professional development and backing from colleagues across health and social care, managers can create a culture of greater spontaneity and responsiveness where positive, informed risks can be taken within a structure of safety and accountability.

Key points about My Home Life are shown in Box 2.2.

Box 2.2: The eight personalisation themes linked to quality of life identified by My Home Life

The best practices that seek to personalise and individualise care by tailoring care to each individual to ensure quality of life are as follows:

* Maintaining identity: working creatively with residents to maintain their sense of personal identity and engage in meaningful activity.

* Sharing decision-making: facilitating informed risk taking and the involvement of residents, relatives and staff in shared decision-making in all aspects of home life.

* Creating community: optimising relationships between and across staff, residents, family, friends and the wider local community. Encouraging a sense of security, continuity, belonging, purpose, achievement and significance for all.

Navigation themes (linked to quality of care), supporting people as they navigate their way through the journey of care:

    *   Managing transitions: supporting people to manage the loss and upheaval associated with going into a home and move forward.

    *   Improving health and health care: ensuring adequate access to health care services and promoting health to optimise residents' quality of life.

    *   Supporting good end of life: valuing the 'living' and 'dying' in care homes and helping residents to prepare for a 'good death' with the support of their families.

Transformation themes (linked to quality of management), concerned with the leadership and management required to transform care into best practice to better meet the changing needs of residents:

    *   Keeping the workforce fit for purpose: identifying and meeting ever-changing training needs within the care-home workforce.

    *   Promoting a positive culture: developing leadership, management and expertise to deliver a culture of care where care homes are seen as a positive option.

SOURCE: DEMOS (2014, P.70).

Researchers have developed instruments and indicators to measure factors that influence person-centred care from patients' and nurses' perspectives (Ross, Tod and Clarke, 2015). These factors include: relationships in the care setting, involvement in decisions about care, and the culture of the care environment. While the focus of these studies is on the individual, many elements have congruence with the relationship-centred approach seen as essential to the Senses framework by Nolan et al. (2004, 2006). This framework was developed specifically to address nursing practice and education in the care of older people. It emphasises the need for each person (patients, family and staff alike) to feel valued and recognised as a person through relationships which are satisfying to all. There has also been a growing realisation of the need to involve family members in care and offering shared decision-making (Sabat, 2005; Sjögren et al., 2011; Van der Steen et al., 2011). The concept of person-centred care has now been fully expanded to include **family-centred care**, which acknowledges the important role of the family or other loved ones in the patient's final days (Teno et al., 2001). This might mean, for example, relieving family members of the burden of being present at all times to advocate for their loved one; or, educating family members so they feel confident enough to care for their loved ones at home. It is also striking that bereaved family members of persons dying from dementia who received hospice treatment reported fewer unmet needs and concerns with quality of care.

Furthermore, McCormack and colleagues have conducted a series of rigorous studies mostly based on the care of older people (McCormack et al., 2012). Their work emphasises the value of the nurse's relationships with the person and their family, but also the need for seeing broader influences on person-centred practice. They identify the importance of elements such as the dynamics of power and control, the effect of institutional discourse, authenticity, the care environment, appropriate skill mix, effective staff relationships and shared values within the team (McCormack and McCance, 2010). These and other concepts drawn from this programme of work have innovatively been used to develop a person-centred framework for nursing, using it as the basis for a series of practice development programmes (McCormack and McCance, 2010).

Barriers to the implementation of person-centred care have been reviewed by the American Geriatrics Society Expert Panel on Person-Centred Care (2016). These include:

» misaligned incentives

» lack of advance care planning

» lack of continuity in health records.

Person-centred care is now thought to be very important in dementia care (Murray and Boyd, 2009). Adaptation of the care process, the staffing models, clinical routines and policies that best meet the needs of the person require a great deal of flexibility in the clinical setting. Thus, the whole organisation of care is an important part of the delivery of person-centred care (Edvardsson, Winblad and Sandman, 2008); this is likely to extend ultimately to the whole health economy.

Consumer-directed care

We are all persons, but the clunky, marketised version of 'consumers' still remains popular, particularly in certain jurisdictions. Many developing countries face the challenge of integrating traditional government health resources with a large and growing private health sector both for profit and not for profit (Kula and Fryatt, 2014). Anticipated upward trends in the number of people with dementia will lead to substantial increases in health and social care spending unless provision is altered or there are somehow major breakthroughs in prevention or disease course (Comas-Herrera et al., 2007). The challenge for programme designers is to develop new structures that allow participants to better articulate their support needs to remain as independent as possible and to make support services more responsive and accountable (Spandler, 2004).

Consumer-directed care (similar notions include 'self-directed care', 'personal budgets' or 'personalisation' in the UK) was introduced to the aged/social care sector of many developed countries in the 1980s and 1990s. It aims to increase clients' service choices and control and ultimately achieve various policy goals, such as improving client outcomes and saving costs (You, Dunt and Doyle, 2015). A new field of 'consumer neuroscience' is now developing, where traditional approaches from sociology, neurology, neuroscience and psychiatry converge to inform how the brains of consumers actually make decisions in varying conditions of risk and reward (Javor et al., 2013).

Co-production

Co-production has historical roots in civil rights and social care movements in the US. The idea was articulated by the 2009 Nobel prize winner for economics, Elinor Ostrom, and her team at Indiana University, who coined the term 'co-production' in a series of studies of the Chicago police in the 1970s (Boyle and Harris, 2009). Ostrom's team defined co-production as the 'process through which inputs used to produce a good or service are contributed by individuals who are not "in" the same organisation' (quoted in Boyle and Harris, 2009, p.13). User involvement in planning and policy decision-making has become the policy of choice for governments as well as health and social care service providers in most democratic countries (Department of Health, 2006). This has become a powerful force for integrated dementia care.

Co-production starts from the idea that no one group or person is more important than any other. Everyone is equal and has assets to bring to the process. The term assets refers to skills, abilities, time and other qualities that people have. This is different from approaches that focus on people's problems and what they cannot do (SCIE, 2013). Co-production refers to participation by stakeholders from civil society and the market in the implementation of public policy, while co-construction refers to participation by those same stakeholders in the design of public policy (Vaillancourt, 2009). Trust is fundamental to effective interpersonal relations and community living (Mechanic and Meyer, 2000). It offers both micro-level benefits for the parties involved in a relationship, and macro-level benefits for the wider society (Stevenson and Scrambler, 2005). Where they are challenged, ways of shifting them to participation and co-production are required (Bovaird, 2007), or else a contrived illusion of participation is fabricated.

—— Human rights-based approaches ——

Human rights, whether conceptualised at an international level or national level, offer powerful frameworks for people to gain fair and equal treatment (Roberts et al., 2015). Public attitudes towards human rights in the UK have, for some time now, been rather confused and contradictory, to some extent resulting from misleading and inaccurate mainstream media coverage, as well as political manipulation (Bell and Cemlyn, 2014). The literature highlights issues such as surrogate decision-making, restraint and 'wandering', where human rights are not routinely considered in decision-making (Robinson et al., 2007).

The Audit Commission's report described the state of human rights in health care in England in 2003. It illustrated why the creation of the Human Rights in Health Care Programme was essential. If health organisations had largely failed to observe the Human Rights Act during a period of relative stability, it was even less likely that human rights would be significantly advanced during the organisational upheaval that was scheduled to occur (Audit Commission, 2003). It is argued that the Human Rights Act[1] has not brought about the cultural change in health services that was originally envisaged.

Examples of potential breaches of human rights are shown in Box 2.3.

Box 2.3: Potential breaches of human rights for care at home

* **Article 8** (right to respect for private and family life): for example, if care interferes with personal dignity or fails to address severe social isolation and a lack of meaningful contact with family, this could be an unjustifiable interference with Article 8 rights.

* **Article 3** (prohibition of inhuman or degrading treatment): for example, in some circumstances, a lack of care, serious neglect or intentional ill-treatment by a care provider may amount to a breach of Article 3.

* **Article 2** (right to life): for example, if an older person who is highly dependent on home care services were to die as a result of care visits being stopped without warning, this could amount to a breach of Article 2.

* **Article 9** (freedom of thought, conscience or religion): for example, if home care services fail to take account of a person's religious observances, this could be an unjustifiable interference with Article 9 rights.

* **Article 14** (on non-discrimination in the enjoyment of other human rights): for example, when compared to younger disabled adults, older people receive

---

1   Available at www.legislation.gov.uk/ukpga/1998/42/contents (accessed 3 Oct 2016).

less generous home care packages which do not support social activity. This could be a breach of Article 14 in conjunction with Article 8 (right to respect for private life).

SOURCE: EQUALITY AND HUMAN RIGHTS COMMISSION (2012).

Human rights are universal in that all people in the world are entitled to them, and these rights are inherent to the dignity of every human. This also applies to people living with dementia and their family carers; however, their rights are often overlooked or even deliberately trampled on. It is therefore important to address the issue of dementia through a **human rights-based approach** (HRBA).[2]

A HRBA views human rights as:

» a set of legal standards and obligations

» a source of principles and practical methods which determine how those standards and obligations are achieved.

Collective narratives, often realised in social policy, create the space within which individuals exercise their citizenship rights (Baldwin and Bradford Dementia Group, 2008). In so doing, they also create formal representations of identity – for example, what constitutes the formal representation of an ageing identity (see, for example, Powell and Edwards, 2002). Service user inclusion is a key component of a human rights-based approach to health care, and models of inclusion are developing rapidly. Co-production, or sharing service design and delivery more equally with service users, has led to outcomes that were initially inconceivable (Roberts, Greenhill and Talbot, 2011). A focus on professionally led approaches to risk assessment and management may also ignore or underplay risks which many service users see as important, such as the disempowering aspects of much mental health provision and the overemphasis on medication to support individuals experiencing mental distress (Langan and Lindow, 2004). A HRBA to development planning and programming can help in addressing unjust distributions of power, bring a focus to the rule of law and make development achievements more sustainable. All human beings are entitled to enjoy their human rights equally without discrimination.

The Sustainable Development Goals (SDGs) have now developed from the WHO. They are a new, universal set of goals, targets and indicators that UN member states will be expected to use to frame their agendas and political policies over the next 15 years. A key one is to ensure healthy lives and promote wellbeing for everyone at all ages (Ford, 2015). Human rights and the SDGs can be implemented in a mutually reinforcing manner, and human rights can strengthen efforts to

---

2   Available at hrbaportal.org (accessed 3 Oct 2016).

achieve the SDGs. Human rights approaches can reinforce the legitimacy of SDG implementation strategies that build on legal obligations in human rights treaties. A key sustainable development goal is to make sure people are in good health and know how to make decisions to stay healthy all through their lives.

The importance of citizenship, or the 'right to belong to some kind of organized community', as a 'right to have rights' (Arendt, 1958, pp.296–297), was highlighted in Arendt's (1958) writing on the plight of stateless people in Europe before, during and after the Second World War. Arendt highlighted the perilous situation of those displaced from one country and accorded no citizenship rights in their new 'home'. Citizenship is commonly referred to as an agreement between the citizens and welfare authorities that typically includes civil, political and social citizenship rights, as well as duties (Marshall and Bottomore, 1950/1992). It is arguably not clear *why* a citizenship lens has not made more of an impact on dementia practice and research. The idea that people with dementia have rights has long been recognised, and the need to treat a person with dementia as an equal has been voiced (Kitwood, 1997). Yet citizenship is rarely if ever explicitly used to theorise the situation of people with dementia; the preferred frame of reference in the literature is invariably personhood (Bartlett and O'Connor, 2007).

Sexual citizenship has many features in common with other claims to wider citizenship. It is about enfranchisement, belonging, equity and justice, and rights balanced by responsibilities. It emerged as a distinct sub-field of citizenship out of a concern for the need to broaden the conceptualisation of citizenship to accommodate not only class and race, but also gender and sexuality (e.g. Cossman, 2007). Sexual citizenship and sexual rights scholarship have made important contributions to broadening citizenship and more fully accommodating rights related to sexuality (Kontos et al., 2016).

From a human rights perspective, it is important to consider whether the protection of public health is potentially also a human right, be it individual or collective in nature (Toebes, 2015).

The Care Act 2014[3] (which came into force in April 2015) is (potentially) very relevant for people with dementia and their carers to consider in terms of securing their rights. The legislation outlines the domains of wellbeing that it pertains to, including protection from abuse, control by the individual over their day-to-day life, physical and mental health, and emotional wellbeing.

---

3   Available at www.legislation.gov.uk/ukpga/2014/23/contents/enacted/data.htm (accessed 3 Oct 2016).

—— Physical restraints

Physical restraints are commonly used in geriatric long-term care in different countries, as shown by several international studies (Hamers, Gulpers and Strik, 2004; Meyer et al., 2009). A European study identified restraint rates in geriatric hospitals at 0% in Austria and Denmark, 0–2% in Germany, 0–3% in Switzerland, 2–12% in the Netherlands, 3% in the Czech Republic, 7% in France and 7–22% in Belgium. The use of bed rails was excluded from the data collection (de Vries et al., 2004).

A physical restraint is commonly defined as:

> Any device, material or equipment attached to or near a person's body and which cannot be controlled or easily removed by the person and which deliberately prevents or is deliberately intended to prevent a person's free body movement to a position of choice and/or a person's normal access to their body. (Joanna Briggs Institute, 2002, p.2)

The commitment to providing quality care and quality of life for residents of an aged care facility is evident. It is important that the concept of risk taking is seen as an integral part of life and is not denied to the older person (Koch, Nay and Wilson, 2006). While nurses accept that the use of restraints infringes on patients' rights, they can also perceive such use as *essential* to protect patients from harm and falls (Johnson, Ostaszkiewicz and O'Connell, 2009).

—— Hidden surveillance

By hidden surveillance one usually means the use of hidden cameras or audio equipment to monitor the actions of staff or others in their interactions with someone under their care. Recent incidents of abusive or neglectful care in care homes and hospitals (e.g. Winterbourne View, Orchid View and Mid-Staffordshire NHS Trust) have prompted a debate about the use of surveillance cameras to deter and detect poor care.

The very organisation of this discussion into a legal and a moral perspective highlights the fundamental conceptual and semantic complexities of capturing all that is subsumed under the rubric of privacy rights. Prominent scholars have dealt with this issue by defining it variously as a value or a moral claim, or as a legal right (Bharucha et al., 2006).

According to the Care Quality Commission (2015) and many others, the use of recording equipment is not a straightforward issue. One perceived benefit of surveillance technology is that it can afford clients more freedom of movement as part of an active policy to reduce the use of traditional physical restraints. But staff might continue to lock certain doors, most often during the night and at the beginning of or during rounds (Niemeijer et al., 2014). There is also concern that 'hidden cameras' do not avoid the problem of cuts in social care budgets, including the 'system-wide problem of chronic understaffing' (Stubbs, 2015).

—— Dementia-friendly environments ——

The notion of the climate or atmosphere of an institution refers to the holistic experience of the environment. Findings from Edvardsson, Fetherstonhaugh and Nay (2010) crucially indicated that the core category of person-centred care was 'promoting a continuation of self and normality'. The analysis further illuminated five content categories contributing to promoting a continuation of self and normality: knowing the person; welcoming family; providing meaningful activities; being in a personalised environment; and experiencing flexibility and continuity. Person-centred care is a best practice concept guiding efforts to improve residents' quality of life in long-term care facilities. The care philosophy recognises that individuals have unique values, personal history and personality (Chaudhury, Hung and Badger, 2013).

In the past decades, there has been an increasing awareness that the physical and psychosocial environment is essential for the quality of life of people with dementia, their family members and the wellbeing of care staff. New care models arose from the idea that people with dementia first needed a safe and familiar environment (Pot, 2013). The restorative effects of places on health and wellbeing are well documented (Lengen, 2015). This has led to the key concept of **therapeutic landscapes** (Gesler, 1992). Gesler's work has emphasised that the positive meanings people attach to place contribute to sustaining health and wellbeing. To this end, place matters in relation to lived experience, emotional ties and meanings (Macintyre, Ellaway and Cummins 2002).

A dementia-friendly environment arguably compensates for disability. It should consider both the importance for the person with dementia of their experiences within the environment and the social, physical and organisational environments which impact on these experiences (Davis et al., 2009). The literature on designing facilities for people with dementia, which has accumulated over the last 35 years, supports the inclusion of a number of features at care homes for people with dementia (Fleming and Purandare, 2010).

In terms of physical environments, designs are sought which provide balanced and controlled stimulation, and features that assist orientation, compensate for disability, and promote involvement in everyday activity (Sawamura, Nakashima and Nakanishi, 2013). The impact of the characteristics of the architectural structure of a nursing home on a resident's wayfinding abilities can be measured by the destinations they were able to reach independently (Marquandt and Schmieg, 2009). When orientation, memory and the ability to understand reality fail, human relations become increasingly valuable to patients' quality of life. The ability of health workers to cooperate with each individual in accordance with his or her needs and remaining resources is imperative (Wogn-Henriksen, 1997). Modern units may incorporate a high-stimulus *Snoezelen* room or a Namaste room. Exercise has proven to be highly efficacious, not only for improving cognition but also for decreasing difficult behaviours (Morley, 2013). *Snoezelen* was developed in the Netherlands in the 1970s; this type of multi-sensory stimulation was first introduced to people with learning difficulties.

—— Quality of care ————————————————

The term quality of care is used aspirationally to describe a goal that health and aged care services should be seeking to provide. However, the concept of quality of care is broad, and many perspectives on its meaning exist. Largely, the focus in the published literature has been on measuring clinical, process or organisational outcomes considered as indicators of good or poor-quality care with the assumption that meeting these indicators will have benefits for the recipients of the care (Castle and Ferguson, 2010). It is important to clearly define 'quality of health care'. Campbell, Roland and Buetow (2000) suggest that there are two principal dimensions of quality of care for individual patients: access and effectiveness. In essence, do users get the care they need, and is the care effective when they get it? Within the term effectiveness, they define two key components: the effectiveness of clinical care and the effectiveness of interpersonal care.

As noted above, people with dementia are users of the physical environment; accordingly, just as quality of care can impact on their experiences, so can the quality of environmental design (Blackman et al., 2003). Quality of care, however, has many dimensions: the environment and the nature of the staff are likely to be most transparent to families and prospective clients. Good medical care may be less visible, despite being crucial to wellbeing, given the complexity of health problems present in the majority of residents today (Donald et al., 2008). Quality of care, and indeed quality of life, for people living with dementia in long-term care, are often underpinned by philosophies of care, such as person-centred care and relationship-centred care (Venturato, Moyle and Steel, 2013).

There is considerable heterogeneity of need in dementia, but it is possible to identify two main streams in dementia care: a 'serious mental illness' stream and an 'early intervention' stream (Banerjee et al., 2007). It is estimated that one-third of people with dementia live in care homes (Prince et al., 2014), and around 70% of care home residents in the UK have dementia or significant memory problems (Prince et al., 2014). Caring for people with dementia can require a high level of specialist attention to mental and physical health needs, important for all care staff to identify (Corbett, Nunez and Thomas, 2013). On top of this, the gist of the quality of overall care has a great deal to do with the wellbeing of the informal carers who provide the glue for this fragile 'house of cards'.

The National Audit Office (2007) identified that 41% of GPs in a survey were unfamiliar with available services to support patients at home, whilst 21% were unsure how to refer patients to such services. Both GPs and care home staff describe that care for residents is affected by inadequate training, insufficient time and uncertainty about who from the health and social care sectors was responsible for key aspects of health care provision, coupled with the fact that the needs of residents are 'complex and unpredictable' (Robbins et al., 2013, p.1). In England, there are 32,937 care homes currently registered with the Care Quality Commission, most privately owned; general practitioners have responsibility for the clinical care of residents, but staffing in care homes varies, often with a few trained nurses supported by a larger pool of health care assistants (Jones et al., 2016).

Quality problems can be broadly grouped into three categories (Chassin and Galvin, 1998):

> » *Overuse* is the provision of a health care service under circumstances in which its potential for harm exceeds the possible benefit.

> » *Underuse* is the failure to provide a health care service when it would have produced a favourable outcome for a patient.

> » With *misuse* an appropriate service is provided, but a preventable complication occurs, and the patient does not receive the full potential benefit of the service.

Examples of overuse can be found right across the NHS – from over-diagnosis and over-prescribing in general practice to the overuse of low-value interventions in acute hospitals. Overuse can lead to unnecessary harm for patients and wasted NHS resources; tackling overuse will improve quality of care and could also result in financial savings for the NHS if unnecessary care is no longer commissioned and delivered (Alderwick et al., 2015).

I return to the issue of quality, in the context of integrated care pathways, in Chapter 14.

—— Care homes ————————————————

Person-centred care has been widely promoted in long-term care settings. It is commonly referred to as a core concept that guides the care philosophy change in long-term care settings from a traditional medical model to a more humanistic approach to care. Long-term institutional residential care in the United Kingdom is provided by care homes. Residents have prevalent cognitive impairment and disability, multiple diagnoses and are subject to polypharmacy. Prevailing models of health care provision (ad hoc, reactive, and coordinated by general practitioners) result in unacceptable variability in care (Gordon et al., 2014).

Every health service in Europe still faces five major problems – variation in quality, waste of resources, poor patient experience, health inequalities and the failure to prevent the preventable (Gray and Ricciardi, 2010). Care homes are a solution in that they provide long-term and end-of-life care for a vulnerable population who would otherwise need hospital care. Interviews with people with direct experience of commissioning, providing and regulating health care provision in care homes and care home residents recently revealed three overlapping approaches to the provision of the NHS that they believed supported access to health care for older people in care homes (Goodman et al., 2015). They are: 1) investment in relational working that fostered continuity and shared learning between visiting NHS staff and care home staff; 2) the provision of age-appropriate clinical services; and 3) the governance arrangements that are used. It is mooted that many of the 280,000 people with dementia living in care homes are currently getting a 'second rate service from the NHS', and having to pay for the privilege, for example as argued recently in the Alzheimer's Society Fix Dementia Care campaign (Alzheimer's Society, 2016).

Facilities that promote socialisation, choice and independence positively impact the quality of life of residents, perhaps suggesting a need to shift from a structured to a more flexible type of care (The Conference Board of Canada, 2011). But we are where we are. We have hospitals, providing acute care, so we are obliged to think about how best to provide care within them for now. Once constructed, the buildings of residents reinforce those values to the inhabitants by guiding their activities through the spatial configurations on a day-to-day basis (Bourdieu, 1990; Shin, 2015). Although nurses claim that they work from a holistic nursing perspective, they admit to a lack of knowledge about how to meet residents' spiritual needs in general, but especially for people with dementia (Ødbehr et al., 2014). Minimum standards are designed to ensure minimum safety and effective care through a number of criteria around inputs (e.g. the living environment, the care workforce and financial solvency), the care process (e.g. user involvement, quality management systems, medication management) and expected outputs (e.g. rights, quality of life) (OECD, 2013).

Older people in care homes are medically complex, and particularly vulnerable to the effects of poor care and poor medicine. They are also a group to whom the NHS seems least committed (Steves, Schiff and Martin, 2009). More integrated working between care homes and primary health services has the potential to improve quality of care in a cost-effective manner, but strategic decisions to create more formal arrangements are required to bring this about (Gage et al., 2012). Commissioners of services for older people need to make use of effective working relationships and address idiosyncratic patterns of provision to care homes (Gage et al., 2012). Internationally, it is recognised that there is a need to focus on the needs of residents in care homes, particularly research that investigates different models of care and their impact on residents' function and wellbeing (Goodman et al., 2015). The pressures on nursing and residential care homes are increasing, with higher levels of dependency among care home residents (Darton, Netten and Forder, 2003) and a significant proportion of people over 65 with dementia residing in a care home rather than in the community (estimated at around one-third; Knapp et al., 2007).

As dementia advances, so can symptom severity, so patients may experience: increasing disorientation, mood and behaviour changes; deepening confusion about events, time and place; unfounded suspicions about family, friends and professional carers; more serious memory loss and behaviour changes; and difficulty speaking, swallowing and walking (Farlow et al., 2015). The other symptoms can actually lessen in severity. The physical aspects of conditions which are common in care home residents are complicated. I will consider some of these in Chapter 3. Basic social skills are important for residents with dementia in nursing homes if they are to optimally engage/interact with staff and others, yet surprisingly little research has been devoted to this area (Chappell, Kadlec and Reid, 2014).

England is too diverse for a 'one size fits all' care model to apply everywhere. But nor is the answer simply to let 'a thousand flowers bloom'. Different local health communities will instead be supported by the national leadership of the NHS to choose from among a small number of radical new care delivery options. NHS England's New Models of Care programme (see Chapter 1), launched in January 2015, as well as examples of outstanding care, will be examined in this book.

—— Introduction to care in hospitals ——

High-quality, dementia-friendly care for people in hospitals exists in certain areas and should be acknowledged; however, not all of these examples reach right across their organisations, and the level of awareness and dementia-friendliness may vary in quality even between wards or individual departments. Care in hospitals can frequently be challenging and disorientating for people with dementia, and more needs to be done to make hospitals dementia-friendly environments. There have been improvements in the awareness of staff in acute hospitals about dementia and the needs of individual patients, following the establishment of senior clinical leads and attempts to create more dementia-friendly environments. For example, the lower use of antipsychotic medications will have reduced the risk of adverse incidents such as falls, Parkinsonism, accelerated cognitive decline and stroke (Black et al., 2015).

The use of quality indicators (QIs) for this purpose is well established in the acute care setting (Panzer et al., 2013). QIs are measurable elements of the process or outcomes of care that are utilised to bring attention to issues that need further investigation or to alert staff to possible opportunities for improvement; they are not direct measures of performance (Giuffrida, Gravelle and Roland, 1999).

— Culture

Organisational culture relates to the assumptions, values, attitudes and beliefs that are shared among significant groups within an organisation (Davies et al., 2007). The organisational change entailed by open innovation is highly pervasive, as it requires a firm to intervene both on the 'hard' aspects of its organisation (e.g. organisational structures or performance evaluation and management systems) as well as the 'soft' ones (e.g. culture, organisational values and individual competencies) (Boscherini et al., 2011). Increasing case loads, documented interprofessional conflicts and tensions between frontline and supervisory staff and task-based approaches to care have contributed to low staff morale, low job satisfaction, high staff turnover rates and absenteeism, and difficulty in recruiting and retaining skilled professionals and strong leaders (Dupuis et al., 2016).

The Lewin model (1946/7) anchors of altering a traditional clinical path or approach (unfreezing), refining the emergent provider behaviours (movement) and reinforcing them through changes in organisational structure (refreezing) have previously been applied to understand how health professions' behaviours become accepted and sustained in a clinical setting (Manchester et al., 2014).

There is a significant literature on how successful change occurs. Familiar themes arise recurrently, both within health and the wider management literature (Allcock et al., 2015).

The seven success factors are:

» Committed and respected leadership that engages staff; particularly a leadership that can engage people with a clear vision for change, centred on patients.

» A culture hospitable to and supportive of change; a healthy culture harnessing the commitment staff have to patient care and engaging clinical staff in change is vital to making successful change.

» Management practices that ensure rigorous execution and implementation; successful change cannot be delivered without effective operational management.

» Data and analytics that measure and communicate impact; detailed, timely data and information are needed at all levels of the system – as well as staff with the skills to interpret them.

» Capabilities and skills to identify and solve problems.

» Resources and support for change; the majority of organisations or health economies committed to change have dedicated teams, in addition to frontline teams dedicated to change.

» An enabling environment which supports and drives change; the environment is a set of factors influencing change beyond the direct control of the unit making changes.

(Allcock et al., 2015, pp.10–11)

When choosing priorities, it often helps to conduct a series of 'safe space' discussions with thoughtful people at different levels throughout your company to learn what behaviours are most affected by the current culture – both positively and negatively (Katzenbach, Steffen, and Pronely, 2012).

Community care is any type of care or assistance with independent living given to functionally impaired persons living in their own home. A variety of services falls under the umbrella term 'community care', including home-delivered meals, personal care, nursing, allied health, cleaning, home modification, transport, day care and case-managed packages of care. There is a range of goals for care, depending on the service. A recent systematic review of community care found that many different outcome measures were used in evaluating services, such as mortality, satisfaction with care, carer confidence in caring and use of other services (Low, Yap and Brodaty, 2011). At present, relatively little is known about models of care, patterns of variation in professional practice, the extent of community-based working and the degree of service integration, particularly with social care, key themes of government policy (Challis et al., 2002).

Culture change as a movement —— in residential settings

Organisational culture is an important characteristic of long-term care. In health care settings, evidence-based practice has been stated as the 'judicious use of current best evidence in conjunction with clinical expertise and patient values to guide health care decisions' (Titler, 2008). Contemporary health care delivery demands a person-centred approach with a focus on values and ethical standards. Nurse leaders play an integral and indispensable role in contributing to the quality of client care, client safety, nurse satisfaction, and nurse recruitment and retention (Bish, Kenny and Nay, 2015).

A strong framework of organisational culture that is often applied in health care research (Scott et al., 2003) is the competing values framework (Cameron and

Freeman, 1991). The competing values framework of organisational culture is a four-quadrant model containing four 'value systems' (see Figure 2.1).

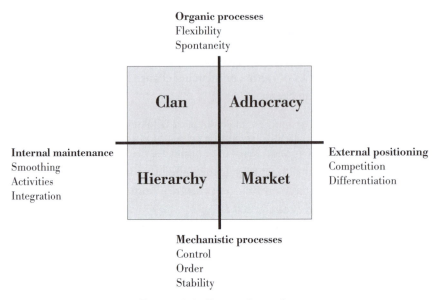

Figure 2.1: Competing values

Clan culture is characterised by shared values and goals, strong cohesion, participation and a sense of 'we-ness'. Adhocracy culture can adapt quickly to new opportunities and is prepared to deal with rapidly changing times. Market culture is highly results-oriented and focuses on profitability, competitiveness and productivity. Hierarchy culture is characterised by structure, rules and centralised decisions. Source: adapted from van Beek and Gerritsen (2010, Fig. 1, p.1275).

There have been growing concerns regarding the inadequacy of the long-term care sector to ensure quality care and quality of life for older adults (Jones, 2011). In the UK, Demos' Commission on Residential Care recommended enshrining a more accurate definition of 'housing with care' throughout government policy; greater co-location of care settings with other community services such as colleges; a possible expansion of the CQC's role in inspecting commissioning practices; and promoting excellence in governance of the caring profession through the introduction of a licence to practise and a living wage (Demos, 2014). Generally there is a growing consensus that the way care is currently delivered, regulated and financed is inadequate to meet the care needs and ensure a high quality of life for the growing numbers of older adults over the next several decades, particularly those living with dementia (Miller, Booth and Mor, 2008). Calls for culture change in long-term conditions including dementia care more generally have sparked a movement away from the medical, institutional model of care towards a relational, community model of living (e.g. Baker, 2007). Culture change is a movement that has been promoted in US nursing homes to create a more home-like environment in the nursing home, empower residents and staff to have a more active role in care, provide a high quality of life and care for residents, and provide a high quality of work life for employees (Eliopoulos, 2013).

Change is a very emotive subjective, for easily understandable reasons. As Schein (2010, p.300) writes, 'Coping, growth, and survival all involve maintaining the integrity of the system in the face of a changing environment that is constantly causing varying degrees of disequilibrium.'

Culture change, when implemented comprehensively, entails the multidimensional reform of care practices, staff procedures, protocols and environmental design. Providing resident-centred care, empowering frontline staff and making environments home-like are the central principles and domains of culture change (Miller et al., 2014).

An approach to cultural change articulated by John Kotter is shown in Figure 2.2.

Establishing a sense of urgency
- Examining market and competitive realities
- Identifying and discussing crises, potential crises or major opportunities

1

Forming a powerful guiding coalition
- Assembling a group with enough power to lead the change effort
- Encouraging the group to work together as a team

2

Creating a vision
- Creating a vision to help direct the change effort
- Developing strategies for achieving that vision

3

Communicating the vision
- Using every vehicle possible to communicate the new vision and strategies
- Teaching new behaviours by the example of the guiding coalition

4

Empowering others to act on the vision
- Getting rid of obstacles to change
- Changing systems or structures that seriously undermine the vision
- Encouraging risk-taking and non-traditional ideas, activities and actions

5

Planning for and creating short-term wins
- Planning for visible performance improvements
- Creating those improvements
- Recognising and rewarding employees involved in the improvements

6

Consolidating improvements and producing still more change
- Using increased credibility to change systems, structures and policies that don't fit the vision
- Hiring, promoting and developing employees who can implement the vision
- Reinvigorating the process with new projects, themes and change agents

7

Institutionalising new approaches
- Articulating the connections between the new behaviours and corporate success
- Developing the means to ensure leadership development and succession

8

Figure 2.2: A framework for cultural change.

Source: after Kotter.

Kitwood and Benson (1995) have contrasted the New and Old Cultures of Dementia Care, examining the underlying beliefs and assumptions about the nature of dementia and the day-to-day behaviours associated with these in practice. Their work emphasises the importance of authentic contact and communication between the person with dementia and the carer, with relationships developing through day-to-day interactions, and these relationships supporting the sense of identity of the person with dementia (Kitwood, 1997). The Eden Alternative is promoted as a comprehensive model for reform and management of aged care facilities. It aims to transform the physical, interpersonal, psychosocial and spiritual environments of an aged care facility as well as the culture of the organisation (Tesh et al., 2002).

—— Leadership and staff development ——

Modern leadership approaches often adopt the position that leadership is not about individuals but about collectives (e.g. teams, shared or distributed leadership) (Edmonstone, 2011). For example, empirical investigations have demonstrated that leadership can be associated with better quality of care, including fewer pressure ulcers, fewer falls and improved pain management (Castle and Decker, 2011). Researchers have also found that nurses working in contexts with a more positive culture, leadership and forms of evaluation reported more research utilisation, staff development and lower rates of patient and staff adverse events (Cummings et al., 2007).

I will resume discussion of this topic in Chapter 9.

—— Essential reading ——

Brooker D, Latham I. 2015. *Person-Centred Dementia Care, Second Edition Making Services Better with the VIPS Framework*, London: Jessica Kingsley Publishers.

Rahman S. 2015. *Living Better with Dementia*, London: Jessica Kingsley Publishers. Chapter 7, Care and Support Networks for Living Better with Dementia, pp.128–163.

Citizenship

Rahman S. 2015. *Living Better with Dementia*, London: Jessica Kingsley Publishers. Chapter 2, Stigma, Citizenship and Living Better with Dementia, pp.68–80.

—— References ——

Alderwick H, Robertson R, Appleby J, Dunn P, Maguire D. 2015. *Better Value in the NHS: The Role of Changes in Clinical Practice*, London: The King's Fund, available at www.kingsfund.org.uk/sites/files/kf/field/field_publication_file/better-value-nhs-Kings-Fund-July%202015.pdf (accessed 2 Oct 2016).

Allcock C, Dromen F, Taunt R, Dixon J. 2015. Constructive Comfort: Accelerating Change in the NHS, Health Foundation, available at www.health.org.uk/sites/health/files/ConstructiveComfortAcceleratingChangeInTheNHS.pdf (accessed 2 Oct 2016).

Alzheimer's Society. 2016. Fix Dementia Care, available at www.alzheimers.org.uk/site/scripts/documents_info.php?documentID=3106 (accessed 3 Oct 2016).

American Geriatrics Society Expert Panel on Person-Centred Care. 2016. Person-centred care: a definition and essential elements. J Am Geriatr Soc, 64(1), 15–18.

Anderson NR, De Dreu CKW, Nijstad BA. 2004. The routinization of innovation research: A constructively critical review of the state-of-the-science. Journal of Organizational Behavior, 25(2), 147–173.

Arendt H. 1958. *The Origins of Totalitarianism*, New York: Meridian Books.

Audit Commission. 2003. *Human Rights: Improving Public Service Delivery*, London: Audit Commission.

Baker B. 2007. *Old age in a new age: The promise of transformative nursing homes*, Nashville, TN: Vanderbilt University Press.

Baldwin C, Bradford Dementia Group. 2008. Narrative, citizenship and dementia: the personal and the political. Journal of Aging Studies, 22, 222–228.

Banerjee S, Willis R, Matthews D, Contell F, Chan J, Murray J. 2007. Improving the quality of care for mild to moderate dementia: an evaluation of the Croydon Memory Service Model. Int J Geriatr Psychiatry, 22(8), 782–788.

Bartlett R, O'Connor D. 2007. From personhood to citizenship: broadening the conceptual base for dementia practice and research. Journal of Aging Studies, 21(2), 107–118.

Bell K, Cemlyn S. 2014. Developing public support for human rights in the United Kingdom: reasserting the importance of socio-economic rights. The International Journal of Human Rights, 18(7–8), 822–841.

Bharucha AJ, London AJ, Barnard D, Wactlar H, Dew MA, Reynolds CF. 2006. Ethical considerations in the conduct of electronic surveillance research. J Law Med Ethics, 34(3), 611–619.

Bish M, Kenny A, Nay R. 2015. Factors that influence the approach to leadership: directors of nursing working in rural health services. J Nurs Manag, 23(3), 380–389.

Black N, Dixon J, Tan S, Knapp M. 2015. Improving health care for people with dementia in England: good progress but more to do. J R Soc Med, 108(12), 478–481.

Blackman T, Mitchell L, Burton E, Jenks M, et al. 2003. The accessibility of public spaces for people with dementia: a new priority for the 'open city'. Disability and Society, 12, 357–371.

Boscherini L, Chiaroni D, Chiesa V, Frattini F. 2010. How to use pilot projects to implement open innovation. International Journal of Innovation Management, 14(6), 1065–1097.

Bourdieu P. 1990. *The Logic of Practice* (R. Nice, trans.), Stanford: Stanford University Press.

Bovaird T. 2007. Beyond engagement and participation: user and community coproduction of public services. Public Administration Review, 67(5), 846–860.

Boyle D, Harris M. 2009. The Challenge of Co-Production: How Equal Partnerships between Professionals and the Public Are Crucial to Improving Public Services (Nesta discussion paper), available at www.nesta.org.uk/sites/default/files/the_challenge_of_co-production.pdf (accessed 3 Oct 2016).

Brooker D. 2007. *Person-Centred Dementia Care*, London: Jessica Kingsley Publishers.

Brooker D, Latham I. 2016. *Person-Centred Dementia Care*, London: Jessica Kingsley Publishers.

Cameron K, Freeman S. 1991. Culture, congruence, strength and type: relationship to effectiveness. Research in Organizational Change and Development, 5, 23–58.

Campbell SM, Roland MO, Buetow SA. 2000. Defining quality of care. Soc Sci Med, 51(11), 1611–1625.

Care Quality Commission. 2015. Thinking about Using a Hidden Camera or Other Equipment to Monitor Someone's Care? Available at www.cqc.org.uk/sites/default/files/20150212_public_surveillance_leaflet_final.pdf (accessed 3 Oct 2016).

Castle NG, Decker FH. 2011. Top management leadership style and quality of care in nursing homes. The Gerontologist, 51(5), 630–642.

Castle NG, Ferguson JC. 2010. What is nursing home quality and how is it measured? The Gerontologist, 50, 426–442.

Challis D, Reilly S, Hughes J, Burns A, Gilchrist H, Wilson K. 2002. Policy, organisation and practice of specialist old age psychiatry in England. Int J Geriatr Psychiatry, 17(11), 1018–1026.

Chappell NL, Kadlec H, Reid C. 2014. Change and predictors of change in social skills of nursing home residents with dementia. Am J Alzheimers Dis Other Demen, 29(1), 23–31.

Chassin MR, Galvin RW. 1998. The urgent need to improve health care quality. Institute of Medicine National Roundtable on Health Care Quality. JAMA, 280(11), 1000–1005.

Chaudhury H, Hung L, Badger M. 2013. The role of physical environment in supporting person-centred dining in long-term care: a review of the literature. Am J Alzheimers Dis Other Demen, 28(5), 491–500.

Cherry B, Carpenter K, Waters C, Hawkins WW, et al. 2008. Social compatibility as a consideration in caring for nursing home residents with dementia. Am J Alzheimers Dis Other Demen, 23(5), 430–438.

Clissett P, Porock D, Harwood RH, Gladman JR. 2013. The challenges of achieving person-centred care in acute hospitals: a qualitative study of people with dementia and their families. Int J Nurs Stud, 50(11), 1495–1503.

Comas-Herrera A, Wittenberg R, Pickard L, Knapp M. 2007. Cognitive impairment in older people: the implications for future demand for long-term care services and their costs. Int J Geriatr Psychiatry, 22(10), 1037–1045.

Corbett A, Nunez K, Thomas A. 2013. Coping with dementia in care homes. Maturitas, 76(1), 3–4.

Cossman B. 2007. *Sexual Citizens: The Legal and Cultural Regulation of Sex and Belonging.* Stanford: Stanford University Press.

Cummings GG, Estabrooks CA, Midodzi WK, Wallin L, Hayduk L. 2007. Influence of organizational characteristics and context on research utilization. Nurs Res, 56, S24–39.

Darton R, Netten A, Forder J. 2003. The cost implications of the changing population and characteristics of care homes. International Journal of Geriatric Psychiatry, 18, 236–243.

Davies HTO, Mannion R, Jacobs R, Powell AE, Marshall MN. 2007. Exploring the relationship between senior management team culture and hospital performance. Medical Care Research and Review, 64, 46–65.

Davis S, Byers S, Nay R, Koch S. 2009. Guiding design of dementia friendly environments in residential care settings: Considering the living experiences. Dementia, 8(2), 185–203.

de Vries OJ, Ligthart GJ, Nikolaus T, European Academy of Medicine of Ageing-Course III. 2004. Differences in period prevalence of the use of physical restraints in elderly inpatients of European hospitals and nursing homes. The Journals of Gerontology Series A Biological Sciences Medical Sciences, 59, M922–M923.

Demos. 2014. *A Report by the Commission on Residential Care: A Vision for Care Fit for the Twenty-First Century,* London: Demos.

Department of Health. 2006. *Our Health, Our Care, Our Say: A New Direction for Community Services,* Norwich: Department of Health, available at www.gov.uk/government/uploads/system/uploads/attachment_data/file/272238/6737.pdf (accessed 3 Oct 2016).

Donald IP, Gladman J, Conroy S, Vernon M, Kendrick E, Burns E. 2008. Care home medicine in the UK – in from the cold. Age Ageing, 37(6), 618–620.

Duin AH, Baer LL. 2010. Shared leadership for a green, global, and Google world. Planning for Higher Education, 39(1), 30–38.

Dupuis S, McAiney CA, Fortune D, Ploeg J, de Witt L. 2016. Theoretical foundations guiding culture change: the work of the Partnerships in Dementia Care Alliance. Dementia, 15(1), 85–105.

Edmonstone J. 2011. Developing leaders and leadership in health care: a case for rebalancing? Leadership in Health Services, 24(1), 8–18.

Edvardsson D, Fetherstonhaugh D, Nay R. 2010. Promoting a continuation of self and normality: person-centred care as described by people with dementia, their family members and aged care staff. J Clin Nurs, 19(17–18), 2611–2618.

Edvardsson D, Winblad B, Sandman PO. 2008. Person-centred care of people with severe Alzheimer's disease: current status and ways forward. Lancet Neurology, 7, 362–367.

Eliopoulos C. 2013. Affecting culture change and performance improvement in Medicaid nursing homes: the Promote Understanding, Leadership, and Learning (PULL) Program. Geriatr Nurs, 34(3), 218–223.

Epp T. 2003. Person-centred dementia care: a vision to be refined. The Canadian Alzheimer Disease Review, 5, 14–18.

Equality and Human Rights Commission (EHRC). 2012. *Older People's Experiences of Home Care in England* (Research Report 79), London: EHRC.

Ettema TP, Dröes R, de Lange J, Mellenbergh GJ, Ribbe MW. 2007. QUALIDEM: development and evaluation of a dementia specific quality of life instrument. Scalability, reliability and internal structure. International Journal of Geriatric Psychiatry, 22, 549–556.

Farlow MR, Borson S, Connor SR, Grossberg GT, Mittelman MS. 2015. Quality improvement in skilled nursing facilities for residents with Alzheimer's disease. Am J Alzheimers Dis Other Demen, 1533317515603501 (e-pub ahead of print).

Fleming R, Purandare N. 2010. Long-term care for people with dementia: environmental design guidelines. International Psychogeriatrics, 22, 1084–1096.

Ford L. 2015. Sustainable Development Goals: All You Need to Know, available at www.theguardian.com/global-development/2015/jan/19/sustainable-development-goals-united-nations (accessed 3 Oct 2016).

Gage H, Dickinson A, Victor C, Williams P, et al. 2012. Integrated working between residential care homes and primary care: a survey of care homes in England. BMC Geriatr, 12, 71.

Gesler W. 1992. Therapeutic landscapes: medical issues in light of the new cultural geography. Soc. Sci. Med, 34(7), 735–746.

Giuffrida A, Gravelle H, Roland M. 1999. Measuring quality of care with routine data: avoiding confusion between performance indicators and health outcomes. British Medical Journal, 319, Article 94.

Gladman JR, Jones RG, Radford K, Walker E, Rothera I. 2007. Person-centred dementia services are feasible, but can they be sustained? Age Ageing, 36(2), 171–176.

Goodman C, Davies SL, Gordon AL, Meyer J, et al. 2015. Relationships, expertise, incentives, and governance: supporting care home residents' access to health care. An interview study from England. J Am Med Dir Assoc, 16(5), 427–432.

Gordon AL, Franklin M, Bradshaw L, Logan P, Elliott R, Gladman JR. 2014. Health status of UK care home residents: a cohort study. Age Ageing, 43(1), 97–103.

Gray M, Ricciardi W. 2010. From public health to population medicine: the contribution of public health to health care services. Eur J Public Health, 20(4), 366–367.

Hamers JP, Gulpers MJ, Strik W. 2004. Use of physical restraints with cognitively impaired nursing home residents. J Adv Nurs, 45(3), 246–251.

Javor A, Koller M, Lee N, Chamberlain L, Ransmayr G. 2013. Neuromarketing and consumer neuroscience: contributions to neurology. BMC Neurol, 13, 13.

Joanna Briggs Institute.2002. Best Practice, available at connect.jbiconnectplus.org/ViewSourceFile.aspx?0=4326 (accessed 3 Oct 2016).

Johnson S, Ostaszkiewicz J, O'Connell B. 2009. Moving beyond resistance to restraint minimization: a case study of change management in aged care. Worldviews Evid Based Nurs, 6(4), 210–218.

Jones CS. 2011. Person-centred care: the heart of culture change. Journal of Gerontological Nursing, 37(6), 18–23.

Jones L, Candy B, Davis S, Elliott M, et al. 2016. Development of a model for integrated care at the end of life in advanced dementia: a whole systems UK-wide approach. Palliat Med, 30(3), 279–295.

Katzenbach JR, Steffen I, Pronely C. 2012. Culture change that sticks. Harvard Business Review, July–August, 110–117.

Kitwood T. 1997. *Dementia Reconsidered: The Person Comes First*, Buckingham: Open University Press.

Kitwood T, Benson S (eds). 1995. *The New Culture of Dementia Care*, London: Hawker Publications.

Knapp M, Prince M, Albanese E, Banerjee S, et al. 2007. *Dementia UK: The Full Report*, London: The Alzheimer's Society.

Koch S, Nay R, Wilson J. 2006. Restraint removal: tension between protective custody and human rights. Int J Older People Nurs, 1(3), 151–158.

Kontos P, Grigorovich A, Kontos AP, Miller KL. 2016. Citizenship, human rights, and dementia: towards a new embodied relational ethic of sexuality. Dementia (London), 15(3), 315–329.

Kula N, Fryatt RJ. 2014. Public–private interactions on health in South Africa: opportunities for scaling up. Health Policy Plan, 29(5), 560–569.

Langan J, Lindow V. 2004. *Living with Risk. Mental Health Service User Involvement in Risk Assessment and Management*, York: Joseph Rowntree Foundation/Policy Press.

Lengen C. 2015. The effects of colours, shapes and boundaries of landscapes on perception, emotion and mentalising processes promoting health and wellbeing. Health Place, 35, 166–177.

Lewin K. 1946. Action Research and Minority Problems. In GW Lewin (ed.), *Resolving Social Conflict*, London: Harper & Row.

Lewin K. 1947. Frontiers in Group Dynamics. In D Cartwright (ed.), *Field Theory in Social Science*, London: Social Science Paperbacks.

Lillekroken D, Hauge S, Slettebø Å. 2015. The meaning of slow nursing in dementia care. Dementia (London), pii: 1471301215625112.

Low LF, Yap M, Brodaty H. 2011. A systematic review of different models of home and community care services for older persons. BMC Health Services Research, 11, 93.

Macintyre S, Ellaway A, Cummins S. 2002. Place effects on health: how can we conceptualise, operationalize and measure them? Soc. Sci. Med, 55, 125–139.

Manchester J, Gray-Miceli DL, Metcalf JA, Paolini CA, Napier AH, Coogle CL, Owens MG. 2014. Facilitating Lewin's change model with collaborative evaluation in promoting evidence based practices of health professionals. Eval Program Plann, 47, 82–90.

Marquardt G, Schmieg P. 2009. Dementia-friendly architecture: environments that facilitate wayfinding in nursing homes. Am J Alzheimers Dis Other Demen, 24(4), 333–340.

Marshall TH, Bottomore TB. 1950/1992. *Citizenship and Social Class*, London: Pluto Press.

Martin GP, Weaver S, Currie G, Finn R, McDonald R. 2012. Innovation sustainability in challenging health-care contexts: embedding clinically led change in routine practice. Health Serv Manage Res, 25(4), 190–199.

McCormack B, McCance T. 2010. *Person-Centred Nursing Theory and Practice*, Oxford: Wiley-Blackwell.

McCormack B, Roberts T, Meyer J, Morgan D, Boscart V. 2012. Appreciating the 'person' in long-term care. Int J Older People Nurs, 7(4), 284–294.

Mechanic D, Meyer S. 2000. Concepts of trust among patients with serious illness. Soc Sci Med, 51(5), 657–668.

Merton RC. 2013. Innovation risk: how to make smarter decisions. Harvard Business Review, April, 48–56.

Meyer G, Köpke S, Haastert B, Mühlhauser I. 2009. Restraint use among nursing home residents: cross-sectional study and prospective cohort study. Journal of Clinical Nursing, 18, 981–990.

Miller EA, Booth M, Mor V. 2008. Assessing experts' views of the future of long-term care. Research on Aging, 30, 450–473.

Miller SC, Lepore M, Lima JC, Shield R, Tyler DA. 2014. Does the introduction of nursing home culture change practices improve quality? J Am Geriatr Soc, 62(9), 1675–1682.

Morley JE. 2013. Future nursing home design: an important component in enhancing quality of life. J Am Med Dir Assoc, 14(4), 227–229.

Murray LM, Boyd S. 2009. Protecting personhood and achieving quality of life for older adults with dementia in the U.S. health care system. Journal of Aging and Health, 21, 350–373.

National Audit Office. 2007. *Improving Services and Support for People with Dementia*, London: National Audit Office.

Nolan M, Brown J, Davies S, Keady J, Nolan J. 2006. *The Senses Framework: Improving Care for Older People through a Relationship-Centred Approach*. Sheffield: University of Sheffield.

Nolan M, Davies S, Brown J, Keady J, Nolan J. 2004. Beyond 'person-centred' care: a new vision for gerontological nursing. International Journal of Older People Nursing, 13, 45–53.

Niemeijer AR, Depla M, Frederiks B, Francke AL, Hertogh C. 2014. Original research: the use of surveillance technology in residential facilities for people with dementia or intellectual disabilities: a study among nurses and support staff. Am J Nurs, 114(12), 28–37.

Nolan MR, Ryan T, Enderby P, Reid D. 2002. Towards a more inclusive vision of dementia care practice. Dementia: The International Journal of Social Research and Practice, 1, 193–211.

Normann HK, Asplund K, Norberg A. 1999. Attitudes of registered nurses towards patients with severe dementia. Journal of Clinical Nursing, 8, 353–359.

Nundy S, Oswald J. 2014. Relationship-centred care: a new paradigm for population health management. Healthc (Amst), 2(4), 216–219.

Ødbehr L, Kvigne K, Hauge S, Danbolt LJ. 2014. Nurses' and care workers' experiences of spiritual needs in residents with dementia in nursing homes: a qualitative study. BMC Nurs, 13, 12.

OECD/European Commission. 2013. A Good Life in Old Age? Monitoring and Improving Quality in Long-Term Care, Paris: OECD Publishing.

Owen T, Meyer J. 2012. My Home Life: Promoting Quality of Life in Care Homes, York: Joseph Rowntree Foundation.

Panzer RJ, Gitomer RS, Greene WH, Webster P, Landry KR, Riccobono CA. 2013. Increasing demands for quality measurement. Journal of the American Medical Association, 310, 1971–1980.

Paparella G. 2016. Person-Centred Care in Europe: A Cross-Country Comparison of Health System Performance, Strategies and Structures, Oxford: Picker Institute.

Pot AM. 2013. Improving nursing home care for dementia: is the environment the answer? Aging Ment Health, 17(7), 785–787.

Powell JL, Edwards MM. 2002. Policy narratives of aging: the right way, the third way or the wrong way? Electronic Journal of Sociology, 6.

Prince M, Knapp M, Guerchet M, McCrone P, et al. 2014. Dementia UK: Update. London: Alzheimer's Society.

Robbins I, Gordon A, Dyas J, Logan P, Gladman J. 2013. Explaining the barriers to and tensions in delivering effective healthcare in UK care homes: a qualitative study. BMJ Open, 3(7), e003178.

Roberts A, Greenhill B, Talbot A. 2011. 'Standing up for my human rights': a group's journey beyond consultation towards co-production. British Journal of Learning Disabilities, 40, 292–301.

Roberts A, Thompson S, Charlesworth A, Gershlick B, Stirling A. 2015. Filling the gap: tax and fiscal options for a sustainable UK health and social care system, available at www.health.org.uk/sites/health/files/FillingTheGap_1.pdf (accessed 29 Nov 2016).

Robinson L, Hutchings D, Corner L, Finch T, et al. 2007. Balancing rights and risks: conflicting perspectives in the management of wandering in dementia. Health, Risk & Society, 9(4), 389–406.

Ross H, Tod AM, Clarke A. 2015. Understanding and achieving person-centred care: the nurse perspective. J Clin Nurs, 24(9–10), 1223–1233.

Sabat SR. 2005. Capacity for decision-making in Alzheimer's disease: selfhood, positioning and semiotic people. Australian and New Zealand Journal of Psychiatry, 39, 1030–1035.

Samet RH. 2011. Exploring the future with complexity science: the emerging models. Futures, 43(8): 831–839.

Sawamura K, Nakashima T, Nakanishi M. 2013. Provision of individualized care and built environment of nursing homes in Japan. Arch Gerontol Geriatr, 56(3), 416–424.

Schein EH. 2010. Organizational Culture and Leadership, San Francisco: Jossey-Bass.

SCIE. 2013. Adults' Services: SCIE Guide 51. Co-Production in Social Care: What It Is and How to Do It, available at www.scie.org.uk/publications/guides/guide51 (accessed 3 Oct 2016).

Scott T, Mannion R, Marshall M, Davies H. 2003. Does organizational culture influence health care performance? A review of the evidence. Journal of Health Services Research & Policy, 82, 105–117.

Shin JH. 2015. Declining body, institutional life, and making home-are they at odds? The lived experiences of moving through staged care in long-term care settings. HEC Forum, 27(2), 107–125.

Sjögren K, Lindkvist M, Sandman PO, Zingmark K, Edvardsson D. 2011. Psychometric evaluation of the Swedish version of the Person-Centered Care Assessment Tool (P-CAT). International Psychogeriatrics, 24, 406–415.

Skaalvik MW, Normann HK, Henriksen N. 2010. Student experiences in learning person-centred care of patients with Alzheimer's disease as perceived by nursing students and supervising nurses. Journal of Clinical Nursing, 19(17/18), 2639–2648.

Spandler H. 2004. Friend or foe? Towards a critical assessment of direct payments. Critical Social Policy, 24, 187–209.

Stevenson F, Scambler G. 2005. The relationship between medicine and the public: the challenge of concordance. Health (London), 9(1), 5–21.

Steves CJ, Schiff R, Martin FC. 2009. Geriatricians and care homes: perspectives from geriatric medicine departments and primary care trusts. Clin Med (Lond), 9(6), 528–533.

Stubbs E. 2015. Hidden cameras in care homes: can they help or hinder British social care? Available at civitas.org.uk/2015/02/12/hidden-cameras-in-care-homes-can-they-help-or-hinder-british-social-care (accessed 3 Oct 2016).

Teno JM, Casey VA, Welch LC, Edgman-Levitan S. 2001. Patient-focused, family-centred end-of-life medical care: views of the guidelines and bereaved family members. J Pain Symptom Manage, 22(3), 738.

Tesh AS, McNutt K, Courts NF, Barba BE. 2002. Characteristics of nursing homes: adopting environmental transformations. Journal of Gerontological Nursing, 28, 28–34.

The Conference Board of Canada. 2011. Elements of an Effective Innovation Strategy for Long-Term Care in Ontario, available at neltoolkit.rnao.ca/sites/default/files/Elements%20of%20an%20Effective%20Innovation%20Strategy%20for%20Long%20Term%20Care%20in%20Ontario%202011.pdf (accessed 3 Oct 2016).

Titler MG. 2008. The Evidence for Evidence-Based Practice Implementation. In RG Hughes (ed.), *Patient Safety and Quality: An Evidence-Based Handbook for Nurses (Vol. 1)*, Rockville, MD: Agency for Health Care Research and Quality.

Toebes B. 2015. Human rights and public health: towards a balanced relationship, The International Journal of Human Rights, 19(4), 488–504.

Uhl-Bien M, Marion R, McKelvey B. 2007. Complexity Leadership Theory: shifting leadership from the industrial age to the knowledge era. The Leadership Quarterly, 18(4), 298–318.

Vaillancourt Y. 2009. Social economy in the co-construction of public policy. Annals of Public and Cooperative Economics, 80(2), 275–313.

van Beek AP, Gerritsen DL. 2010. The relationship between organizational culture of nursing staff and quality of care for residents with dementia: questionnaire surveys and systematic observations in nursing homes. Int J Nurs Stud, 47(10), 1274–1282.

Van Der Steen JT, Van Soest-Poortvliet MC, Achterberg WP, Ribbe MW, De Vet HC. 2011. Family perceptions of wishes of dementia patients regarding end-of-life care. International Journal of Geriatric Psychiatry, 26, 217–220.

van Hoof J, Kort HS, van Waarde H, Blom MM. 2010. Environmental interventions and the design of homes for older adults with dementia: an overview. Am J Alzheimers Dis Other Demen, 25(3), 202–232.

Venturato L, Moyle W, Steel A. 2013. Exploring the gap between rhetoric and reality in dementia care in Australia: could practice documents help bridge the great divide? Dementia (London), 12(2), 251–267.

Wogn-Henriksen K. 1997. *Siden blir det vel verre*. Norway: INFO-banken.

You EC, Dunt D, Doyle C. 2015. How would case managers' practice change in a consumer directed care environment in Australia? Health Soc Care Community, doi:10.1111/hsc.12303 (e-pub ahead of print).

Zhao Y. 2014. Interpreting Innovation Dynamics with Complexity Theory International Journal of Innovation and Technology Management, 11(5), 1–18.

Chapter 3

CARING WELL: PHYSICAL HEALTH AND MEDICATION REVIEWS

Learning objectives

In this chapter, you will:

> » see the case for enhancing health in care homes
>
> » understand in more detail features of 'complexity'
>
> » acknowledge fully 'multimorbidity'
>
> » be able to outline important features of the following clinical issues: mobility, falls, visual and hearing impairments, hand hygiene, hip fractures, frailty, medication and polypharmacy, infections, diabetes, chronic pain
>
> » have an awareness of issues of polypharmacy for people with dementia

—— Introduction ——————————————————————

In England, commercial companies and not-for-profit organisations are the main formal providers of long-term care (in care homes, with and without on-site nursing) for older people. In the UK as of 2014 there were 17,688 (12,535 residential care and 5153 nursing homes) care homes for older people and 433,000 residents with approximately 405,000 aged 65+; the vast majority (90% across the UK) of care homes are independently owned, either by private companies or charitable organisations (Laing and Buisson, 2015). In March 2012, there were 13,134 residential care homes with 247,824 beds in England, and 4672 nursing homes with 215,463 beds (Care Quality Commission, 2013). The majority of residents are female, in their mid-80s, with multiple morbidities and diverse health needs. They have a median life expectancy of two to three years in residential care and one to two years in nursing homes (Davies et al., 2014). At roughly the same time as this publication, the mean consensus estimates of the prevalence of dementia in different care settings in residential homes and nursing homes are thought to be 57.9% and 73.0% respectively, according to the second edition of the Dementia UK report published in September 2014 (Prince et al., 2014).

In this chapter, I wish to look at the evidence base for due attention to the physical health needs of persons with dementia – including in care homes. Care homes are particularly fascinating, as they provide a crucial role in supporting a vulnerable, frail population. Services commissioned for care are insufficiently comprehensive (e.g. podiatry or dentistry might 'fall through the gaps'), coordinated or expert (limited access to specialist expertise in old age psychiatry and geriatric medicine) (Iliffe et al., 2016).

When you've met one person with dementia, you've done just that – met *just one* person with dementia. You should not allow the diagnostic label to overwhelm your appreciation of other health needs, whether physical or mental. And because of parity of esteem, which I discussed in Rahman (2015, pp.206–207), mental health needs should not be considered 'inferior' to physical health ones.

This chapter will look at physical health needs.

Tom Kitwood could not have been clearer. In *Dementia Reconsidered*, Kitwood (1997, p.33) remarks:

> There is a wide range of conditions related to physical health which can cause dementia-like conditions. When primary dementia is present, these tend to enhance the symptoms, and can lead to false estimates of a person's genuine impairments.

The topics of this chapter include:

- » mobility
- » falls
- » visual and hearing impairment
- » hand hygiene
- » hip fractures
- » frailty
- » medications and polypharmacy
- » infections

» diabetes

» chronic pain.

Mental health needs are considered in Chapter 4.

—— Enhancing health ————————————————

There are numerous approaches to providing health care for this population of care home residents. General practitioners have a statutory obligation towards care home residents registered with their practices, but fulfil this obligation in various ways (Goodman et al., 2014). The International Association of Gerontology and Geriatrics has called for increased research into nursing homes to help improve the quality of life of the residents, while recognising that there are *major qualitative differences in nursing homes in different parts of the world* (Kaehr et al., 2015).

The norm in dementia is **complexity** and **comorbidity**. Coincident factors such as symptoms of other diseases, the adverse effects of medications, pain, depression or features of the social and physical environment can aggravate declining function associated with dementia. Some of these factors are potentially modifiable, and failing to recognise and address them results in disability *in excess of* that due purely to dementia progression (Slaughter and Hayduk, 2012). The privatisation of care since the 1980s has led to a number of adverse effects in terms of the involvement of NHS clinicians in care homes, including the withdrawal of NHS specialist clinicians, a lack of clarity around NHS obligations, a NHS aimed at the working-age population with single conditions (not frail older people with comorbidity), and the assumption that ordinary general practice is sufficient. This has led to an extremely unfortunate belief that care homes are, at best, left as 'islands of care', or at worst left as separate 'fortresses'.

People with dementia living in residential care tend to have complex needs, and this must be factored into any consideration of their psychological wellbeing (Martin et al., 2002). An unmet need may be described as a situation where an individual has significant problems for which there is an appropriate intervention which could potentially meet that need (Stevens and Gabbay, 1991; Orrell and Hancock, 2004). Chronic illness has been shown to be less well managed in care homes than in the community (Fahey et al., 2003). Care home residents may have poor access to external specialist resources, and effective assessment procedures are important both at the point of entry and after admission to a care home to ensure that residents' health and social care needs are identified and addressed, and to ensure that resources are used appropriately (Worden et al., 2008).

The definition of a care home is provided by section 3 of the Care Standards Act 2000:[1]

(1) For the purposes of this Act, an establishment is a care home if it provides accommodation, together with nursing or personal care, for any of the following persons.

(2) They are –

(a) persons who are or have been ill;

(b) persons who have or have had a mental disorder;

(c) persons who are disabled or infirm;

(d) persons who are or have been dependent on alcohol or drugs.

(3) But an establishment is not a care home if it is –

(a) a hospital;

(b) an independent clinic; or

(c) a children's home,

or if it is of a description excepted by regulations.

Care homes typically include homes with and without 24-hour on-site nursing staff, known as residential and nursing homes respectively (Gordon et al., 2014). In addition to routine GP services, there are payment schemes for enhanced GP services free at the point of contact through the NHS, outreach clinics, care home specialist nurses or support teams, pharmacist-led services, designated NHS hospital beds and enhanced services (Goodman et al., 2014). Iliffe and colleagues comment that 'there is a strong case to establish what is and what is not covered by the General Medical Service contract for general practice, to consider means of assuring compliance with the contract, as well as considering the adequacy of the contractual obligations' (p.135).

Recent landmark research has begun to give us a clearer picture of residents' needs and has provided some indications as to how services can most effectively respond (Gordon et al., 2014). Gordon and colleagues (2014) completed a 180-day longitudinal cohort study of 227 residents across 11 UK care homes, five nursing and six residential, selected to be representative of nursing/residential status and dementia registration. Residents had impaired mobility and transfers, and a high prevalence of incontinence, implying a need for access to physiotherapy, occupational therapy and specialist nursing.

---

1   Available at www.legislation.gov.uk/ukpga/2000/14/contents (accessed 3 Oct 2016).

The International Covenant on Economic, Social and Cultural Rights[2] is the most pertinent document for health. Article 12 calls for countries to recognise the right of everyone to enjoy the highest attainable standard of physical and mental health. The management of long-term conditions is one of the key challenges facing the health and social care system.

The imperative to promote health in care homes is intimately linked to the area of reducing avoidable admissions in hospitals (which I discuss in Chapter 10). There are, as you would expect, innovations being swiftly developed in this area – for example, the Better Health in Residents in Care Homes (BHiRCH) study.[3] This was funded by a grant from the National Institute for Health Research programme and started on 1 June 2015. It aims to develop clinical guidance and a decision-support system, comprised of several assessment steps, to screen and provide a more detailed assessment of the resident. Two key components of the BHiRCH intervention are an early warning tool and a care pathway. These components will facilitate the early detection and intervention of four key conditions (UTI, CHF, dehydration and lower respiratory tract infection) that commonly lead to unplanned hospitalisations.

—— Complex adaptive systems ——

The health and social care system is not simple. Far from it, in fact.

A complex adaptive system is 'a collection of individual agents with freedom to act in ways that are not always totally predictable, and whose actions are interconnected so that one agent's actions changes the context for other agents' (Plesk and Greenhalgh, 2001, p.625). Complex patients can be found with acute or chronic medical, neurological, obstetrical or surgical condition(s), including patients with unexplained physical conditions, and psychiatric comorbidity and psychiatric disorders, which are the direct consequence of primary medical conditions, such as organic psychiatric disorders and substance abuse (Gitlin, Levenson and Lyketsos, 2004).

Insights from complexity science show that the natural state of things is not a state of equilibrium. New opportunities are always being created by the system (McDaniel Jr, Jordan and Fleeman, 2003). Complex systems typically have fuzzy boundaries.

The organisational structure enacted through the Health and Social Care Act 2012 has created a system where more national bodies share responsibility for leading work to improve quality. A lack of clarity about the roles and responsibilities of different national bodies in relation to quality is not a new issue, but the reforms

---

2   Available at www.ohchr.org/EN/ProfessionalInterest/Pages/CESCR.aspx (accessed 3 Oct 2016).
3   Available at www.bradford.ac.uk/health/dementia/research/bhirch (accessed 3 Oct 2016).

undertaken in the last parliament appear to have exacerbated the situation (Molloy et al., 2016).

Health can only be maintained (or re-established) through a holistic approach that accepts unpredictability and builds on subtle emergent forces within the overall system (Wilson, Holt and Greenhalgh, 2001). A complexity approach would suggest that attempts to reduce or rigidly control complexity and uncertainty may fail, as the agents in the systems – service providers, patients and policymakers – are aware and able to learn and take action to affect outcomes (Matlow et al., 2006).

—— Multimorbidity (comorbidity) ——

Multimorbidity (comorbidity) has been defined as the co-occurrence of multiple chronic or acute diseases and medical conditions within one person. Multimorbidity is not just a condition of old age, and studies must begin to investigate multimorbidity across the life-course (Barnett et al., 2012).

Dementia never travels alone, but there are regional variations internationally in the relative proportions of multimorbidity (see Figure 3.1).

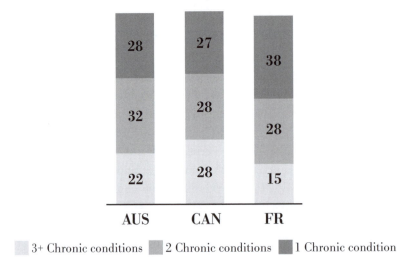

Figure 3.1: Variation in the relative proportions of comorbidity conditions
Source: Sarnak and Ryan (2016).

It is not unreasonable for policy to have turned its attention to comorbidity and dementia relatively late.

As Sube Banerjee (2015, p.587) has commented in *The Lancet*:

Research, policy, and action have transformed our ability to prevent infant mortality, to prevent and treat infectious diseases, and to prevent and treat the great killers in midlife such as heart disease and cancer. This is a fantastic success. But such success brings consequences – increased longevity is accompanied by complexity and multimorbidity (two or more long-term disorders).

Current guidelines are not designed to consider the cumulative impact of treatment recommendations on people with several conditions, nor to allow for comparing relative benefits or risks; this arguably leads to 'a focus on diseases not people' (Hughes, McMurdo and Guthrie, 2013).

It is therefore not surprising that there has been talk of a fresh approach to multimorbidity. The new NICE guidance 'Multimorbidity: Clinical Assessment and Management' (NICE, 2016) is intended to provide guidance on the optimum management of people with multimorbidity who need an approach to care that takes account of their multimorbidity because the combination of their conditions or the complexity of their treatments and health care appointments significantly affects their lives (Farmer, O'Flynn and Guthrie, 2016).

The management of the rising prevalence of long-term disorders is the main challenge facing governments and health care systems worldwide. Multimorbidity is, therefore, not simply a problem of chronological ageing, or randomly distributed in the population. For example, a recent analysis of nearly 200,000 patients registered with over 300 GP practices in Scotland has shown that multimorbidity is the norm for people with chronic disease and, although its prevalence increases with age, more than half of all people with multimorbidity are younger than 65 years of age (Mercer and Watt, 2007).

Case management as a model aims to improve the coordination of different services, such as health and social care, and has become a way of intervening in a fragmented health system that is moving towards non-optimal care for older persons (Gustafsson et al., 2013). Polypharmacy can be an important consequence of following guidelines in people with multimorbidity. Polypharmacy can be appropriate, but it is quite often associated with riskier prescribing and is often particularly problematic in people who are physically frail or have cognitive impairment (Guthrie et al., 2012).

Comorbidity among people with dementia presents particular challenges for both primary and secondary care and integrated care as a whole. Certain comorbid medical conditions may exacerbate the progression of dementia. For example, cognitive decline may be accelerated in older people with type 2 diabetes (Bunn et al., 2014). Comorbidity seems to increase with dementia severity, and has been related to cognition in several cross-sectional studies. However, the association between comorbidity and cognitive decline over time is still unclear, as medical conditions are often considered separately (Solomon et al., 2011).

—— Clinical issues ————————————————

Mobility

Person-centred care is often equated with quality nursing home care and involves the consideration of residents' choice, autonomy, independence and control. The mobility of older adults with dementia often declines after admission to a nursing home. Sedentary behaviour and limited mobility, common among older adults in nursing homes, can contribute to disability in terms of activities of daily living and the increased need for personal care (Slaughter et al., 2015). The assessment and management of mobility impairment are an integral part of the clinical management of residents in residential aged care because, in this population, mobility is an important risk factor for adverse health events such as respiratory tract infections, falls and fractures. Further, mobility limitation leads to increased health care utilisation, pressure sores, muscle atrophy, bone loss, pneumonia, incontinence, constipation and general functional decline (Williams et al., 2005).

Beyond adverse health outcomes for residents, mobility impairment increases the need for physical assistance, which increases the risk of staff injury (Barker et al., 2008). Many health care issues in older adults (e.g. falls, fractures and cognitive decline) are accompanied by forms of care including health and social care (Davis et al., 2015). Many residents require some form of staff assistance (referred to as mobility care) to achieve activities of daily living, but any staff promotion of residents' autonomy, independence and control during mobility is frequently absent (Taylor et al., 2015).

Falls

Falls are common in care homes, where rates vary from three to 13 falls per 1000 bed days (Burns and Nair, 2014).

Dementia has been acknowledged as a major risk factor for falls and bone fractures for decades. In 1988, Tinetti and colleagues demonstrated in 336 subjects aged 75 years and over who were monitored for a period of one year that cognitive impairments increased the risk of falling by five times (Tinetti, Speechley and Ginter, 1988). Another study of falls and fractures in 157 patients with dementia demonstrated that 50% of patients fell or were unable to walk during the three-year follow-up period (Buchner and Larson, 1987). Oliver and colleagues (2007) have helpfully identified many gaps in the evidence that deserve further investigation – for example, interventions specifically for those with cognitive impairment or dementia; the reproducibility of interventions within and between different types of service setting; the cost-effectiveness of interventions; and the effect of a range of single interventions, such as medication review, the use of alarms, or changes or differences in the physical environment.

A number of features of the physical environment are highly relevant to whether this happens (see Box 3.1).

Box 3.1: Universal recommendations: the environment

AREAS THAT SHOULD BE CONSIDERED

* **Flooring:** nonslip surfaces; prompt cleaning up of spills and urine, quick-dry and low-shine cleaning methods; avoiding flooring patterns that create the illusion of slopes or steps for people with visual impairment; visible highlighting of steps.

* **Lighting:** adequate and even lighting, including stairs; avoiding glare; way-finding night lighting to the toilet; making sure night lighting is used consistently and safely.

* **Observation:** improving lines of sight from staff to patients through dispersed nursing stations, observation windows or mirrors.

* **Threats to mobilising:** promptly reducing clutter and other trip hazards in patients' rooms and wards; installing handrails; prompt assessment for walking aids of the correct height and type and that are well maintained and kept within easy reach.

* **Signposting:** ensuring toilets are easy to find, with signage suitable for those with visual impairment, cognitive problems or language barriers.

* **Personal aids and possessions:** spectacles or hearing aids kept clean, working and available; drinks, tissues or other personal possessions within easy reach; call bells in reach for patients able to use them; catheters, intravenous lines and oxygen tubing secure and not trailing.

* **Furniture:** chairs available in a range of heights; beds kept at the correct height for safe standing for mobile patients; beds kept at the lowest height for non-mobile patients (including low-low beds); furniture should be stable for handhold walking; brakes applied to beds and wheeled chairs.

* **Footwear:** unsafe footwear can further compound fall risk, especially in those with gait, balance, lower limb and proprioceptive problems. In addition, a failure to act on environmental hazards is not only a risk in itself, but is likely to demotivate staff and adversely affect any other efforts for fall prevention.

SOURCE: ADAPTED FROM OLIVER, HEALEY AND HAINES (2010, BOX 2, P.683).

Falls are three times more frequent in care home residents than in older adults living in the community and outside long-term care (Rapp et al., 2012). Falls can lead to significant injury, with one in ten care home residents who fall sustaining a fracture (Rapp et al., 2009). Falls account for 40% of all injury deaths in care homes (Rubenstein, 2006). This can lead to a fear of falling in care home residents, with subsequent activity restriction and associated depressive symptoms, muscular atrophy and weakness (Gillespie and Friedman, 2007). The Guide to Action Care Home Falls Prevention Intervention is a multifactorial risk factor checklist for falls, with suggested actions to reverse or modify fall-risk factors. It was co-produced by care home staff, clinical staff and researchers (Walker et al., 2015).

Risk management must be balanced up against the need to promote functional independence and respect autonomy. Up to 45% of A&E department attendees over 65 years of age have fallen, and up to 10% of falls in community-dwelling older persons result in significant injury (Campbell et al., 1990). Recurrent falls lead to loss of confidence to perform functional activities, social isolation, increased hospitalisation and an increased likelihood of early admission to nursing care. Recurrent falls are also associated with increased mortality, unlike single falls (Davison et al., 2005).

Research findings have shown that factors contributing to falls are multifactorial, complex, interrelated and can be fixed or transient (Quigley et al., 2010). Nursing home residents fall at three times the rate of community-dwelling older adults (Rubenstein, Josephson and Osterweil, 1996), and 50–75% of nursing home residents fall each year. The physical, psychological and social consequences of falls are considerable (Thapa et al., 1996). There is tremendous pressure on the staff of aged care facilities, leaving them little time to concentrate on programmes such as falls injury prevention.

Recent meta-analyses of research into falls in care homes have reported a beneficial effect from hip protectors in reducing the rate of hip fracture by one-third (Oliver et al., 2007). Falls often indicate underlying frailty or illness and thus require a broad approach to assessment and management. In recognising that risk factors for falls are multifactorial and interacting, providers require guidance on the components, intensity, dose and duration for an effective fall and fall injury prevention programme (Quigley et al., 2010).

Most falls in hospital result from synergistic interactions between person-specific risk factors, the physical environment, the riskiness of a person's behaviour and the interactions between the patient and hospital staff (Koh et al., 2009). During hospitalisation for acute illness, these synergistic interactions are magnified and falls become a major concern for older people, their carers, the hospital and the health care system (Basic and Hartnell, 2015). Most evidence about successful prevention strategies, however, is derived from less frail and more clinically stable people living in their own homes (Gillespie et al., 2006). Hip protectors can lower the risk of a fall-related hip fracture by reducing the impact of the fall on the greater trochanter. Since hip fracture rates are exceptionally high in residents of nursing homes, the use of hip protectors seems to be particularly appealing in this group of people (Klenk et al., 2011). Several studies have demonstrated that hip protectors can be beneficial in an institutional setting, but poor compliance with treatment is still common and may be a reason for therapeutic failure (Marinker and Shaw, 2003). A Cochrane review of hip protectors used in care home residents found that fracture rates may not be reduced because of problems with adherence to treatment (Gillespie, Gillespie and Parker, 2010).

There are also many barriers to using potentially effective strategies (Ward et al., 2010). Nonetheless, promising research continues.

Visual and hearing impairments

Older people move to a care home when they are no longer able to live independently in the community. In the UK, care homes are facilities that provide personal, nursing and social care in a residential environment. The move to a care home therefore involves relocation to a new environment and a change in living arrangements. In this setting the older person is in close continuous contact with other people who require care and support with their daily activities (Cook, Brown-Wilson and Forte, 2006). They may share few or no common interests with these people, other than their need for assistance. Together these factors have a significant impact on the types and quality of social relationships that residents experience.

Visual and hearing impairments are associated with higher rates of common clinical problems among nursing home residents, independent of functional disability, cognitive impairment and depressive symptoms. Effective communication is challenging when working with individuals with dementia and hearing loss, and the challenges are exacerbated when dementia and hearing loss co-occur (Gallacher, 2004; Gallacher et al., 2012). The incidence of dementia has been associated with the severity of hearing loss, and among nursing home residents hearing loss and dementia both have a high prevalence: the prevalence of hearing loss has been estimated at approximately 90% and the prevalence of dementia at approximately 60% (Slaughter et al., 2014).

The combination of a hearing impairment and dementia may exacerbate agitation in nursing home residents, possibly increasing their loneliness and feelings of isolation, resulting in a poorer quality of life (Jupiter, 2012). In addition, individuals with other medical conditions who have hearing loss need to be identified so that physicians can provide effective treatment and the patients can understand and comply with the treatment (Weinstein, 2011). Hearing loss can be an important target for treatment if it is identified by carers. A range of interventions can be useful to facilitate communication, including the manner of speaking, the removal of cerumen from the ear canal, environmental approaches and assistive technology (Slaughter et al., 2014).

Hand hygiene

Healthy employees are the most important resource for a healthy business. Nonetheless, little is known about hand hygiene adherence rates and similar challenges in nursing homes (Mody, 2009). Despite the importance of hand hygiene practices, challenges such as adherence rates for using appropriate practices exist across many health care providers (Castle, Handler and Wagner, 2013). In nursing homes, infectious risk is high, making infection control using approaches such as hand hygiene a major issue. A recent study from the US presented information from 4211 nurse aides working in a nationally representative sample of 767 nursing homes (Castle et al., 2013). Overall, they found that compliance with hand washing by nurse aides is probably less than optimal.

Hip fractures

Osteoporosis is a common condition estimated to affect >200 million people worldwide (Cooper, 1999). It is characterised by the progressive loss of bone mineral content and consequently an increased risk of fracture. A large Finnish study reported that 94% of all pelvic fractures in people aged over 60 years of age were attributable to osteoporosis (Kannus et al., 2000). The most cost-effective strategy to reduce hip fracture costs is to prevent it in the first place. Two recent meta-analyses have shown a reduction in hip fracture risk with calcium and vitamin D supplementation, although for one of the meta-analyses, the effects were only significant in subjects living in institutions (Sahota, Morgan and Moran, 2012). Current research appears insufficient to determine the best ways to care for people with dementia after a hip fracture operation, so further research is needed to establish what the best strategies are to improve the care of people with dementia following a hip fracture (Smith et al., 2015). Fracture of the hip is a frequent condition in the elderly, and it has been estimated that the lifetime risk for an 80-year-old man or woman to sustain a hip fracture is 9% and 19% respectively (Kannus et al., 2000).

Hip fractures are one of the most debilitating injuries caused by falls, often bringing excess mortality, decline in functional independence, diminished quality of life and psychological distress (e.g. delirium, depression, anxiety and fear) (Korrall et al., 2015). This is mostly explained by limited user adherence in the wearing of hip protectors, resulting in a large number of falls (and subsequently, hip fractures) (Parker, Gillespie and Gillespie, 2005). However, when comparisons are drawn from analyses of protected vs unprotected falls, the relative risk of hip fracture is reduced by between 69% and 80% when a hip protector is in place at the time of a fall (Cameron et al., 2003). Thus, despite the observation of good biomechanical efficacy (more than equivalent to the best osteoporosis pharmaceutical treatments) (Liberman et al., 2006), poor adherence causes the intervention to appear ineffective.

Hip fractures overall are associated with high morbidity and mortality despite advances in surgical and regional anaesthesia techniques (Parker, Handoll and Griffiths, 2004). Up to 50% of patients do not regain their pre-fracture functional status, as judged by their ability to walk and their need for ambulatory aids at home (Wehren and Magaziner, 2003). Long-term dependency and institutional care placement explain much of the economic cost of this injury (Cumming, Kineberg and Katelaris 1996; Dolan and Torgerson, 1998). Acute care in-hospital mortality following hip fractures remains high and is consistent across academic and community hospitals (Alzahrani et al., 2010). Because of the greater prevalence of frailty, older persons living in long-term care facilities are more prone to fall than their peers living in a community setting and, thus, more likely to suffer the consequences. Fractures that are sustained in these populations have worse outcomes compared with age-matched controls living in community settings. Accordingly, this situation places this population at a high need for specific interventions aimed to improve their physical condition, decrease the number of falls and avoid injuries (Silva, Eslick and Duque, 2013).

Frailty

Frail older people are the core users of NHS care. The available physical frailty phenotypes are difficult to test for in the nursing home, creating a need for a simpler frailty scale. Sarcopenia is a geriatric syndrome associated with ageing that is characterised by a progressive loss of skeletal muscle mass and muscle function. It is known to increase the risk of disability, falls and fall-related injuries, loss of independence, hospitalisation and mortality (Senior et al., 2015).

In the recent NICE guidance 'Dementia, Disability and Frailty in Later Life – Mid-Life Approaches to Delay or Prevent Onset', there is a focus on delaying the onset of dementia, disability and frailty, increasing the amount of time that people can be independent, healthy and active in later life (*successful ageing*) (NICE, 2015); the notion of 'successful ageing' is explored in more detail in Chapter 13. This guidance suggested helping people stop smoking, be more active, reduce alcohol consumption, improve their diet and, if necessary, lose weight and maintain a healthy weight, and increasing people's resilience, for example by improving their social and emotional wellbeing.

Examples of frailty measures are shown in Table 3.1.

Table 3.1: A comparison of three validated measures of frailty

	Description and classification	Pros	Cons
Fried's Frailty Phenotype	Frail = >/= 3 characteristics Pre-frail = >/= 2 characteristics Robust = none	Four of the five items are objective (performance can be measured). Extensively validated to predict health outcomes. Correlation with physiological markers of poor health outcomes including haemoglobin and pro-inflammatory markers.	The phenotype definition for frailty can be insensitive and non-specific (especially in relation to Parkinson's disease, dementia and some cancers). It does not readily grade degrees of frailty. Does not stage degrees of frailty.
Clinical Frailty Scale	Classification on ordinal scale according to global clinical assessment. In this approach, the health professional considers information about cognition, mobility, function and comorbidities based on the history and physical examination to assign a frailty level from one (very fit) to nine (terminally ill with a life expectancy <6 months).	Clinically feasible.	Requires additional data on feasibility and validity in clinical settings.
Frailty Index	Number of health deficits present/number of possible health deficits, using a pre-specified list of health conditions.	Precise measurement. Reproducible across populations and disease states.	Usually cumbersome to use in clinical settings, but note the potential impact of electronic patient records.

SOURCE: ADAPTED FROM MOORHOUSE AND ROCKWOOD (2012, TABLE 3).

The clinical syndrome of frailty is characterised by poor muscle strength, vulnerability to infections because of impaired immunity and failures of the endocrine system resulting in a critically reduced homeostatic capacity to withstand any insult (whether from infection, organ impairment, etc.) (Burns and Nair, 2014). It is a condition characterised by the loss of biological reserves across multiple organ systems and vulnerability to physiological decompensation after a stressor event (Clegg et al., 2013). Common comorbidities such as dementia also contribute to frailty. About 750,000 people in the UK currently have dementia, and the number is expected to double in the next 30 years (Department of Health, 2009).

A small insult can result in a catastrophic loss of function (Rockwood and Hubbard, 2004). The characteristic response of the frail person to such an insult is to fall, become immobile or suffer a delirium. The effects of frailty on older people attending hospital can be easily seen in any medical admissions unit, but they are often inadequately recognised. This leads to harmful diagnoses such as 'off-legs', acopia or UTI, a collection of terms which identify the likely presence of the frailty syndrome, but without an attempt to find the stressor that has resulted in the decline (Wyrko, 2015).

Care home residents are substantially frail, and developments in the treatment of frailty and its prevention will undoubtedly be of key interest to those who care for care home residents. Early evidence points to the importance of exercise (including chair-based) and nutrition in reducing the impact of frailty (Clegg et al., 2012).

The current focus on person-centred care arguably runs the risk of over-emphasising independence and stigmatising dependence and interdependence – both of which are facts of life for many older patients (Gordon and Oliver, 2015). When carers are involved, relationship-centred care should be the goal. A recent Cochrane review investigated whether specialist, organised and coordinated geriatric care (normally referred to as comprehensive geriatric assessment or CGA) is better for patient outcomes than conventional care in a hospital setting (Ellis et al., 2011).

The CGA may have a role in providing health care to care home residents. The Proactive Healthcare for Older People in Care Home (PEACH) study aims to consider how and whether CGA helps address this in greater detail. Quality improvement collaboratives, representing health and social care commissioners, providers, care home organisations, NHS frontline staff and lay representatives will work to align health care to care homes more fully with the principles of CGA across four Care Commissioning Groups in South Nottinghamshire.[4]

Frailty is associated with a higher risk of poor health outcomes after health interventions, including prolonged hospital stay, delirium, permanent functional decline, the need for long-term care, adverse drug reactions and death (Moorhouse and Rockwood, 2012). The British Geriatrics Society (BGS), working with the Royal College of General Practitioners and Age UK, have published *Fit for Frailty*, advice aimed at all levels of health and social care professionals encountering older people living with frailty in community and outpatient settings. The second part of this work features guidance directed at senior clinicians, managers and commissioners on the development of services for those who may be frail.

---

4   See the excellent blogpost by Adam Gordon on the BGS website (3 March 2016), available at https://britishgeriatricssociety.wordpress.com/2016/03/03/can-comprehensive-geriatric-assessment-make-a-difference-to-care-home-residents.

Frailty is a good example of a condition which tends to show a particular 'trajectory'. These trajectories are relevant to the organisation of care – for example, Chapter 12 considers a discussion of whether dementia is a terminal illness (refer to Figure 3.2).

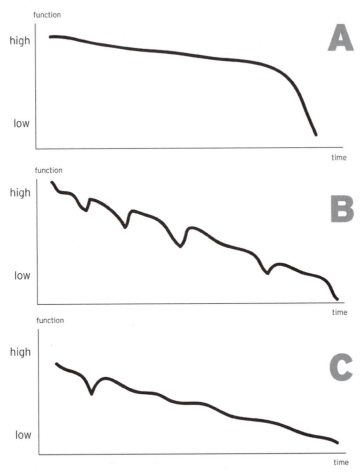

Figure 3.2: Different disease trajectories

A: short period of evident decline (e.g. cancer).
B: long-term limitations with intermittent various episodes (e.g. heart and lung failure).
C: prolonged dwindling (e.g. frailty, dementia).
Source: adapted from Lynn and Adamson (2005, Fig. 3, p.8).

Medication and polypharmacy

As just one example, over one-third of care home residents receive antidepressants, sometimes for longer than necessary; the use of these among older adults can be associated with serious adverse events, including serious bleeding, paradoxical aggression, falls and fractures (Jordan et al., 2014).

NICE have made some very important recommendations about what should be in care home policy ('Checklist for Health and Social Care Staff Developing and Updating a Care Home Medicines Policy Implementing the NICE Guideline on Managing Medicines in Care Homes' (NICE, 2014)).

The care home sector is an increasingly important provider of long-term care for older people. A review of the international literature has recently identified that research in the areas of quality and safety is lacking, especially for residential homes which have no on-site nursing staff (Szczepura, Nelson and Wild, 2008). Medication use is considered optimal when prescribed drugs have a clear indication, based on scientific evidence, and are well tolerated. Inappropriate prescribing (i.e. an unfavourable ratio of the risk for adverse drug events relative to potential benefits) frequently leads to negative health outcomes (Kröger et al., 2015).

Polypharmacy is common in this population: data from US and European samples showed that nursing home residents with dementia receive an average of seven to eight drugs every day (Onder et al., 2013). Polypharmacy, furthermore, increases the risk of potentially inappropriate drug prescribing, which may lead to adverse drug events, such as falls and hospitalisation (Cool et al., 2014). It presents challenges for those providing care and exposes residents to an increased risk of adverse drug events. Polypharmacy has considerable workforce and management implications for providers of long-term care (Jokanovic et al., 2015).

Medication safety is a pressing concern for residential aged care facilities (RACFs). Retrospective studies in RACF settings identify inadequate communication between RACFs, doctors, hospitals and community pharmacies as the major cause of medication errors (Tariq, Georgiou and Westbrook, 2013). Medication management in RACFs differs from acute care settings due to its extended duration and the long-term relationships between the residents and the care providers (Field et al., 2008). Health care technology is meant to reduce medication errors, and yet a considerable proportion of all incidents were technology-related. Most errors were due to socio-technical issues. Unintended and unanticipated errors may occur when using technologies. Therefore, when using technologies, system improvement, awareness, training and monitoring are needed to minimise medication errors (Samaranayake et al., 2012). But it is clear that there are other factors at work in heightening the risk of prescribing errors in RACFs. For example, based on work in Australia, Tariq and colleagues (2016) also identified 'team factors' (or 'human factors') which included the 'lack of established lines of responsibility, inadequate team communication and limited participation of doctors in multidisciplinary initiatives like medication advisory committee meetings'.

Brulhart and Wermeille (2011) recommended multidisciplinary medication reviews and reported that the pharmacist working with the physician and nursing staff reduced the medication burden and identified potential adverse drug reactions in care home residents. However, a recent Cochrane review examined interventions designed to optimise prescribing for older people in care homes. The authors commented on the heterogeneous nature of the studies which tested several types of intervention with mixed results. They reported no clear benefit on adverse drug reactions, mortality, hospital admissions or quality of life. Some studies reported a benefit for medicine costs, but this effect was not consistent (Alldred et al., 2013).

Deprescribing is not only feasible, but associated benefits include reduced polypharmacy, positive clinical outcomes and increased adherence. Individual physician practices vary widely. Limited data from palliative care and advanced dementia settings demonstrate considerable variation and inadequate structures for deprescribing (Ní Chróinín, Ní Chróinín and Beveridge, 2015). UK care home residents with type 2 diabetes had an increased burden of comorbidities and prescriptions. The majority of these patients were prescribed potentially inappropriate medicines. Validation by a care home physician supported the clinical applicability of the medicines optimisation tool (Andreassen et al., 2016). Medication mismanagement can result in several adverse health outcomes for older patients, along with higher medical costs (Bhuyan et al., 2015). One study reported that such improper use of medications could also lead to adverse drug events (ADEs), which accounted for over 30% of hospitalisations among the elderly populations (Chan, Nicklason and Vial, 2001).

The prevalence of inappropriate prescribing is particularly high in nursing homes. Over the past ten years, several studies have been conducted to identify interventions that can increase appropriate prescribing in this specific setting (Anrys et al., 2016).

There have been a number of exciting initiatives in the area of medication reviews.

The objective of the Care Homes' Use of Medicines Study (CHUMS) was to determine the prevalence and potential harm of prescribing, monitoring, dispensing and administration errors in UK care homes and to identify their causes. The themes identified included: doctors who were not accessible, did not know the residents and lacked information in homes when prescribing; the high workload of the home's staff, a lack of medicines training and drug-round interruptions; a lack of team work between home, practice and the pharmacy; inefficient ordering systems; inaccurate medicine records and the prevalence of verbal communication; and medication administration systems that were difficult to fill and check (Barber et al., 2009). Possible solutions might include the potential of IT to improve systems and enhance safety, unified access to a single care record, a lead GP for each home and regular reviewing of prescribing (comprehensive medication review – CMR).[5]

---

5   See David Alldred's presentation at the King's Fund: www.kingsfund.org.uk/sites/files/kf/media/David%20Alldred%20pres.pdf.

Medication Safety in Care Homes is an ambitious cross-sector partnership project aiming to improve the medicines pathway for residents in care homes.[6] The partnership, led by the National Care Forum on behalf of the Care Provider Alliance, was formed to try and address some of the issues raised by CHUMS and ongoing concerns about safety and standards related to medication prescribing, administration and management in care homes. Furthermore, as medicines' use in care homes has been shown to be suboptimal, it has been suggested that, to address this, one person should assume overall responsibility for medicines management in a care home. The Care Homes Independent Pharmacist Prescribing Study (CHIPPS) is a five-year, NIHR-funded research programme.[7] It proposes that a suitable model for appropriate medicines management in care homes is a Pharmacist Independent Prescriber. He or she would assume responsibility for repeat prescriptions' monitoring and authorising and, overall, the management of medicines in the care home. CHIPPS is developing this innovative new model of care and then testing it in a feasibility study before completing a randomised controlled trial.

Infections

The delay or failure to provide necessary care is an emerging area of concern in nursing. Necessary but incomplete nursing care activities, commonly labelled 'missed care', are indicators of impaired nursing processes and overall poor care quality (Nelson and Flynn, 2015). Infections are a crucial aspect of this.

Nursing facilities, in general, have less physician involvement in direct patient care than hospitals and are characterised by a lack of an organised medical staff. Defining the diagnostic work-up that is appropriate in nursing homes for a clinical syndrome is problematic (Beier, 1999). The rate of growth in the elderly population around the world has led to the estimate that 40% of adults around the world will reside in a long-term care facility for some time before death, over the next 30 years (Furman, Rayner and Tobin, 2004). Infections are common in residents of long-term care facilities. The high frequency of infection is attributed to ageing-associated physiologic changes, multiple comorbidities, functional impairment and the increased opportunities for transmission of organisms in an institutional setting. The increasing use of invasive devices for residents of some of these facilities also contributes to infection (Nicolle, 2014).

It has previously been shown that infections are the most common causes of hospital admissions from nursing homes; the most frequent infections in nursing homes have been urinary tract infections (UTIs), respiratory tract infections and skin/soft tissue infections (described in Krüger et al., 2011).

---

6   Available at www.nationalcareforum.org.uk/project-medication.asp (accessed 3 Oct 2016).
7   Available at www.uea.ac.uk/chipps/summary (accessed 4 Oct 2016).

UTIs are the most common reason for prescribing antibiotics in long-term care (LTC) facilities. Of systemic antimicrobial courses, 25% to 70% are used for UTI treatments (Rummukainen et al., 2012). A UTI is arguably the most common infection in the long-term care setting. Making the diagnosis of UTI and deciding when to initiate treatment with antimicrobial therapy are challenging to all long-term care providers. *Asymptomatic bacteriuria* is commonly found among elderly long-term care residents (Nicolle, 2001). The widespread prevalence of asymptomatic bacteriuria, the lack of an accepted clinical or laboratory gold standard to start antibiotics for UTI and a high prevalence of cognitive impairment in the long-term care population all contribute to this challenge (Nace, Drinka and Crnich, 2014). Owing to the unique nature of the LTC setting, clinicians rarely evaluate residents personally before diagnosing UTI (Levy et al., 2006). Remaining options then appear to be to prescribe an antimicrobial agent, or to simply observe and monitor.

Pneumonia represents 13–48% of all infections in nursing home settings (Mehr et al., 1998). Several patient characteristics predispose nursing home patients to pneumonia, including chronic diseases, impaired functional abilities, malnourishment, diminished cough reflex, lack of elastic tissue and decreased immunoglobulin A (Dhawan et al., 2015). Pneumonia is a common event in nursing home residents with dementia. The illness may be associated with severe discomfort, irrespective of whether antibiotics are used (van der Steen et al., 2015). Treatment of pneumonia in dementia involves specific challenges, because patients are not always able to verbalise symptoms (van der Maaden et al., 2015).

Diabetes

More than a quarter of care home residents have diabetes, much of the care for which may be inadequate, and a large amount remains undiagnosed. A 150% increase in care home residents is indeed expected over the next 50 years (Yarnall et al., 2011). Although the association between T2DM and dementia is well established, it is less clear which factors account for the increased dementia risk in diabetes (Exalto et al., 2012). Although knowledge in the prevention and treatment of diabetes in the general population is increasing, there remains currently a relative paucity in research examining the management of diabetes in long-term care, including for example the impact of lifestyle interventions on health and quality of life (Hager, Loprinzi and Stone, 2013). Symptoms of hypoglycaemia in the elderly are often unspecific and less marked compared to those in younger patients, and may be mistaken for symptoms of their cognitive or functional impairment, or even stroke (Andreassen et al., 2014).

Inadequate procedures and training in diabetes care may compromise the rationale for capillary blood glucose measurements in nursing homes, and hence the residents' safety. These concerns should be addressed together with the possibility of involving and empowering residents by exploring their ability and wish to manage their own disease (Andreassen et al., 2016). Specific attention should be paid to the needs of the nursing home population, with aims to maintain or improve quality of life. Medical care is organised around specific disease entities, but with frail, dependent patients suffering from multiple health problems, the focus switches to a more global approach and clinical decisions are made with the holistic objectives of enhancing quality of life, maintaining function, preventing as much further loss as possible and avoiding complications that might necessitate hospital admission (Benetos et al., 2013). Consequently, future studies in long-term care examining the association between diabetes management and mood, depression and quality of life are warranted.

Chronic pain

Chronic pain is highly prevalent in the ageing population. Individuals with neurological disorders such as dementia are susceptible patient groups in which pain is frequently under-recognised, underestimated and undertreated (Hadjistavropoulos et al., 2014). Results from neurophysiological and neuroimaging studies showing that elderly adults are particularly susceptible to the negative effects of pain are of additional concern. The inability to successfully communicate pain in severe dementia is a major barrier to effective treatment. Pain is common in older people, particularly those in residential aged care facilities and those with dementia. People with severe dementia have multiple potential sources of pain, such as genitourinary infection, fall-related injuries, pressure ulcers, contractures and gastrointestinal and cardiac pain, compounding the generic musculoskeletal and cancer-related pain associated with ageing per se (Peisah et al., 2014). Improving pain management, particularly in long-term care facilities, should be considered as a high priority for health care services. A prerequisite for improvement is to understand patterns of pain and factors that may influence its onset and treatment.

Nursing home residents with dementia gradually lose the ability to process information so that they are less likely to express pain in typical ways. These residents may express pain through distressed responses because they cannot appropriately verbalise their pain experience. Poor management of pain in people with dementia has been attributed, in part, to the difficulty in accurately assessing the presence and intensity of pain, especially as a person's cognitive and communication abilities worsen (Barry et al., 2015). Care home staff may have to increasingly rely on surrogate reports or behavioural indicators of pain (Hadjistavropoulos et al., 2007). Although knowledge about the differences in pain prevalence between dementia subtypes is scarce, it has been suggested that differences in neuropathology between dementia subtypes could be of vital importance in the treatment of pain (Benedetti et al., 2006).

The organisation of long term-care

A key concern of residents in care homes is making sure that they have the right care, at the right time, at the right place.

The organisation and day-to-day running of long-term care facilities differ significantly between countries, although resident cohorts are very similar in terms of the types of care they require (Tolson et al., 2013). If effective health care support to care homes is to be established and sustained, it is important to understand what makes different interventions effective in their own settings and to seek to identify differences and commonalities between them. This is the aim of the Optimal Study (Gordon et al., 2014).

I will resume discussion of care homes in integrated care in Chapter 10.

Essential reading

Baker C. 2014. *Developing Excellent Care for People Living with Dementia in Care Homes*, London: Jessica Kingsley Publishers.

Antipsychotics

Rahman S. 2015. *Living Better with Dementia*, London: Jessica Kingsley Publishers, pp.321–334.

Delirium

Rahman S. 2015. *Living Better with Dementia*, London: Jessica Kingsley Publishers, pp.118–123.

References

Alldred DP, Raynor DK, Hughes C, Barber N, Chen TF, Spoor P. 2013. Interventions to optimise prescribing for older people in care homes. Cochrane Database Syst Rev, 2, CD009095.

Alzahrani K, Gandhi R, Davis A, Mahomed N. 2010. In-hospital mortality following hip fracture care in southern Ontario. Can J Surg, 53(5), 294–298.

Andreassen LM, Granas AG, Sølvik UØ, Kjome RL. 2016. 'I try not to bother the residents too much' – the use of capillary blood glucose measurements in nursing homes. BMC Nurs, 15, 7.

Andreassen LM, Sandberg S, Kristensen GB, Sølvik UØ, Kjome RL. 2014. Nursing home patients with diabetes: prevalence, drug treatment and glycemic control. Diabetes Res Clin Pract, 105(1), 102–109.

Anrys P, Strauven G, Boland B, Dalleur O, et al. 2016. Collaborative approach to Optimise MEdication use for Older people in Nursing homes (COME-ON): study protocol of a cluster controlled trial. Implement Sci, 11, 35.

Banerjee S. 2015. Multimorbidity – older adults need health care that can count past one. Lancet, 385(9968), 587–589.

Barber ND, Alldred DP, Raynor DK, Dickinson R, et al. 2009. Care homes' use of medicines study: prevalence, causes and potential harm of medication errors in care homes for older people. Qual Saf Health Care, 18(5), 341–346.

Barker AL, Nitz JC, Low Choy NL, Haines TP. 2008. Clinimetric evaluation of the physical mobility scale supports clinicians and researchers in residential aged care. Arch Phys Med Rehabil, 89(11), 2140–2145.

Barnett K, Mercer SW, Norbury M, Watt G, Wyke S, Guthrie B. 2012. Epidemiology of multimorbidity and implications for health care, research, and medical education: a cross-sectional study. Lancet, 380, 37–43.

Barry HE, Parsons C, Passmore AP, Hughes CM. 2015. Pain in care home residents with dementia: an exploration of frequency, prescribing and relatives' perspectives. Int J Geriatr Psychiatry, 30(1), 55–63.

Basic D, Hartwell TJ. 2015. Falls in hospital and new placement in a nursing home among older people hospitalized with acute illness. Clin Interv Aging, 10, 1637–1643.

Beier MT. 1999. Management of urinary tract infections in the nursing home elderly: a proposed algorithmic approach. Int J Antimicrob Agents, 11(3–4), 275–284.

Benedetti F, Arduino C, Costa S, Vighetti S, et al. 2006. Loss of expectation-related mechanisms in Alzheimer's disease makes analgesic therapies less effective. Pain, 121, 133–144.

Benetos A, Novella JL, Guerci B, Blickle JF, et al. 2013. Pragmatic diabetes management in nursing homes: individual care plan. J Am Med Dir Assoc, 14(11), 791–800.

Bhuyan SS, Chandak A, Powell MP, Kim J, et al. 2015. Use of information technology for medication management in residential care facilities: correlates of facility characteristics. J Med Syst, 39(6), 70.

Brulhart M, Wermeille J. 2011. Multidisciplinary medication review: evaluation of a pharmaceutical care model for nursing homes. Int J Clin Pharmacol, 33, 549–557.

Buchner DM, Larson EB. 1987. Falls and fractures in patients with Alzheimer-type dementia. JAMA, 257(11), 1492–1495.

Bunn F, Burn AM, Goodman C, Rait G, et al. 2014. Comorbidity and dementia: a scoping review of the literature. BMC Med, 12, 192.

Burns E, Nair S. 2014. New horizons in care home medicine. Age Ageing, 43(1), 2–7.

Cameron ID, Cumming RG, Kurrle SE, Quine S, et al. 2003. A randomised trial of hip protector use by frail older women living in their own homes. Inj Prev, 9(2), 138–141.

Campbell AJ, Borrie MJ, Spears GF, Jackson SL, Brown JS, Fitzgerald JL. 1990. Circumstances and consequences of falls experienced by a community population 70 years and over during a prospective study. Age Ageing, 19, 136–141.

Care Quality Commission. 2013. The State of Health Care and Adult Social Care in England in 2012/13, available at www.cqc.org.uk/sites/default/files/documents/cqc_soc_report_2013_lores2.pdf (accessed 3 Oct 2016).

Castle N, Handler S, Wagner L. 2013. Hand hygiene practices reported by nurse aides in nursing homes. J Appl Gerontol (e-pub ahead of print).

Chan M, Nicklason F, Vial J. 2001. Adverse drug events as a cause of hospital admission in the elderly. Intern Med J, 31, 199–205.

Clegg A, Logan PA, Jones RG, Forrester-Paton C, Mamo JP. 2012. A systematic mapping review of randomized controlled trials (RCTs) in care homes. BMC Geriatr, 12, 31–46.

Clegg A, Young J, Iliffe S, Rikkert MO, Rockwood K. 2013. Frailty in elderly people. Lancet, 381(9868), 752–762.

Cook G, Brown-Wilson C, Forte D. 2006. The impact of sensory impairment on social interaction between residents in care homes. Int J Older People Nurs, 1(4), 216–224.

Cool C, Cestac P, Laborde C, Lebaudy C, et al. 2014. Potentially inappropriate drug prescribing and associated factors in nursing homes. J Am Med Dir Assoc, 15(11), 850.e1–9.

Cooper C. 1999. Epidemiology of osteoporosis. Osteoporosis Int, 9(Suppl 2), S2–8.

Cumming RG, Klineberg R, Katelaris A. 1996. Cohort study of risk of institutionalisation after hip fracture. Aust NZ J Public Health, 20, 579–582.

Davies SL, Goodman C, Manthorpe J, Smith A, Carrick N, Iliffe S. 2014. Enabling research in care homes: an evaluation of a national network of research ready care homes. BMC Med Res Methodol, 14(47).

Davis JC, Best JR, Bryan S, Li LC, et al. 2015. Mobility is a key predictor of change in wellbeing among older adults who experience falls: evidence from the Vancouver falls prevention clinic cohort. Arch Phys Med Rehabil, 96(9), 1634–1640.

Davison J, Bond J, Dawson P, Steen IN, Kenny RA. 2005. Patients with recurrent falls attending Accident & Emergency benefit from multifactorial intervention – a randomised controlled trial. Age Ageing, 34(2), 162–168.

Department of Health. 2009. *Living Well with Dementia: A National Dementia Strategy*, London: Department of Health, available at www.gov.uk/government/uploads/system/uploads/attachment_data/file/168220/dh_094051.pdf (accessed 3 Oct 2016).

Dhawan N, Pandya N, Khalili M, Bautista M, et al. 2015. Predictors of mortality for nursing home-acquired pneumonia: a systematic review. Biomed Res Int, 285983.

Dolan P, Torgerson DJ. 1988. The cost of treating osteoporosis in the United Kingdom female population. Osteoporos Int, 8, 611–617.

Ellis G, Whitehead MA, O'Neill D, Langhorne P, Robinson D. 2011. Comprehensive geriatric assessment for older adults admitted to hospital. Cochrane Database of Systematic Reviews, 7, Art. No. CD006211.

Exalto LG, Whitmer RA, Kappele LJ, Biessels GJ. 2012. An update on type 2 diabetes, vascular dementia and Alzheimer's disease. Exp Gerontol, 47(11), 858–864.

Fahey T, Montgomery AA, Barnes J, Protheroe J. 2003. Quality of care for elderly residents in nursing homes and elderly people living at home: controlled observational study. British Medical Journal, 326, 580–584.

Farmer C, Fenu E, O'Flynn N, Guthrie B. 2016. Clinical assessment and management of multimorbidity: summary of NICE guidance. BMJ, 354, i4843.

Field TS, Rochon P, Lee M, Gavendo L, Subramanian S, Hoover S, Baril J, Gurwitz J. 2008. Costs associated with developing and implementing a computerized clinical decision support system for medication dosing for patients with renal insufficiency in the long-term care setting. J Am Med Inform Assoc, 15(4), 466–472.

Furman CD, Rayner AV, Tobin EP. 2004. Pneumonia in older residents of long-term care facilities. American Family Physician, 70(8), 1495–1500.

Gallacher J. 2004. Hearing, cognitive impairment and aging: a critical review. Rev Clin Gerontol, 14, 199–209.

Gallacher J, Ilubaera V, Ben-Shlomo Y, Bayer A, et al. 2012. Auditory threshold, phonologic demand, and incident dementia. Neurology, 79(15), 1583–1590.

Gillespie LD, Gillespie WJ, Robertson MC, Lamb SE, Cumming RG, Rowe BH. 2006. Interventions for preventing falls in elderly people. Cochrane Database Syst Rev, 4, CD0003402.

Gillespie SM, Friedman SM. 2007. Fear of falling in new long-term care enrollees. J Am Med Directors Assoc, 8, 307–313.

Gillespie WJ, Gillespie LD, Parker MJ. 2010. *Hip Protectors for Preventing Hip Fractures in Older People (Review)*, Cambridge: Wiley and Sons Ltd.

Gitlin DF, Levenson JL, Lyketsos CG. 2004. Psychosomatic medicine: a new psychiatric subspecialty. Acad. Psychiatry, 28, 4–11.

Gordon AL, Franklin M, Bradshaw L, Logan P, Elliott R, Gladman JR. 2014. Health status of UK care home residents: a cohort study. Age Ageing, 43(1), 97–103.

Goodman C, Gordon AL, Martin F, Davies SL, et al. 2014. Effective health care for older people resident in care homes: the optimal study protocol for realist review. Syst Rev, 3, 49.

Gordon AL, Oliver D. 2015. Commentary: frameworks for long-term conditions must take account of needs of frail older people. BMJ, 350, h370.

Gordon AL, Franklin M, Bradshaw L, Logan P, Elliott R, Gladman JR. 2014. Health status of UK care home residents: a cohort study. Age Ageing, 43(1), 97–103.

Gustafsson M, Kristensson J, Holst G, Willman A, Bohman D. 2013. Case managers for older persons with multi-morbidity and their everyday work – a focused ethnography. BMC Health Serv Res, 13, 496.

Guthrie B, Payne K, Alderson P, McMurdo ME, Mercer SW. 2012. Adapting clinical guidelines to take account of multimorbidity. BMJ, 345, e6341.

Hadjistavropoulos T, Herr K, Prkachin KM, Craig KD, et al. 2014. Pain assessment in elderly adults with dementia. Lancet Neurol, 13(12), 1216–1227.

Hadjistavropoulos T, Herr K, Turk DC, Fine PG, et al. 2007. An interdisciplinary expert consensus statement on assessment of pain in older persons. Clin J Pain, 23(1 Suppl), S1–43.

Hager KK, Loprinzi P, Stone D. 2013. Implementing diabetes care guidelines in long-term care. J Am Med Dir Assoc, 14(11), 851.e7–15.

Hughes LD, McMurdo ME, Guthrie B. 2013. Guidelines for people not for diseases: the challenges of applying UK clinical guidelines to people with multimorbidity. Age Ageing, 42(1), 62–69.

Iliffe S, Davies SL, Gordon AL, Schneider J, et al. 2016. Provision of NHS generalist and specialist services to care homes in England: review of surveys. Prim Health Care Res Dev, 17(2), 122–137.

Jokanovic N, Tan EC, Dooley MJ, Kirkpatrick CM, Bell JS. 2015. Prevalence and factors associated with polypharmacy in long-term care facilities: a systematic review. J Am Med Dir Assoc, 16(6), 535.e1–12.

Jordan S, Gabe M, Newson L, Snelgrove S, et al. 2014. Medication monitoring for people with dementia in care homes: the feasibility and clinical impact of nurse-led monitoring. Scientific World Journal, 843621.

Jupiter T. 2012. Cognition and screening for hearing loss in nursing home residents. J Am Med Dir Assoc, 13(8), 744–747.

Kaehr E, Visvanathan R, Malmstrom TK, Morley JE. 2015. Frailty in nursing homes: the FRAIL-NH Scale. J Am Med Dir Assoc, 16(2), 87–89.

Kannus P, Palvanen M, Niemi S, Parkkari J, Järvinen M. 2000. Epidemiology of osteoporotic pelvic fractures in elderly people in Finland: sharp increase in 1970–1997 and alarming projections for the new millennium. Osteoporos Int, 11(5), 443–448.

Kitwood T. 1997. *Dementia Reconsidered*, Buckingham: Open University Press.

Klenk J, Kurrle S, Rissmann U, Kleiner A, Heinrich S, König HH, Becker C, Rapp K. 2011. Availability and use of hip protectors in residents of nursing homes. Osteoporos Int, 22(5), 1593–1598.

Koh SL, Hafizah N, Lee JY, Loo YL, Muthu R. 2009. Impact of a fall prevention programme in acute hospital settings in Singapore. Singapore Med J, 50(4), 425–432.

Korall AM, Feldman F, Scott VJ, Wasdell M, Gillan R, Ross D, Thompson-Franson T, Leung PM, Lin L. 2015. Facilitators of and barriers to hip protector acceptance and adherence in long-term care facilities: a systematic review. J Am Med Dir Assoc, 16(3), 185–193.

Kröger E, Wilchesky M, Marcotte M, Voyer P, et al. 2015. Medication use among nursing home residents with severe dementia: identifying categories of appropriateness and elements of successful intervention. J Am Med Dir Assoc, 16(7), 629.e1–17.

Krüger K, Jansen K, Grimsmo A, Eide GE, Geitung JT. 2011. Hospital admissions from nursing homes: rates and reasons. Nurs Res Pract, 247623.

Laing W, Buisson E. 2015. *Care of Older People – 27th Edition*, London: Laing and Buisson.

Levy CR, Eilertsen T, Kramer AM, Hutt E. 2006. Which clinical indicators and resident characteristics are associated with health care practitioner nursing home visits or hospital transfer for urinary tract infections? J Am Med Dir Assoc 2006;7: 493e498

Liberman UA, Hochberg MC, Chattopadhyay, A, Geusens P. 2006. Hip and nonspine fracture risk reductions differ among antiresorptive agents: evidence from randomised controlled trials. Int J Clin Pract, 60, 1394–1400.

Lynn J, Adamson DM. 2005. *Living Well at the End of Life: Adapting Health Care to Serious Chronic Illness in Old Age*, Pittsburgh: Rand Health, available at https://www.rand.org/content/dam/rand/pubs/white_papers/2005/WP137.pdf (accessed 28 Oct 2016).

Marinker M, Shaw J. 2003. Not to be taken as directed. BMJ, 326, 348–349

Martin MD, Hancock GA, Richardson B, Simmons P, et al. 2002. An evaluation of needs in elderly continuing-care settings. Int Psychogeriatr, 14, 379–404.

Matlow AG, Wright JG, Zimmerman B, Thomson K, Valente M. 2006. How can the principles of complexity science be applied to improve the coordination of care for complex pediatric patients? Qual Saf Health Care, 15(2), 85–88.

McDaniel RR Jr, Jordan ME, Fleeman BF. 2003. Surprise, surprise, surprise! A complexity science view of the unexpected. Health Care Manage Rev, 28(3), 266–278.

Mehr DR, Zweig SC, Kruse RL, Popejoy J, et al. 1998. Mortality from lower respiratory infection in nursing home residents: a pilot prospective community-based study, Journal of Family Practice, 47(4), 298–304.

Mercer SW, Watt GC. 2007. The inverse care law: clinical primary care encounters in deprived and affluent areas of Scotland. Ann Fam Med, 5(6), 503–510.

Mody L. 2009. Infection Control Programmes in Nursing Homes. In D. Norman, T. Yoshikawa (eds), *Infectious Disease in the Aging: A Clinical Handbook*, New York: Humana Press.

Molloy A, Martin S, Gardner T, Leatherman S. 2016. *A clear road ahead: Creating a coherent quality strategy for the English NHS*. NHS Health Foundation, available at www.health.org.uk/sites/health/files/AClearRoadAhead.pdf (accessed 29 Nov 2016).

Moorhouse P, Rockwood K. 2012. Frailty and its quantitative clinical evaluation. J R Coll Physicians Edinb, 42(4), 333–340.

Nace DA, Drinka PJ, Crnich CJ. 2014. Clinical uncertainties in the approach to long-term care residents with possible urinary tract infection. J Am Med Dir Assoc, 15(2), 133–139.

Nelson ST, Flynn L. 2015. Relationship between missed care and urinary tract infections in nursing homes. Geriatr Nurs, 36(2), 126–130.

Ní Chróinín D, Ní Chróinín C, Beveridge A. 2015. Factors influencing deprescribing habits among geriatricians. Age Ageing, 44(4), 704–708.

NICE. 2015. Dementia, Disability and Frailty in Later Life – Mid-Life Approaches to Delay or Prevent Onset, available at www.nice.org.uk/guidance/ng16 (accessed 3 Oct 2016).

NICE. 2016. Multimorbidity: Clinical Assessment and Management, NICE guideline [NG56], available at https://www.nice.org.uk/guidance/indevelopment/gid-cgwave0704 (accessed 29 Nov 2016).

Nicolle LE. 2001. The SHEA long-term-care committee: urinary tract infections in long-term-care facilities. Infect Control Hosp Epidemiol, 22, 167–175.

Nicolle LE. 2014. Infection prevention issues in long-term care. Curr Opin Infect Dis, 27(4), 363–369.

Oliver D, Connelly JB, Victor CR, Shaw FE, et al. 2007. Strategies to prevent falls and fractures in hospitals and care homes and effect of cognitive impairment: systematic review and meta-analyses. BMJ, 334(7584), 82.

Oliver D, Healey F, Haines TP. 2010. Preventing falls and fall-related injuries in hospitals. Clin Geriatr Med, 26(4), 645–692.

Onder G, Liperoti R, Foebel A, Fialova D, et al. 2013. Polypharmacy and mortality among nursing home residents with advanced cognitive impairment: results from the SHELTER study. J Am Med Dir Assoc, 14(6), 450.e7–12.

Orrell M, Hancock G. 2004. *Camberwell Assessment of Need for the Elderly, CANE*, London: Gaskell.

Parker MJ, Gillespie WJ, Gillespie LD. 2005. Hip protectors for preventing hip fractures in older people. Cochrane Database Syst Rev, 3, CD001255.

Parker MJ, Handoll HH, Griffiths R. 2004. Anaesthesia for hip fracture surgery in adults. Cochrane Database Syst Rev, 4, CD000521.

Peisah C, Weaver J, Wong L, Strukovski JA. 2014. Silent and suffering: a pilot study exploring gaps between theory and practice in pain management for people with severe dementia in residential aged care facilities. Clin Interv Aging, 9, 1767–1774.

Plesk PE, Greenhalgh T. 2001. Complexity science: the challenge of complexity in health care. BMJ, 323(7313), 625–628.

Prince M, Knapp M, Guerchet M, McCrone P, et al. 2014. *Dementia UK: Update (Second Edition)*, London: Alzheimer's Society UK, available at www.cfas.ac.uk/files/2015/07/P326_AS_Dementia_Report_WEB2.pdf (accessed 29 Nov 2016).

Quigley P, Bulat T, Kurtzman E, Olney R, Powell-Cope G, Rubenstein L. 2010. Fall prevention and injury protection for nursing home residents. J Am Med Dir Assoc, 11(4), 284–293.

Rahman S. 2015. Living Better with Dementia, London: Jessica Kingsley Publishers.

Rapp K, Becker C, Cameron ID, König H-H, Büchele G. 2012. Epidemiology of falls in residential aged care: analysis of more than 70,000 falls from residents of Bavarian nursing homes. J Am Med Directors Assoc, 13, 187e1–e6.

Rapp K, Lamb SE, Klenk J, Kleiner A, et al. 2009. Fractures after nursing home admission: Incidence and potential consequences. Osteop Inter, 20, 1775–1783.

Rockwood K, Hubbard R. 2004. Frailty and the geriatrician. Age and Ageing, 33, 429–430.

Rubenstein LZ. 2006. Falls in older people: epidemiology, risk factors and strategies for prevention. Age Ageing, 35, ii37–ii41.

Rubenstein LZ, Josephson KR, Osterweil D. 1996. Falls and fall prevention in the nursing home. Clin Geriatr Med, 12, 881–902.

Rummukainen ML, Jakobsson A, Matsinen M, Järvenpää S, Nissinen A, Karppi P, Lyytikäinen O. 2012. Reduction in inappropriate prevention of urinary tract infections in long term care facilities. Am J Infect Control, 40(8), 711–714.

Sahota O, Morgan N, Moran CG. 2012. The direct cost of acute hip fracture care in care home residents in the UK. Osteoporos Int, 23(3), 917–920.

Samaranayake NR, Cheung ST, Chui WC, Cheung BM. 2012. Technology-related medication errors in a tertiary hospital: a 5-year analysis of reported medication incidents. Int J Med Inform, 81(12), 828–833.

Sarnak DO, Ryan J. 2016. How High-Need Patients Experience the Health Care System in Nine Countries, The Commonwealth Fund, available at www.commonwealthfund.org/publications/issue-briefs/2016/jan/high-need-patients-nine-countries (accessed 3 Oct 2016).

Senior HE, Henwood TR, Beller EM, Mitchell GK, Keogh JW. 2015. Prevalence and risk factors of sarcopenia among adults living in nursing homes. Maturitas, 82(4), 418–423.

Silva RB, Eslick GD, Duque G. 2013. Exercise for falls and fracture prevention in long-term care facilities: a systematic review and meta-analysis. J Am Med Dir Assoc, 14(9), 685–689.e2.

Slaughter SE, Hayduk LA. 2012. Contributions of environment, comorbidity, and stage of dementia to the onset of walking and eating disability in long-term care residents. J Am Geriatr Soc, 60(9), 1624–1631.

Slaughter SE, Hopper T, Ickert C, Erin DF. 2014. Identification of hearing loss among residents with dementia: perceptions of health care aides. Geriatr Nurs, 35(6), 434–440.

Slaughter SE, Wagg AS, Jones CA, Schopflocher D, et al. 2015. Mobility of Vulnerable Elders Study: effect of the sit-to-stand activity on mobility, function, and quality of life. J Am Med Dir Assoc, 16(2), 138–143.

Smith TO, Hameed YA, Cross JL, Henderson C, Sahota O, Fox C. 2015. Enhanced rehabilitation and care models for adults with dementia following hip fracture surgery. Cochrane Database Syst Rev, 6, CD010569.

Solomon A, Dobranici L, Kåreholt I, Tudose C, Lăzărescu M. 2011. Comorbidity and the rate of cognitive decline in patients with Alzheimer dementia. Int J Geriatr Psychiatry, 26(12), 1244–1251.

Stevens A, Gabbay J. 1991. Needs assessment, needs assessment. Health Trends, 23, 20–23.

Szczepura A, Nelson S, Wild D. 2008. *Models for Providing Improved Care in Residential Care Homes: A Thematic Literature Review*, York: Joseph Rowntree Foundation.

Tariq A, Georgiou A, Raban M, Baysari MT, Westbrook J. 2016. Underlying risk factors for prescribing errors in long-term aged care: a qualitative study. BMJ Qual Saf, 25(9), 704–715.

Tariq A, Georgiou A, Westbrook J. 2013. Medication errors in residential aged care facilities: a distributed cognition analysis of the information exchange process. Int J Med Inform, 82(5), 299–312.

Taylor J, Barker A, Hill H, Haines TP. 2015. Improving person-centred mobility care in nursing homes: a feasibility study. Geriatr Nurs, 36(2), 98–105.

Thapa PB, Gideon P, Brockman KG, Fought RL, Ray WA. 1996. Clinical and biomechanical measures of balance as fall predictors in ambulatory nursing home residents. J Gerontol, A: Biol Sci Med Sci, 51, M239–246.

Tinetti ME, Speechley M, Ginter SF. 1988. Risk factors for falls among elderly persons living in the community. N Engl J Med, 319(26), 1701–1707.

Tolson D, Rolland Y, Katz PR, Woo J, Morley JE, Vellas B. 2013. An international survey of nursing homes. J Am Med Dir Assoc, 14(7), 459–462.

van der Maaden T, van der Steen JT, de Vet HC, Achterberg WP, et al. 2015. Development of a practice guideline for optimal symptom relief for patients with pneumonia and dementia in nursing homes using a Delphi study. Int J Geriatr Psychiatry, 30(5), 487–496.

van der Steen JT, Sampson EL, Van den Block L, Lord K, et al. 2015. Tools to assess pain or lack of comfort in dementia: a content analysis. J Pain Symptom Manage, 50(5), 659–675.e3.

Walker GM, Armstrong S, Gordon AL, Gladman J, et al. 2015. The falls in care home study: a feasibility randomized controlled trial of the use of a risk assessment and decision support tool to prevent falls in care homes. Clin Rehabil, 0269215515604672 (e-pub ahead of print).

Ward JA, Harden M, Gibson RE, Byles JE. 2010. A cluster randomised controlled trial to prevent injury due to falls in a residential aged care population. Med J Aust, 192(6), 319–322.

Wehren LE, Magaziner J. 2003. Hip fracture: risk factors and outcomes. Curr Osteoporos Rep, 1, 78–85.

Weinstein BE. 2011. Screening for otologic functional impairments in the elderly: whose job is it anyway? Audiol Res, 1, 41–48.

Williams SW, Williams CS, Zimmerman S, Sloane PD, Preisser JS, Boustani M, Reed PS. 2005. Characteristics associated with mobility limitation in long-term care residents with dementia. Gerontologist, 1(1), 62–67.

Wilson T, Holt T, Greenhalgh T. 2001. Complexity science: complexity and clinical care. BMJ,0 323(7314), 685–688.

Worden A, Challis D, Hancock G, Woods R, Orrell M. 2008. Identifying need in care homes for people with dementia: the relationship between two standard assessment tools. Aging Ment Health, 12(6), 719–728.

Wyrko Z. 2015. Frailty at the front door. Clin Med (Lond), 15(4), 377–381.

Yarnall AJ, Hayes L, Hawthorne GC, Candlish CA, Aspray TJ. 2012. Diabetes in care homes: current care standards and residents' experience. Diabet Med, 29(1), 132–135.

— Chapter 4 —

CARING WELL: MENTAL HEALTH AND WELLBEING

Learning objectives

In this chapter, you will:

» appreciate the following threats to mental health and wellbeing: delirium, agitation and aggression, anxiety and depression, and apathy

» be introduced to the relevance of awareness and insight

» be introduced to mindfulness-based cognitive therapy

» begin to understand how sleep might be disturbed by dementia and dementia care

Introduction

The WHO made a bold offer in 1948. Their definition of health is *not merely the absence of disease or infirmity but a state of complete physical, mental and social wellbeing.*[1] The Five Year Forward View on Mental Health emphasises that one in five older people living in the community and 40% of older people living in care homes are affected by depression (NHS England, 2016).

In a document from the Mental Health Foundation entitled *The Interface between Dementia and Mental Health: An Evidence Review*, mental health problems are defined as a general term covering the range of negative mental health states

---

1   See www.who.int/about/mission/en (accessed 4 Oct 2016).

including mental disorder, mental health problems meeting the criteria for psychiatric diagnosis and mental health problems which fall short of a diagnostic criteria threshold (Regan, 2016). Meanwhile, so-called 'neuropsychiatric symptoms' occur frequently in people with dementia. These symptoms, which can be divided into psychiatric symptoms (delusions, hallucinations, depressive symptoms, anxiety, euphoria) and behavioural symptoms (agitation, aggression, apathy, disinhibition), have prevalence rates of about 80% in nursing home residents with dementia (Selbaek, Engedal and Bergh, 2013).

There are six important quality statements for the mental wellbeing of older people in care homes from NICE Quality Standard 50 (published December 2013).[2]

Some key topics I intend to cover in this chapter are:

» delirium

» agitation and aggression

» anxiety and depression

» apathy

» awareness and insight

» mindfulness-based cognitive therapy

» sleep.

—— Threats to mental health and wellbeing ——

Delirium

The role of anticipatory care of the clinical features of endstage dementia in reducing hospital admission is less important. However, delirium, which often precipitates hospital admission, is generally known to be partially preventable (Young and Inouye, 2007) and requires vigilance.

Clegg and colleagues (2014) reviewed the evidence about the effectiveness of interventions for preventing delirium in older people living in long-term care. Some people with delirium become quiet and sleepy, but others become agitated and disorientated, so it can be a very distressing condition.

Delirium has been linked to quality of care (Inouye, Schlesinger and Lydon, 1999). Delirium (or an acute confusional state) is a serious illness common in older people, in which a person's thinking and perceptions may be affected. It is

---

2   Available at https://www.nice.org.uk/guidance/qs50 (accessed 28 Oct 2016).

associated with increased morbidity, mortality, functional decline, hospitalisation and significant health care costs (Leslie et al., 2008). Delirium prevalence in the care home population has been estimated to be 14% and 33% for residents with advanced dementia (Siddiqi et al., 2016). Reducing delirium is important because of the considerable distress it causes, and the poor outcomes associated with it, such as increased admissions to hospital, falls, mortality and costs to the NHS (Heaven et al., 2014). Most research on delirium has focused on hospital patients. Another high-risk group is residents of care homes for older people (Wittenberg, 2001). Preventing delirium is possible using multicomponent interventions; successful interventions in hospitals have reduced it by one-third.

However, there is little research to guide practice in care homes, where it is common because of the clustering of known risk factors (older age, frailty and dementia) (Bowman, Whistler and Ellerby, 2004). As detection of delirium depends on observing changes from usual behaviour, care home staff are best placed to make such observations (Cody, Beck and Svarstad, 2002). Individuals admitted to hospital from long-term care have higher rates of delirium (Kelly et al., 2001). In previous work a multicomponent intervention has been developed to prevent delirium in care homes, called 'Stop Delirium!' (see Figure 4.1). The intervention was based upon evidence from the research literature relating to the prevention of delirium and upon strategies to change professional practice (Siddiqi et al., 2011).

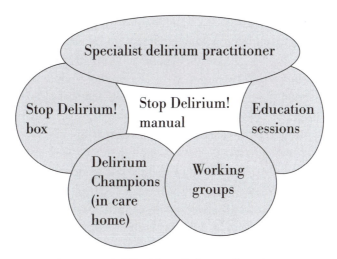

Figure 4.1: The 'Stop Delirium!' project
Source: redrawn from Heaven et al. (2014, Fig. 1, p.2).

The study intervention has been described extensively elsewhere (e.g. Siddiqi et al., 2016). It comprises a multifaceted enhanced educational package incorporating multiple strategies to change practice delivered to each care home over 16 months.

Generally, the training of staff for delirium prevention has not kept pace with the changing demands of care homes (Fitzpatrick and Roberts, 2004), and there is poorer management of medical conditions, increasing the need for unplanned hospital admissions and GP consultations (Heaven et al., 2014). Surprisingly, in the UK, there are no statutory requirements for nurses to demonstrate specialist skills to meet the health and social care needs of older people in care homes (Siddiqi et al., 2011).

Agitation and aggression

The assumption has been that there is little that professional carers can do other than control the person's behaviour with tranquillising medication or restraint. There has thankfully been a profound change in culture here. The person-centred paradigm, by contrast, sees meaning in the person's behaviour, regarding expressions of aggression, as 'poorly communicated need' (Stokes, 2000). Agitation has been defined as 'inappropriate verbal, vocal, or motor activity that is not judged by an outside observer to result directly from apparent needs or confusion of the agitated individual' (Cohen-Mansfield and Billig, 1986, p.712). In spite of a plethora of studies that have begun to increase understanding of agitation, there is no commonly accepted consensus description of this common clinical phenomenon (Laughren, 2001; Cummings et al., 2015).

Pain and agitation are common and frequently persistent in residents with dementia during nursing home stays, but symptom management intensifies only at the end of life. Symptom control may be suboptimal even from the time of assessment and admission (Hendriks et al., 2015). More severe dementia may be associated with more pain and more agitation (Zuidema et al., 2009). Optimal symptom control needs a holistic approach because symptoms may be interrelated; for example, pain may be associated with agitation (Ahn and Horgas, 2013). It is frequently said that agitation in persons with dementia is manifested in a wide variety of verbal and physical behaviours that deviate from social norms, including irrelevant vocalisations, screaming, cursing or restlessness (De Jonghe and Kat, 1996). Discomfort, definition-wise, seems to underlie the impact of several factors, such as pain, depression, sleep disturbances, restraint and social isolation, on verbal agitation (Lemay and Landreville, 2010).

In recent decades, person-centred dementia care (PCC) has been suggested as an intervention to develop quality of dementia care and further prevent or mitigate neuropsychiatric symptoms (NPS) (Rokstad et al., 2013). A main focus in PCC is the need to preserve the patient's personhood through the course of the disease and in spite of cognitive decline (Kitwood, 1997) (see Chapter 2). Using the PCC approach, the impact of the social environment is considered important for the wellbeing of the patient. The basic psychological needs for comfort, identity, occupation, attachment and inclusion need to be met in all stages of dementia. According to Dawn Brooker, PCC is the sum of the four essential elements described as the VIPS framework: Valuing people with dementia (V), Individualised care (I), understanding the world from the Patient's Perspective (P), and providing a Social environment that Supports the needs of the patient (S) – that is, PCC = V + I + P + S (Brooker and Latham, 2016).

Agitation in people living with dementia can be reduced effectively using even elementary nursing interventions, such as avoiding noise. In order to select a promising intervention, nurses need to know the individual resident's needs and skills, as well as the range of possible specific interventions (Oppikofer and Geschwindner, 2014). This fact should be recognised in daily nursing practice. Nurses who are aware of these facts have the prerequisites to recognise settings that promote agitation and to introduce the corresponding nursing intervention. Non-pharmacological interventions have been used to address the unmet needs of the agitated individual and to avoid the drawbacks of pharmacological interventions such as medication interactions and side effects. Examples of commonly reported neuropsychiatric inventories include music, physical activity, horticulture, hand massage, multi-sensory rooms and pet therapy (Janzen et al., 2013). I will return to these at various points in this book, including in Chapters 7 and 13.

The original Focused Intervention Training and Support (FITS) programme (Fossey et al., 2006) was implemented as a research intervention to enable care home staff to deliver effective person-centred care for people with dementia. A cluster randomised controlled trial revealed that, compared with usual care, the FITS programme reduced the prescribing of antipsychotics for people with dementia by over 40% (Fossey et al., 2014; Brooker et al., 2015). In addition, the implementation of psychosocial approaches to enable people living with dementia in care homes to connect with others and to have a good quality of life relies on a wide range of factors such as staff skills, job roles, tailored interventions, staff time and attitudes (Lawrence et al., 2012). Cohen-Mansfield (2016) argues that a more thoughtful paradigm is needed. Rather than examining each specific intervention, we need to develop and test algorithms that match interventions to unmet needs, personal abilities and preferences, and the environment. The whole issue of antipsychotics in care homes still causes considerable concern. For example, a recent UK study examined the long-term impact of a national policy initiative on antipsychotic prescribing in care homes, but found that prescribing rates, antipsychotic agent type (including unlicensed antipsychotics) and the length of treatment were unchanged; antipsychotic prescribing patterns in UK care homes are not open to public scrutiny or routinely reported by regulatory inspection (Szczepura et al., 2016).

It has been suggested that aggression management in residential care in the UK involves the overuse of controlling strategies such as tranquillising medication

(All Party Parliamentary Group on Dementia, 2008). Recent findings may even appear to contradict reports in the UK of the overuse of controlling strategies, such as tranquillising medication (Pulsford, Duxbury and Hadi, 2011). Staff and relative perspectives on patient aggression in dementia care units are seriously under-researched in the UK. Any work that has been conducted has relied upon quantitative studies. Qualitative research on aggression management in older people's services is rare (Duxbury et al., 2013). According to Voyer and colleagues, persons with dementia often have elevated rates of aggressive behaviours (Voyer et al., 2005). This is not surprising given that persons with cognitive impairment often have reduced tolerance levels and can be vulnerable to stimulation overload (Hall and Buckwalter, 1987).

Resident–resident physical aggression (RRA) is an interesting focus of interest in agitation in care homes. While RRA can be evidenced as a form of common assault and battery, the issue of 'intent' in this context is contentious as the presence of cognitive impairment in residents means that it is often not possible to establish whether the actions of the person exhibiting the aggression were conscious, voluntary and intended to result in harm to the target of aggression (Ferrah et al., 2015). RRA represents a collective organisational and social failure to protect and preserve the rights of vulnerable older people in nursing homes. Any form of assault leads to increased morbidity and mortality in an older person (Krug et al., 2002). Another commonly mentioned trigger was territoriality and the challenges of communal living, discussed in 75% of focus groups and by 39% of participants. Conflict may arise between residents because of competition for a preferred chair in a television lounge or dining room, for example (Rosen et al., 2008).

Dementia Care Mapping (DCM) is an observational tool that has been used in formal dementia care settings since 1992, both as an instrument for developing person-centred care practice, and as a tool in evaluative research (Brooker and Surr, 2006). DCM has been designed to be used in a series of developmental evaluations over time to help care teams identify ways in which they could improve the quality of person-centred care. Bradford University Dementia Group and Leeds University's Clinical Trials Research Unit are among a number of centres collaborating to undertake a cluster randomised controlled trial looking at enhancing person-centred care delivery to care home residents with dementia. The EPIC trial will investigate whether DCM, as an observational tool and a practice development cycle, is more effective than usual care (UC) in supporting the implementation of person-centred care in care homes.[3] The project started on 1 September 2013 and will end on 30 September 2017. The protocol states clearly that the primary objective is 'To determine if DCM plus UC (i.e. the intervention) is (i) more effective in reducing agitation as measured by the total Cohen-Mansfield Agitation Inventory (CMAI)

---

3   See www.leedsbeckett.ac.uk/pages/epic-trial (accessed 4 Oct 2016).

score, and (ii) more cost-effective than UC alone (i.e. the control), 16 months after randomisation of care homes' (p.19).[4]

Anxiety and depression

'Residential care facilities' is a broad term used to refer to congregational living settings for older adults. Conn and colleagues (2008) have reported rates of mental health disorders in older adults living in residential care facilities of between 80% and 90%, with depression being the most common (Snowdon, 2010). Anxiety and depression are common in people with dementia and mild cognitive impairment (MCI). Estimates of the prevalence of depressive symptoms in people with dementia range between 10% and 62%, with substantially lower rates when employing strict criteria for major depression (Orgeta et al., 2015). Creighton, Davison and Kissane (2015), from a total of 2249 articles, reviewed that the rate of overall anxiety disorders was found to range from 3.2% to 20%, with the highest-quality studies estimating a prevalence rate of 5% to 5.7%. Generalised anxiety disorder and specific phobias were found to be the most common anxiety disorders among aged care residents, while clinically significant anxiety symptoms were found to be more frequent (6.5% to 58.4%) than threshold disorders.

Depression is one of the most common of all chronic health problems worldwide and yet one that is consistently overlooked (WHO, 2004). In nursing homes, where prevalence rates are the highest, a number of individual and organisational factors have been associated with resident depression in US nursing homes. Rates of depression have been reported to be particularly high in older nursing home residents and, in 2009, an estimated 31% of Australian nursing home residents with dementia also had a diagnosis of depression or mood disorder recorded, while the number of residents with symptoms of depression has been reported to be as high as 41.6% (Travers, 2015). Some physical complaints from patients with depressive symptoms are medically unexplained, and correspondingly boosted costs due to the high utilisation of health services (Luo et al., 2015). Higher rates have been identified among younger residents, female residents, non-Hispanic white residents, married residents, those with higher educations, those with some impairments in daily living activities and those with better cognitive function (Cassie and Cassie, 2012).

There is currently only limited understanding of factors that are associated with late-life depression among people who have undergone the major transition of relocating to a residential facility (Davison et al., 2013). Research with older people who have not yet made the transition to care has consistently demonstrated an association between chronic physical illness and depression, with depression found to be more common among those with at least two serious physical illnesses (Osborn et al., 2003). Staff training in depression, supplemented with a protocol for routine screening and guidelines on referring residents, can improve pathways to care. However, strategies to overcome barriers to the appropriate subsequent treatment of depression are required for staff-focused initiatives to translate into better outcomes for depressed older adults (Davison et al., 2013). Results from regression analysis show that taking greater amounts of medication and living in a less independent environment were both associated with greater depression, while using alcohol was associated with less depression (Stroud, Steiner and Iwuagwu, 2008).

Treating depression in dementia is therefore a clinical priority with the potential to improve the wellbeing, quality of life and level of function of people with dementia; it might also have an effect on costs (Romeo et al., 2013). A trial by Banerjee and colleagues (2011) clearly suggested that antidepressants, given with normal care, are not clinically effective when compared with placebo for the treatment of clinically significant depression in dementia. Such an absence of efficacy of antidepressants in the dementia population raises questions about whether there are different pathogenic mechanisms at play in depression in Alzheimer's disease (Brodaty, 2011). In one recent study, although depression was prevalent in recently admitted long-term care patients, documented diagnostic initiatives were sparse after admission, and screening tools for depression which can be applied by trained nurses should be mandatory on admission (Iden et al., 2014).

The psychosocial and medical management of depressed aged care residents might be improved by increasing access to specialist mental health consultation (McSweeney et al., 2012). Support around diagnosis, person-centred care, fostering good relationships and engagement in meaningful activity are of great importance to people with dementia and those who care for them. Yet in clinical practice, people with dementia suffering from anxiety may receive no help or else be given medication due to a lack of understanding of what else might help. Developing evidence-based psychological treatments for anxiety in dementia, to improve care and quality of life, should be a priority (Qazi, Spector and Orrell, 2010). There is very little literature examining the causes of anxiety, perhaps because it tends to fluctuate and is often related to the situation. Anxiety is common in those with mild dementia, particularly those who retain insight (Shankar et al., 1999).

Apathy

Apathy can be more formally assessed and quantified using several different rating scales. Clinician-rated or carer-rated scales are usually more reliable than self-report questionnaires, because apathy is usually accompanied by a lack of insight

(Stanton and Carson, 2010). Levy and Dubois (2006) have defined apathy as an observable behavioural syndrome consisting of a quantitative reduction in self-generated voluntary and purposeful behaviours. Recent studies identified apathy as a significant and most frequently occurring symptom, particularly in nursing home residents living with dementia, with prevalence of up to 81.6% (Treusch et al., 2015). The existence of apathy has some bearing on participation in therapeutic activities for older people with dementia living in nursing homes (Ellis, Doyle and Selvarajah, 2014). Based on a sample of 90 residents, with residents participating in six activities per week, those residents who were involved in the most activities had the lowest levels of apathy.

There are some simple strategies for trying to deal with apathy in the residents of care homes (Box 4.1).

Box 4.1: Simple strategies for reducing the impact of apathy symptoms

Create a regular daily routine with more varied activities but fewer choices for the patient to make.

Open discussion and reassurance from the patients themselves that they are not distressed may be all that is required in this situation.

Use frequent prompts to remind the patient to start activities: these could be set as alarms on a mobile phone rather than always having to come verbally from a carer.

Get out of the house every day, even if only to the local shops. For patients with dementia in nursing homes, there is some evidence for interventions designed to 'increase the reward potential of the environment'.

If motor or cognitive symptoms limit participation in previous interests, think carefully about how these could be adapted with advice from an occupational therapist.

Encourage carers to take up regular respite care without guilt.

SOURCE: ADAPTED FROM STANTON AND CARSON (2016, BOX 2).

—— Awareness and insight ——

Legal and ethical issues clearly exist in the social sphere of the dementia experience, and as such are likely to have an effect on both the expression of awareness and the subjective experience of living with dementia (Woods and Pratt, 2005). One may ask why coping with dementia has rarely been the subject of systematic empirical research (in contrast to coping with other chronic diseases, such as cancer) and why the voice of people with dementia has not been adequately listened to (Dröes, 2007). Clare writes that there is a 'great deal of confusion about predictors and correlates of unawareness' (2002, p.275), and this lack of conclusive findings from the biomedical approach indicates that new and different directions must be developed so debates and research into insight may be pursued.

The term anosognosia was first introduced by Babinski in 1914 to describe subjects who denied their left hemiplegia, with the condition considered to be related to a brain lesion in the right parietal lobe (Kashiwa et al., 2005). Anosognosia is a major problem in patients affected by dementia because of its implications in various aspects of patient care, such as treatment compliance, personal safety and carer distress (Rosen, 2011). Clare (2004) argues that awareness is best understood in the context of the interaction of cognitive functioning, individual psychological responses and the influence of social context. In contrast, the unawareness of impairment is manifested in several domains, including memory and other cognitive functions as well as psychological and behavioural functions.

Poor insight has been described as a clinical feature in a number of somatic, neurological and psychiatric disorders. The concepts used for this feature vary according to context and approach. The latter may, for instance, be neuropsychological/biological, psychological or socio-psychological (Robertsson, Nordström and Wijk, 2007). Cognitive insight is defined as a patient's current capacity to evaluate his or her anomalous experiences and atypical interpretations of events. It is difficult to discriminate between cognitive and clinical insight, but it can be concluded that clinical insight constitutes only a part of cognitive insight and is invaluable for the formulation and treatment of patients (Riggs et al., 2012). Insight is, however, always partial and relative. The term suggests a discrepancy between the subject's view of reality and that of others (in the case of dementia, that of professionals and carers) (Howorth and Saper, 2003).

While the term 'insight' is widely used in everyday language and that of health professionals, Bond and colleagues (2002) suggest there is a lack of clarity within medical discourses as to what insight means; they argue that a claimed lack of insight is a judgement made by a health care professional, based within the medicalisation of dementia. In the medical approach, insight refers to the degree to which people express awareness of the nature and extent of their deficits (Sabat, 2002). Sabat (2002) created a model of insight where he identified, in addition to the organic effects of the disease, three other factors that affect a person with dementia's insight that must be taken into account in any understanding of awareness. These are: the person's reaction to the effects of the disease; the behaviour and reactions of others to it; and the reactions of the person with Alzheimer's disease to the behaviours of others in his or her social world. Lower awareness can be associated with greater carer stress and the poorer perceived quality of relationships. A lack of awareness of social functioning has important implications for relationship quality and levels of carer stress (Nelis et al., 2011).

The perception of awareness and insight provides clues about the nature of the 'self' in dementia (see Figure 4.2).

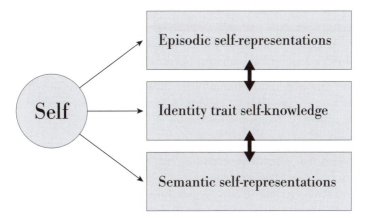

Figure 4.2: Organisation of the structural self according to the neuropsychological literature

Note: The self-structure merges three self-representation systems: episodic self-representations and semantic self-representations, grounded in episodic and semantic autobiographical memory, and identity trait self-knowledge relying on highly abstract personal conceptual memory. Source: redrawn from Duval et al. (2012, Fig. 1).

—— Mindfulness-based cognitive therapy ——

The relationship between mindfulness and wellbeing is crucially important (see Box 4.2).

A specific class of contemplative approaches may transform the way we envision dementia care. These are mindfulness-based interventions, such as mindfulness-based cognitive therapy (MBCT; Segal, Williams and Teasdale, 2012). Mindfulness involves learning to notice what is occurring in one's present moment experience, with an attitude of openness and non-judgemental acceptance (e.g. Larouche, Hudon and Goulet, 2015). Future investigations should clarify what the precise potential benefits and harms are. Arguably, evidence in mindfulness in dementia is generally weak and very preliminary so far. Expert professional advice must always be sought in this field.

Box 4.2: Mindfulness and wellbeing: the evidence

There is strong evidence linking mindfulness with a range of benefits including better concentration, greater calmness and reduced emotional reactivity, reduced stress and improved immune functioning, and better overall wellbeing and life satisfaction.

Mindfulness has been shown to improve physical as well as mental health: for example, by reducing blood pressure and helping people to manage long-term conditions including chronic pain, diabetes and cardiovascular disease.

Although the evidence base on mindfulness in schools is still relatively new, studies suggest that it can improve both children's mental health and wellbeing and their ability to pay attention, problem-solve and learn.

There may also be particular benefits for children with special needs or difficulties: one study found that mindfulness training helped adolescents with attention deficit hyperactivity disorder (ADHD) to control their symptoms; another found that it helped reduce aggressive behaviour in boys; and a third found that it led to reduced anxiety and improved academic performance among children with learning disabilities.

Finally, there is some evidence that mindfulness programmes can improve teachers' sense of wellbeing and self-efficacy, as well as their ability to manage classroom behaviour and establish and maintain supportive relationships with students.

SOURCE: REPRODUCED UNDER A CREATIVE COMMONS LICENCE FROM THE SOURCE: NEF (2014).

—— Sleep ——

Sleep is a complex phenomenon that is rooted in neurologic function. It is an active process generated and modulated by a complex set of neural systems located mainly in the hypothalamus, brainstem and thalamus. Sleep serves a restorative function in the brain and has a critical role in cognitive functions (Cipriani et al., 2015). Persons with dementia often have trouble sleeping. Disordered sleep is also prevalent in older persons (Foley et al., 2004) and has been shown to have significant cognitive, physical and psychological consequences (Misra and Malow, 2008).

Not all persons with dementia develop sleep problems. According to Guarnieri and colleagues (2012), insomnia frequency appears identical in Alzheimer's disease and persons with frontotemporal dementia but higher in vascular dementia or diffuse Lewy body dementia. However, persons with disordered sleep have a range of sleep problems which include the following: hypersomnia (e.g. sleep apnoea and narcolepsy), parasomnia (e.g. confusional arousal, night terrors, restless leg syndrome and sleep walking), insomnia (e.g. difficulty falling and/or staying asleep) and sleep–wake cycle disturbances. These symptoms all share the common outcome of non-restorative sleep (Brown et al., 2013).

Institutionalisation itself seems to be an aggravating factor, as it accelerates degradation in sleep quality even more. It seems to exacerbate the tendency towards age-related alterations, predisposing the elderly to poor sleep quality (Nóbrega et al., 2014). Changes in the amount and quality of sleep affect approximately 70% of aged institutionalised individuals when compared with community-dwelling older adults (cited in Nóbrega et al., 2014), and this occurs primarily because of a high prevalence of cognitive impairment, low level of physical activity, adjusting to daily routines with defined activity times, and a large amount of time spent indoors (Gordon and Gladman, 2010).

—— Essential reading ——

Baker C. 2014. *Developing Excellent Care for People Living with Dementia in Care Homes*, London: Jessica Kingsley Publishers.

Brooker D, Latham I. 2015. *Person-Centred Dementia Care, Second Edition: Making Services Better with the VIPS Framework*, London: Jessica Kingsley Publishers.

Rezek C. 2015. *Mindfulness for Carers: How to Manage the Demands of Caregiving While Finding a Place for Yourself*, London: Jessica Kingsley Publishers.

—— References ——

Ahn H, Horgas A. 2013. The relationship between pain and disruptive behaviors in nursing home residents with dementia. BMC Geriatr, 13, 14.

All Party Parliamentary Group on Dementia. 2008. Always a Last Resort – Inquiry into the Prescription of Antipsychotic Drugs to People with Dementia Living in Care Homes, available at www.alzheimers.org.uk/site/scripts/documents_info.php?documentID=1583&pageNumber=4 (accessed 3 Oct 2016).

Banerjee S, Hellier J, Dewey M, Romeo R, et al. 2011. Sertraline or mirtazapine for depression in dementia (HTA-SADD): a randomised, multicentre, double-blind, placebo-controlled trial. Lancet, 378(9789), 403–411.

Bond J, Corner L, Lilley A, Ellwood C. 2002. Medicalization of insight and caregivers' response to risk in dementia. Dementia: The International Journal of Social Research and Practice, 1(3), 313–328.

Bowman C, Whistler J, Ellerby M. 2004. A national census of care home residents. Age Aging, 33, 561–566.

Brodaty H. 2011. Antidepressant treatment in Alzheimer's disease. Lancet, 378(9789), 375–376.

Brooker DJ, Latham I. 2016. *Person-Centred Dementia Care: Making Services Better* (second edition), London: Jessica Kingsley Publishers.

Brooker DJ, Surr C. 2006. Dementia Care Mapping (DCM): initial validation of DCM 8 in UK field trials. Int J Geriatr Psychiatry, 21(11), 1018–1025.

Brooker DJ, Latham I, Evans SC, Jacobson N, et al. 2015. FITS into practice: translating research into practice in reducing the use of anti-psychotic medication for people with dementia living in care homes. Aging Ment Health, July, 1–10 (e-pub ahead of print).

Brown CA, Berry R, Tan MC, Khoshia A, Turlapati L, Swedlove F. 2013. A critique of the evidence base for non-pharmacological sleep interventions for persons with dementia. Dementia (London), 12(2), 210–237.

Cassie KM, Cassie WE. 2012. Organizational and individual conditions associated with depressive symptoms among nursing home residents over time. Gerontologist, 52(6), 812–821.

Cipriani G, Lucetti C, Danti S, Nuti A. 2015. Sleep disturbances and dementia. Psychogeriatrics, 15(1), 65–74.

Clare L. 2002. Editorial – awareness in dementia: new directions. Dementia: The International Journal of Social Research and Practice, 1(3), 275–278.

Clare L. 2004. The construction of awareness in early-stage Alzheimer's disease: a review of concepts and models. British Journal of Clinical Psychology, 43, 155–175.

Clegg A, Siddiqi N, Heaven A, Young J, Holt R. 2014. Interventions for preventing delirium in older people in institutional long-term care. Cochrane Database Syst Rev, 1, CD009537.

Cody M, Beck C, Svarstad BL. 2002. Challenges to the use of nonpharmacological interventions in nursing homes. PsychiatrServ, 53, 1402–1406.

Cohen-Mansfield J. 2016. Non-pharmacological interventions for agitation in dementia: various strategies demonstrate effectiveness for care home residents; further research in home settings is needed. Evid Based Nurs, 19(1), 31.

Cohen-Mansfield J, Billig N. 1986. Agitated behaviors in the elderly. I. A conceptual review. J Am Geriatr Soc, 34, 711–721.

Conn D, Gibson M, and the Canadian Coalition for Seniors' Mental Health. 2008. Guidelines for the assessment and treatment of mental health issues in LTC: Focus on mood and behaviour symptoms. Canadian Nursing Home, 19, 24–35.

Creighton AS, Davison TE, Kissane DW. 2015. The prevalence of anxiety among older adults in nursing homes and other residential aged care facilities: a systematic review. Int J Geriatr Psychiatry, doi: 10.1002/gps.4378.

Cummings J, Mintzer J, Brodaty H, Sano M, et al. 2015. Agitation in cognitive disorders: International Psychogeriatric Association provisional consensus clinical and research definition. Int Psychogeriatr, 27(1), 7–17.

Davison TE, Karantzas G, Mellor D, McCabe MP, Mrkic D. 2013. Staff-focused interventions to increase referrals for depression in aged care facilities: a cluster randomized controlled trial. Aging Ment Health, 17(4), 449–455.

De Jonghe JFM, Kat MG. 1996. Factor structure and validity of the Dutch version of the Cohen-Mansfield Agitation Inventory (CMAI-D). Journal of the American Geriatrics Society, 44(7), 888–889.

Dröes RM. 2007. Insight in coping with dementia: listening to the voice of those who suffer from it. Aging Ment Health, 11(2), 115–118.

Dröes RM, van Mierlo LD, van der Roest HG, Meiland FJM. 2010. Focus and effectiveness of psychosocial interventions for people with dementia in institutional or care settings from the perspective of coping with the disease. Non-Pharmacological Therapies in Dementia, 1(2), 139–161.

Duval C, Desgranges B, de La Sayette V, Belliard S, Eustache F, Piolino P. 2012. What happens to personal identity when semantic knowledge degrades? A study of the self and autobiographical memory in semantic dementia. Neuropsychologia, 50(2), 254–265.

Duxbury J, Pulsford D, Hadi M, Sykes S. 2013. Staff and relatives' perspectives on the aggressive behaviour of older people with dementia in residential care: a qualitative study. J Psychiatr Ment Health Nurs, 20(9), 792–800.

Ellis JM, Doyle CJ, Selvarajah S. 2014. The relationship between apathy and participation in therapeutic activities in nursing home residents with dementia: evidence for an association and directions for further research. Dementia (London), March (e-pub ahead of print).

Ferrah N, Murphy BJ, Ibrahim JE, Bugeja LC, et al. 2015. Resident-to-resident physical aggression leading to injury in nursing homes: a systematic review. Age Ageing, 44(3), 356–364.

Fitzpatrick JM, Roberts JD. 2004. Challenges for care homes: education and training of health care assistants. Br J Nurs, 13, 1258–1261.

Foley D, Ancoli-Israel S, Britz P, Walsh J. 2004. Sleep disturbances and chronic disease in older adults: results of the 2003 National Sleep Foundation Sleep in America Survey. J Psychosom Res, 56(5), 497–502.

Fossey J, Ballard C, Juszczak E, James I, Alder N, Jacoby R, Howard R. 2006. Effect of enhanced psychosocial care on antipsychotic use in nursing home residents with severe dementia: A cluster randomised trial. British Medical Journal, 332(7544), 756–758.

Fossey J, Masson S, Stafford J, Lawrence V, Corbett A, Ballard C. 2014. The disconnect between evidence and practice: A systematic review of person-centred interventions and training manuals for care home staff working with people with dementia. International Journal of Geriatric Psychiatry, 29(8), 797–807.

Gordon AL, Gladman JRF. 2010. Sleep in care homes. Rev Clin Gerontol, 20, 309–316.

Guarnieri B, Adorni F, Musicco M, Appollonio I, et al. 2012. Prevalence of sleep disturbances in mild cognitive impairment and dementing disorders: a multicenter Italian clinical cross-sectional study on 431 patients. Dement Geriatr Cogn Disord, 33, 50–58.

Hall G, Buckwalter K. 1987. Progressively lowered stress threshold: a conceptual model for care of adults with Alzheimer's disease. Archives of Psychiatric Nursing, 1, 339–406.

Heaven A, Cheater F, Clegg A, Collinson M, et al. 2014. Pilot trial of Stop Delirium! (PiTStop) – a complex intervention to prevent delirium in care homes for older people: study protocol for a cluster randomised controlled trial. Trials, 15, 47.

Hendriks SA, Smalbrugge M, Galindo-Garre F, Hertogh CM, van der Steen JT. 2015. From admission to death: prevalence and course of pain, agitation, and shortness of breath, and treatment of these symptoms in nursing home residents with dementia. J Am Med Dir Assoc, 16(6), 475–481.

Howorth P, Saper J. 2003. The dimensions of insight in people with dementia. Aging Ment Health, 7(2), 113–122.

Iden KR, Engedal K, Hjorleifsson S, Ruths S. 2014. Prevalence of depression among recently admitted long-term care patients in Norwegian nursing homes: associations with diagnostic workup and use of antidepressants. Dement Geriatr Cogn Disord, 37(3–4), 154–162.

Inouye SK, Schlesinger MJ, Lydon TJ. 1999. Delirium: a symptom of how hospital care is failing older persons and a window to improve quality of hospital care. Am J Med, 106, 565–573.

Janzen S, Zecevic AA, Kloseck M, Orange JB. 2013. Managing agitation using nonpharmacological interventions for seniors with dementia. Am J Alzheimers Dis Other Demen, 28(5), 524–532.

Kashiwa Y, Kitabayashi Y, Narumoto J, Nakamura K, Ueda H, Fukui K. 2005. Anosognosia in Alzheimer's disease: association with patient characteristics, psychiatric symptoms and cognitive deficits. Psychiatry Clin Neurosci, 59(6), 697–704.

Kelly KG, Zisselman M, Cutillo-Schmitter T, Reichard R, Payne D, Denman SJ. 2001. Severity and course of delirium in medically hospitalized nursing facility residents. J Am Geriatr Psychiatr, 9, 72–77.

Kitwood T. 1997. *Dementia Reconsidered: The Person Comes First*, Buckingham, Open University Press.

Krug EG, Mercy JA, Dahlberg LL, Zwi AB. 2002. The world report on violence and health. Lancet, 360(9339), 1083–1088.

Larouche E, Hudon C, Goulet S. 2015. Potential benefits of mindfulness-based interventions in mild cognitive impairment and Alzheimer's disease: an interdisciplinary perspective. Behav Brain Res, 276, 199–212.

Laughren T. 2001. A regulatory perspective on psychiatric syndromes in Alzheimer's disease. American Journal of Geriatric Psychiatry, 9, 340–345.

Lawrence V, Fossey J, Ballard C, Moniz-Cook E, Murray J. 2012. Making psychosocial interventions work: improving quality of life for people with dementia in care homes. British Journal of Psychiatry, 201, 344–351.

Lemay M, Landreville P. 2010. Review. Verbal agitation in dementia: the role of discomfort. Am J Alzheimers Dis Other Demen, 25(3), 193–201.

Leslie DL, Marcantonio ER, Zhang Y, Leo-Summers L, Inouye SK. 2008. One-year health care costs associated with delirium in the elderly population. Arch Intern Med, 168, 27–32.

Levy R, Dubois B. 2006. Apathy and the functional anatomy of the prefrontal cortex-basal ganglia circuits. Cereb Cortex, 16, 916–928.

Luo H, Tang JY, Wong GH, Chen CC, et al. 2015. The effect of depressive symptoms and antidepressant use on subsequent physical decline and number of hospitalizations in nursing home residents: a 9-year longitudinal study. J Am Med Dir Assoc, 16(12), 1048–1054.

McSweeney K, Jeffreys A, Griffith J, Plakiotis C, Kharsas R, O'Connor DW. 2012. Specialist mental health consultation for depression in Australian aged care residents with dementia: a cluster randomized trial. Int J Geriatr Psychiatry, 27(11), 1163–1171.

Misra S, Malow BA. 2008. Evaluation of sleep disturbances in older adults. Clin Geriatr Med, 24(1), 15–26, v.

NEF. 2014. Wellbeing in Four Policy Areas – Report by the All-Party Parliamentary Group on Wellbeing Economics, September.

Nelis SM, Clare L, Martyr A, Markova I, et al. 2011. Awareness of social and emotional functioning in people with early-stage dementia and implications for carers. Aging Ment Health, 15(8), 961–969.

NHS England. 2016. *The Five Year Forward View for Mental Health: A Report from the Independent Mental Health Taskforce to the NHS in England*, London: NHS England.

Nóbrega PV, Maciel AC, de Almeida Holanda CM, Oliveira Guerra R, Araújo JF. 2014. Sleep and frailty syndrome in elderly residents of long-stay institutions: a cross-sectional study. Geriatr Gerontol, 14(3), 605–612.

Oppikofer S, Geschwindner H. 2014. Nursing interventions in cases of agitation and dementia. Dementia (London), 13(3), 306–317.

Orgeta V, Qazi A, Spector A, Orrell M. 2015. Psychological treatments for depression and anxiety in dementia and mild cognitive impairment: systematic review and meta-analysis. Br J Psychiatry, 207(4), 293–298.

Osborn DP, Fletcher AE, Smeeth L, Stirling S, et al. 2003. Factors associated with depression in a representative sample of 14217 people aged 75 and over in the United Kingdom: results from the MRC trial of assessment and management of older people in the community. Int J Geriatr Psychiatry, 18(7), 623–630.

Pulsford D, Duxbury JA, Hadi M. 2011. A survey of staff attitudes and responses to people with dementia who are aggressive in residential care settings. J Psychiatr Ment Health Nurs, 18(2), 97–104.

Qazi A, Spector A, Orrell M. 2010. User, carer and staff perspectives on anxiety in dementia: a qualitative study. J Affect Disord, 125(1–3), 295–300.

Regan M. 2016. *The Interface between Dementia and Mental Health: An Evidence Review*, London: Mental Health Foundation.

Riggs SE, Grant PM, Perivoliotis D, Beck AT. 2012. Assessment of cognitive insight: a qualitative review. Schizophr Bull, 38(2), 338–350.

Robertsson B, Nordström M, Wijk H. 2007. Investigating poor insight in Alzheimer's disease: a survey of research approaches. Dementia, 6(1), 45–61.

Rokstad AM, Røsvik J, Kirkevold Ø, Selbaek G, Saltyte Benth J, Engedal K. 2013. The effect of person-centred dementia care to prevent agitation and other neuropsychiatric symptoms and enhance quality of life in nursing home patients: a 10-month randomized controlled trial. Dement Geriatr Cogn Disord, 36(5–6), 340–353.

Romeo R, Knapp M, Hellier J, Dewey M, et al. 2013. Cost effectiveness analyses for mirtazapine and sertraline in dementia: randomised controlled trial. Br J Psychiatry, 202, 121–128.

Rosen HJ. 2011. Anosognosia in neurodegenerative disease. Neurocase, 17, 231.

Rosen T, Lachs MS, Bharucha AJ, Stevens SM, et al. 2008. Resident-to resident aggression in long-term care facilities: insights from focus groups of nursing home residents and staff. J Am Geriatr Soc, 56(8), 1398–1408.

Sabat S. 2002. Epistemological issues in the study of insight in people with Alzheimer's disease. Dementia: The International Journal of Social Research and Practice, 1(3), 279–293.

Segal ZV, Williams JMG, Teasdale JD. 2012. *Mindfulness-Based Cognitive Therapy for Depression*, New York: Guilford Press.

Selbaek G, Engedal K, Bergh S. 2013. The prevalence and course of neuropsychiatric symptoms in nursing home patients with dementia: a systematic review. J Am Med Dir Assoc, 14, 161–169.

Shankar KK, Walker M, Frost D, Orrell MW. 1999. The development of a valid and reliable scale for rating anxiety in dementia (RAID). Ageing and Mental Health, 3(1), 39–49.

Siddiqi N, Cheater F, Collinson M, Farrin A, et al. 2016. The PiTSTOP study: a feasibility cluster randomized trial of delirium prevention in care homes for older people. Age Ageing, May, afw091 (e-pub ahead of print).

Siddiqi N, Young J, House AO, Featherstone I, et al. 2011. Stop Delirium! A complex intervention to prevent delirium in care homes: a mixed-methods feasibility study. Age Ageing, 40, 90–98.

Snowdon J. 2010. Review: depression in nursing homes. International Psychogeriatrics, 22, 1143–1148.

Stanton BR, Carson A. 2016. Apathy: a practical guide for neurologists. Pract Neurol, 16(1), 42–47.

Stokes G. 2000. *Challenging Behaviour in Dementia*. London: Speechmark Publications.

Stroud JM, Steiner V, Iwuagwu C. 2008. Predictors of depression among older adults with dementia. Dementia, 7(1), 127–138.

Szczepura A, Wild D, Khan AJ, Owen DW, et al. 2016. Antipsychotic prescribing in care homes before and after launch of a national dementia strategy: an observational study in English institutions over a 4-year period. BMJ Open, 6(9), e009882.

Travers C. 2015. Increasing enjoyable activities to treat depression in nursing home residents with dementia: a pilot study. Dementia (London), May, 1471301215586069 (e-pub ahead of print).

Treusch Y, Majic T, Page J, Gutzmann H, Heinz A, Rapp MA. 2015. Apathy in nursing home residents with dementia: results from a cluster-randomized controlled trial. Eur Psychiatry, 30(2), 251–257.

Voyer P, Verault R, Azizah GM, Desrosiers J, Champoux N, Bedard A. 2005. Prevalence of physical and verbal aggressive behaviours and associated factors among older adults in long-term care facilities. BMC Geriatrics, 5, 13.

WHO. 2004. *The Global Burden of Disease: 2004 Update*, Geneva: WHO, available at www.who.int/healthinfo/global_burden_disease/GBD_report_2004update_full.pdf (accessed 3 Oct 2016).

Wittenberg R. 2001. Demand for long-term care for older people in England to 2031. National Statistics Quarterly, 12, 5–16.

Woods B, Pratt R. 2005. Awareness in dementia: ethical and legal issues in relation to people with dementia. Aging Ment Health, 9(5), 423–429.

Young J, Inouye S. 2007. Delirium in older people. BMJ, 334, 842–846.

Zuidema SU, de Jonghe JF, Verhey FR, Koopmans RT. 2009. Predictors of neuropsychiatric symptoms in nursing home patients: influence of gender and dementia severity. Int J Geriatr Psychiatry, 24, 1079–1086.

— Chapter 5 ————————————————————————————

COGNITIVE APPROACHES AND LIFE STORY

Learning objectives ————————————————————————

In this chapter, you will:

» understand the growing importance of social prescribing

» be able to understand and evaluate critically the evidence for cognitive training, cognitive stimulation therapy, reality orientation, multi-sensory stimulation, cognitive neurorehabilitation and reminiscence therapy

» be given a very brief introduction to validation therapy

» be introduced to the controversial areas of 'therapeutic lying' and 'covert medication'

» understand the importance of life story work and its relevance to supporting effective communication

——— Introduction ————————————————————————

Cognitive health is a fundamental determinant of independent living and successful ageing (WHO, 2002), and an urgent societal challenge considering the higher risk of cognitive decline and dementia with ageing (Sachs et al., 2011; WHO, 2012; Prince et al., 2013). It is likely that if a group of people were asked to define cognition, they would provide a variety of answers. However, at their heart, most definitions would be likely to focus on attending to, processing and responding to information.

Cognitive approaches can be usefully conceptualised as follows (Aguirre et al., 2013):

» **cognitive stimulation** as engagement in a range of activities and discussions (usually in a group) aimed at general enhancement of cognitive and social functioning

» **cognitive training** as guided practice on a set of standard tasks designed to reflect particular cognitive functions with a range of difficulty levels to suit the individual's level of ability

» **cognitive rehabilitation** as an individualised approach where personally relevant goals are identified, and the therapist works with the person and their family to devise strategies to address these.

In the early stages of Alzheimer's disease, declarative memory is affected the most, while instrumental functions such as language, gnoses, praxies and visuospatial abilities are affected later on, followed by executive functions (Bouchard and Rossor, 1996). Institutionalisation is associated with an impoverished environment, as well as reduced sensorimotor and cognitive stimulation, social interactions and physical activity which contribute to a sedentary lifestyle (De Oliveira et al., 2014).

The current limits of the effectiveness of pharmacotherapies highlight the value and the significant role of non-pharmacological interventions in delaying the progression of the disease and the functional decline (Mapelli et al., 2013).

Famously, it was said about a decade ago: 'Psychosocial interventions are emerging as potentially important therapies for primary care, partly to fill a therapy "vacuum" and partly because the evidence base for their effectiveness is growing' (Iliffe, Wilcock and Haworth, 2006, p.327).

Psychosocial treatment can be described as the aid or care that is offered to reduce or prevent the mental and behavioural problems that occur in the process of adaptation to the consequences of dementia; in other words, offering assistance in coping with the various consequences of dementia (Dröes et al., 2011).

Several data suggest that physical activity and cognitive stimulation have a positive effect on the quality of life (QoL) of people with Alzheimer's disease, slowing the decline due to the disease (Maci et al., 2012). Urie Bronfenbrenner described these respectively as the **exosystem**, **microsystem** and **mesosystem**. He also outlined a **macrosystem**, which for gerontological dementia care relates to the contributions of epidemiological trends in ageing and the sociopolitical ideologies that underpin policies and attitudes (Bronfenbrenner, 2004). Cognition-focused interventions are interventions that directly or indirectly target cognitive functioning, as opposed to interventions that focus primarily on behavioural (e.g. wandering), emotional (e.g. anxiety) or physical (e.g. sedentary lifestyle) function (Bahar-Fuchs, Clare and Woods, 2013). Considering the millions of people worldwide with Alzheimer's disease and the corresponding societal costs in terms of management and care, there is a significant lack of funding for the systematic research of non-pharmacological therapy (Olazarán et al., 2010). It is necessary to factor in the vast majority of this research that is most apt for the cognitive features of Alzheimer's disease, rather than other common dementias – this bias will need addressing at some stage.

Taking further perspectives in care and treatment is illustrated in Figure 5.1.

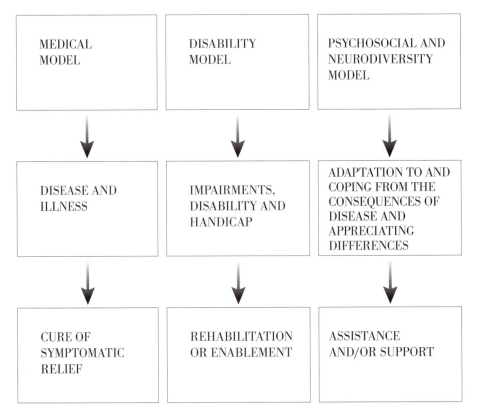

Figure 5.1: Taking further perspectives in care and treatment
Source: adapted from Dröes et al. (2010, Fig. 2).

Psychological treatments for dementia, such as reality orientation, have been in use for nearly half a century (Taulbee and Folsom, 1966). The term **psychosocial** implies human interactive behaviour (Bates, Boote and Beverley, 2004), and a definition of such intervention therefore fits well within the notion of 'shared partnerships of care' (Harris and Keady, 2006). A recent review of qualitative research focused on psychosocial interventions delivered in residential settings for people with dementia (Lawrence et al., 2012). It found that beneficial interventions enabled people with dementia to connect with others, make a meaningful contribution and reminisce. Successful implementation of the approach depended on factors such as the engagement of staff and family, flexibility, the provision of individualised care and the allocation of sufficient staff time. (The reader at this point is strongly advised to consult the excellent contribution from the British Psychological Society: *A Guide to Psychosocial Interventions in Early Stages of Dementia* – see 'Essential reading' at the end of this chapter.)

Social prescribing

To make sense of how these tools can be placed in an overall care pathway, it is worth noting that the infrastructure for delivering them would benefit from their harmonisation across different care settings – an 'interoperability' of sorts.

Social prescribing has been defined as:

> …options that make available new life opportunities that can add meaning, form new relationships, or give the patient a chance to take responsibility or be creative. Usually these services need to be available locally and often within the voluntary, community, and social enterprise sector ('third sector')… (Brandling and House, 2009, p.454)

Continuing to medicalise society's problems is unsustainable. Cross-sector collaboration has been promoted by government policies in the United Kingdom and many Western welfare states for decades. Literature on joint working has focused predominantly on the strategic level, neglecting the role of individual practitioners in putting 'joined-up working' into practice (White, Cornish and Kerr, 2015).

There is a genuine feeling that there are unmet needs because of policy: 'On the face of it, empowering our communities to attend to some of our more intransigent health problems seems to be an obvious approach and is in line with stated government policy, including joint projects between health and social care' (Brandling and House, 2009, p.455).

Cognitive training

The Cochrane review of 11 randomised controlled trials (RCTs) was unable to find a positive effect of cognitive training in patients with dementia (Bahar-Fuchs et al., 2013). Cognitive training typically involves guided practice on a set of standardised tasks designed to reflect particular cognitive functions, such as memory, attention or problem solving. There has been huge interest in cognitive reserve and brain training as preventive or remediating factors for cognitive decline (Valenzuela and Sachdev, 2009). Cognitive training is designed to improve performance within specific domains such as short-term memory or attention using well-designed cognitive tasks (Clare et al., 2004). Tasks may be presented in paper-and-pencil or computerised form or may involve analogues of activities of daily living (e.g. Heiss et al., 1993).

Surprisingly little attention has been devoted to quantifying the cognitive benefits of the interaction of individuals with their geographical environment in everyday activities (Wu, Prina and Brayne, 2015), arguably the most pervasive and complex form of cognitive training or stimulation (Cassarino and Setti, 2015). Furthermore, the various methodological aspects of the various studies carried out so far are not entirely exempt from criticism (the absence of or low-quality RCTs, poorly specified interventions, the absence of a theoretical model) (Clare et al., 2003). One assumption underlying cognitive training is that practice has the potential to improve or at least maintain functioning in the given domain. An additional assumption is that any effects of practice will generalise beyond the immediate training context, although this latter assumption has not often been supported by evidence (Papp, Walsh and Snyder, 2009). Techniques usually associated with cognitive training such as the repeated exercising of standardised cognitive tests of increasing difficulty, targeting specific cognitive domains, tend to reflect restorative principles and 'thrive on the lure of neuroplasticity' (Rabipour and Raz, 2012, p.2). Evidence in support of this comes from a functional magnetic resonance imaging (fMRI) study that reported increased memory-related brain activation following cognitive training in several brain regions of individuals at high risk of dementia due to mild cognitive impairment (Belleville et al., 2011).

—— Cognitive stimulation ——————————————

An introduction

The central assumption underlying cognitive stimulation is that a lack of cognitive stimulation can increase the decline in both normal ageing and dementia (Salthouse, 2006). Support for this assumption comes from increasing evidence that activation of neurons may enhance neuronal function and survival, though possibly in a limited way (Swaab et al., 1998), often couched in the meme *use it or lose it*. The development of cognitive interventions designed to slow the progression of dementia and improve the behaviour/quality of life of those with the condition is not new (Malec and Basford, 1996; Basford and Malec, 2015).

In 1999, in response to this need, INTERDEM (Early and Timely INTERventions in DEMentia), the European network of dementia care researchers, was established (Moniz-Cook et al., 2008, 2011). Its mission was to move forward from the seemingly lacklustre and often fragmented research studies, by supporting a critical mass of expertise and developing high-quality pan-European research in timely interventions in dementia care from early recognition to end-of-life care. The new generation of psychosocial interventions for dementia has been characterised by great improvements in methodology and high-quality randomised controlled trials, including cost-effectiveness analyses (Orrell, Woods and Spector, 2012).

Cognitive stimulation therapy

Cognitive stimulation therapy (CST) is an evidence-based intervention for people with mild-to-moderate dementia, involving themed activities to stimulate cognitive function. It is both effective and cost-effective when delivered biweekly over seven weeks (Woods et al., 2012). Following Breuil and colleagues (1994), the term 'cognitive stimulation' is now widely used to describe approaches, including 'reality orientation', which have a general cognitive focus. This builds on the positive aspects of reality orientation, while ensuring that it is implemented in a coherent, person-centred and sensitive manner (Spector et al., 2001; Woods, 2002).

Clare and Woods (2004) have provided a definition which stated that cognitive stimulation:

» targets cognitive and/or social function

» has a social element – usually in a group or with a family carer

» includes cognitive activities which do not primarily consist of practice on specific cognitive modalities

» may be described as reality orientation sessions or classes.

Quality of life is now seen as a key outcome in many aspects of dementia care. As reported by Woods and colleagues (2006), 201 people with dementia living in residential homes or attending day centres participated in a study using the Quality of Life–Alzheimer's Disease (QOL-AD) scale and a range of measures of cognition, dementia level, mood, dependency and communication. This was to assess the effect of the intervention programme of CST. Their results suggested that, while QoL in dementia appears to be independent of the level of cognitive function, interventions aimed at improving cognitive function can, nonetheless, have a direct effect on QoL.

Although the cognitive benefits of CST have now been well established, the mechanisms of change remain unclear (Spector et al., 2006). It is thought to provide an optimum learning environment, with the continuity and consistency between sessions supporting the formation of memories. Key principles include using implicit learning rather than explicit teaching, and a focus on opinion rather than facts (Spector, Gardner and Orrell, 2011). Different types of interventions for people with dementia may be more or less effective depending on the nature of the relationship between the carer and the care recipient. It may be that a cognitive-based intervention delivered by a family carer such as individualised CST may be of greater success in positively influencing both partners (Orrell, Woods and Spector, 2012).

Family carers are also affected due to the practical impact of memory problems on everyday life and the strain and frustration that can result (Zarit and Edwards, 1996). In a pilot study, Moniz-Cook and colleagues (1998) found that a home-based memory management programme involving the family carer led to improvements in memory in the person with dementia, improvements in carer wellbeing and a reduction in care home admissions at 18 months' follow-up. Future studies need to further explore and compare the effects that CST might bring to family carers of people with dementia attending the intervention (Aguirre et al., 2014).

While CST groups are being integrated into NHS services nationally, and further research is underway into the implementation and maintenance of CST in practice, for those unable to participate in groups due to local service constraints, personal preferences or health or mobility issues, an individualised carer-led version of CST would arguably be beneficial (Yates et al., 2015). It is increasing in popularity in the UK and worldwide, and a number of research teams have examined its effectiveness in other contexts and cultures. However, it is necessary to develop clear evidence-based guidelines for cultural modification of the intervention, and to consider what the options are for CST being fruitfully applied to dementias other than Alzheimer's disease.

Reality orientation

One of the first established non-pharmacological interventions for dementia that focused on improvement of cognitive abilities was reality orientation (Taulbee and Folsom, 1966). It involves presenting the patient with continuous memory and orientation information related to personal issues and the patient's environment.

Numerous ways of implementing reality orientation have been described (Spector, Orrell and Woods, 2010). For example, it has included, among other interventions, classroom sessions, normally held daily for 30 minutes, where a small group of participants was presented with basic personal and current information and a variety of materials, such as individual calendars, word games, building blocks and large-piece puzzles (Aguirre et al., 2013). These sessions also provide practical help with memory management and activities of daily living (Clare et al., 2004). Encouraging the patient to engage socially, especially when this is based on his or her personal interests, is also a very important part of the therapy (Spector et al., 2000).

Reality orientation is a means to alleviate potential distress, and is achieved by orientating the person living with dementia to their current place, date and time. It can be achieved directly through communication between health care providers and people living with dementia. Arguably, more subtle reality orientation approaches are also as effective, for example, with adaptations to a care environment, such as prominently displaying clocks or calendars throughout a unit.

There are some genuine methodological concerns. Unlike with drug trials, in reality orientation and skills training interventions (both psychological interventions) it is arguably impossible to completely blind patients and staff to treatment (Carrion et al., 2013).

Validation therapy

Validation therapy is described by Naomi Feil (1993), and has been a popular approach in dementia care. It centres on the idea of acceptance of another's reality and is about providing a high level of empathy as care partners and health care professionals to understand a person's entire frame of reference. A Cochrane review entitled 'Validation Therapy for Dementia' reviewed the evidence in 2000 and concluded that the analysis of the data at that stage failed to reveal statistically significant results, although there were trends towards favouring validation therapy for some outcomes (Neal and Briggs, 2000).

The senses

Multi-sensory stimulation

Multi-sensory stimulation interventions may well be operating through their effects on the senses, whether smell, sight, hearing or touch, or a combination of many in multi-sensory stimulation (Behrman, Chouliaras and Ebmeier, 2014). Multi-sensory stimulation, previously known as *Snoezelen*, is a therapy developed in the field of leisure facilities for people with learning difficulties (Hulsegge and Verheul, 1987). The technique involves the stimulation of multiple senses by the patient's exploration of an environment including light effects, calming sounds, smells and tactile stimulation.

It is worth emphasising that sensory interventions may not only be part of a specific therapy but may have a role in orientating people with dementia and minimising distress from confusion. Overall, good practice in caring for patients with dementia includes furnishing them with appropriate sensory aids (glasses, hearing aid) and maintaining orientation with appropriate lighting for the time of day, along with prominent windows, clocks and calendars. A Cochrane review of four studies found insufficient evidence to make any recommendations (Chung et al., 2002). Kovach suggests that older adults with dementia experience an imbalance of sensory input due to prolonged periods of a lack of stimuli or sensory deprivation, and other periods of high stimulus (i.e. in a large, noisy communal room). She proposes that this imbalance (or lack of sensoristasis) leads to discomfort which presents itself as agitation and decline in social and cognitive function (Kovach, 2000).

Specific senses

Light therapy has been proposed as a strategy for maintaining stable circadian rhythms by stimulating the suprachiasmatic nucleus. This has been attempted by increasing ambient light in care facilities (Barrick et al., 2010).

Hearing loss has an impact on the quality of life in older adults, and in particular it is associated with a significant impairment of measures of activities of daily living (Dalton et al., 2003). NICE currently recommends the use of aromatherapy for the behavioural and psychological symptoms of dementia (NICE, 2012), although it has been pointed out that, as olfaction tends to decline in dementia, this may not be an appropriate intervention (Vance, 2003).

It is worth noting, however, that the current main NICE guidance on dementia was under revision at the time of preparation of this book.

—— Cognitive neurorehabilitation ——

To sustain quality of life, timely intervention and support for people with dementia are an internationally emphasised priority given the expansive global prevalence (WHO, 2002, 2012; Prince et al., 2013). It has been suggested that cognitive rehabilitation (CR) provides a useful overarching conceptual framework for the care and support of people with dementia and for the design of interventions to meet their needs (Cohen and Eisdorfer, 1986). Given rather conflicting evidence, Yamagami and colleagues (2012) have suggested that the principles of intervention are much more important than each technique of intervention because intersubjectivity between participants and therapists/care staff has a much greater influence than each technique used. Aiming to reduce functional disability and increase wellbeing is likely to be a more realistic and helpful goal than aiming to reduce underlying impairment; evaluations of outcome need to be consistent with this goal, and the measures used must be such as to offer the chance of demonstrating that the goal has been met (Clare and Woods, 2004).

Both cognitive training and rehabilitation may be accompanied by psychoeducational activities aimed at facilitating an understanding of cognitive strengths and difficulties and by supportive discussion relating to individual emotional reactions or other needs (Bahar-Fuchs et al., 2013). CR, on the other hand, helps the patient regain specific skills for practical activities such as food preparation and shopping to maintain independence. The aims of CR for the person with dementia include optimising functioning and wellbeing, minimising the risk of excess disability, and preventing the development of a 'malignant social psychology' (Kitwood, 1997) within the person's family system and social environment. (I will return to malignant positioning in a different context in Chapter 14.)

The purpose of cognitive rehabilitation is 'to enable clients or patients, and their families, to live with, manage, by-pass, reduce or come to terms with cognitive deficits precipitated by injury to the brain' (Wilson, 1989, p.117). The emphasis is not on enhancing performance on cognitive tasks as such but on improving functioning in the everyday context. Defining rehabilitation as 'a process of active change' aimed at enabling people who are disabled by injury or disease to 'achieve an optimal level of physical, psychological, and social function' (McLellan, 1991, p.785) implies a focus on maximising functioning across a whole range of areas including physical health, psychological wellbeing, living skills and social relationships.

Although the concept continues to evolve, cognitive rehabilitation generally now refers to an individualised approach to helping people with cognitive impairments, by which those affected, and their families, work together with health care professionals to identify personally relevant goals and devise strategies for addressing these (Wilson, 2002).

In their formulation of the goal-oriented cognitive rehabilitation in early-stage dementia (GREAT) study protocol for a multi-centre, single-blind, randomised controlled trial, Linda Clare and colleagues (2013) argue that central to the practice of rehabilitation is the identification of realistic and personally meaningful individual rehabilitation goals for each client and the development of tailored interventions to address these. Goal-based approaches have been applied in numerous conditions, including brain injury, stroke, neurological illness, physical disability and chronic pain, as well as for frail, older people.

More recent views of rehabilitation include a deeper appreciation of the complex interplay between disease and the ability to function. A disability may persist even once the disease that triggered it has been eliminated, and equally, disability can be reduced in the face of permanent injury or even chronic disease (Koehler, Wilhelm and Shoulson, 2011). Participants are taught restorative techniques to build on residual abilities to help learning, such as errorless learning (Clare and Jones, 2008), spaced retrieval (Dröes et al., 2011) and verbal labelling (Miyahara, 2003). There is an emphasis on compensatory approaches by using strategies and aids. The programme may also include psychoeducation and supportive discussion related to the needs of participants (Bahar-Fuchs et al., 2013), including families (Tardif and Simard, 2011). Traditionally, cognitive rehabilitation has been offered individually, allowing each person living with cognitive impairment to receive full attention and individualised treatment from a therapist (Moebs et al., 2015). (This is worth bearing in mind in discussions of community-based rehabilitation – see Chapter 13.)

—— Reminiscence therapy ——————————————

Reminiscence therapy (RT) has the potential to benefit individuals with dementia as well as family carers, and to improve staff care.

Box 5.1 provides some cues for managers on how they might use reminiscence therapy to best effect.

Box 5.1: Reminiscence and staff development

First, communication and coordination of care is key.

Second, even though a person lacks capacity to make decisions regarding care planning, the person remains an individual with specific values and wishes. As far as is possible, these need to be respected. It is important for all those working with people with dementia to work towards enabling them to be as involved in their care as much as possible.

Third, planning in advance ensures that, as and when the person deteriorates, everybody knows what is happening. Partnership working is imperative. For example, older people who live in extra care housing have the full legal rights of occupation associated with being tenants or homeowners, in combination with access to 24-hour on-site care, which is delivered flexibly according to a person's changing needs.

Finally, people with dementia can have an extended period of time when they are receiving end-of-life care. People with advanced dementia may not necessarily be able to articulate clearly their thoughts, fears and anxieties. However, by acknowledging and validating a person's feelings behind the words or behaviours, carers can help a person with dementia feel safe and secure.

SOURCE: BASED ON SKILLS FOR CARE (2013, PP.13–15).

The therapeutic purposes of RT for people with dementia include reducing social isolation, offering an enjoyable and stimulating activity, promoting self-worth and providing a way to sustain relationships with loved ones (Gibson, 2004). Although reminiscence often involves pleasant memories to promote enjoyment, it can also involve serious or sad memories for therapeutic or cathartic purposes (Parker, 2006). Reminiscence is an activity which involves remembering and retelling past memories and events from one's life, often aided by looking at materials from a particular time. It is more general than, and different from, life story work and life review therapy (British Psychological Society, 2014).

Reminiscence therapy has been popular and widely used across Europe for a number of years, promoting communication and wellbeing for people with dementia through stimulating earlier memories which are often intact. It consists of recollections and discussions of past events in one's life with the aid of materials that invoke memories, and it is classified into two methods: the individual reminiscence and group reminiscence approaches (Wang, 2007). This encourages social inclusion, increased levels of wellbeing, pleasure and cognitive stimulation (Woods et al., 2005). Reminiscence is the process of recalling personal events or experiences from one's past that are memorable to the person (Lin, Dai and Hwang, 2003). Interest in reminiscence has been further stimulated by Erikson's lifespan developmental theory where the last psychosocial task of life, being the achievement of 'integrity', is described as 'the acceptance of one's one and only life cycle as something that has to be and that, by necessity, permitted of no substitutions' (Erikson, 1963, in Coleman, 2005, p.260).

A Cochrane systematic review of reminiscence therapy in dementia showed that there was some evidence of an improvement in cognition and mood in people with dementia, as well as a decrease in carer strain (Woods et al., 2005). However, the four studies included in that review were small in scale and incorporated diverse forms of reminiscence, resulting in inconclusive and limited evidence on their overall effectiveness (O'Shea et al., 2014). To advance dementia care within nursing homes, there is an urgent need to develop evidence-based psychosocial interventions and equip nursing home teams with the knowledge and skills to implement and make informed decisions about approaches to intervention delivery (Van Bogaert et al., 2013).

Cognitive behavioural therapy, counselling and psychotherapy

Cognitive behavioural therapy (CBT) is a term used to describe a number of talking therapies which are used to overcome emotional and psychological problems. CBT is commonly used to treat stress, anxiety and depression (British Psychological Society, 2014).

Counselling and psychotherapy provide a means of helping participants to resolve emotional threats and play an active role in their lives. Consequently, psychotherapy is increasingly used within dementia care. There are different types of counselling and psychotherapy to choose from. The therapist aims to help you understand your particular problems so that you can work to overcome or manage these differently (British Psychological Society, 2014). Cheston and Ivanecka (2016) published a systematic review of the English-language literature and concluded that the strongest evidence supported the use of short-term group therapy after diagnosis and an intensive, multifaceted intervention for nursing home residents.

But this area is definitely a work in progress. Spector and colleagues (2015) have reported on their initiative to develop a CBT manual for anxiety in dementia and determine its feasibility through a randomised controlled trial involving participants with dementia. The authors found in their pilot trial that there were significant improvements in depression at 15 weeks after adjustment (–5.37, 95% CI, –9.50 to –1.25). Improvements remained significant at six months. CBT was cost neutral. The conclusion of this study was that CBT was feasible (in terms of recruitment, acceptability and attrition) and effective. A fully powered RCT is now required.

For a much more detailed introduction to this topic, the reader is reminded to consult the document from the British Psychological Society in 'Essential reading'.

—— Therapeutic lying and covert medication ——

There is no agreement on this issue in the UK or elsewhere, and there are no static views among people with dementia or their paid or informal carers regarding the acceptability of lying. A number of years ago, a UK study found that 96% of care staff reported using lies when caring for residents with dementia (James et al., 2003). As discussed, there was an overwhelming sense of 'paralysis' among staff about how to respond when faced with a situation in which they could use truth or deception with a person with dementia. This was caused by the identified factors and ethical frameworks which sometimes contradicted and overrode each other, for example a staff member may deem that lying is in a person's best interests but they may then feel the need to tell the truth in the presence of relatives due to personal ethical frameworks (Turner et al., 2016).

In the context of lying to a resident with dementia, lying is conceptualised as therapeutic (hence the term **therapeutic lying**). Understood by reference to compassion, the care provider's intent is to eliminate harm and also control behaviour. Currently, no official guidelines in the UK justify 'lying' or 'not telling the truth' to any patients or to people living with more severe dementia (Culley et al., 2013). The Nursing and Midwifery Council (2008, p.2) urges nurses and midwives to 'be open and honest, act with integrity and uphold the reputation of your profession', and warns that 'failure to comply with this code may bring your fitness to practise into question and endanger your registration' (Nursing and Midwifery Council, 2008, p.2). In addition, the most recent regulations of the General Medical Council underline that as a professional a doctor must 'be honest and trustworthy in all your communication with patients and colleagues'.[1]

How decision-making can go awry to produce therapeutic lying is of considerable interest (see Figure 5.2).

---

1   General Medical Council (2013), para. 68, available at www.gmc-uk.org/guidance/good_medical_practice/20463.asp (accessed 3 Oct 2016).

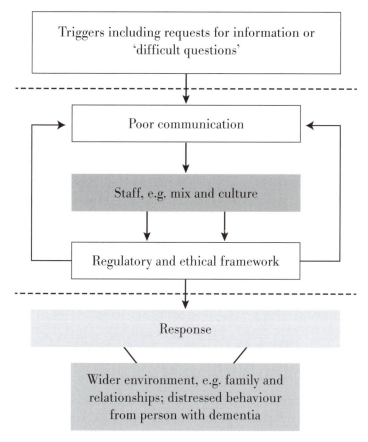

Figure 5.2: A process map for public decision-making and lying
Source: adapted from Turner et al. (2016, Fig. 1).

Despite the absence of any formalised published guidelines on circumstances where not telling 'the truth' to people living with dementia may be justifiable, studies of people with dementia (Day et al., 2011), nurses and staff (Wood-Mitchell et al., 2006, 2007), psychiatrists (Culley et al., 2013) and informal carers (Hughes et al., 2002) show that lying is pervasive and sometimes considered justifiable in dementia care by people living with dementia and their family carers. Examples of untruths include not telling someone that their loved one was dead when they asked for them, or colluding with delusions to reduce distress and agitation and thus avoid behaviour that challenges (e.g. agitation, aggression) (Mental Health Foundation, 2014).

Covert medication administration, also known as surreptitious or concealed medication administration, is a controversial practice whereby medication is given to patients without their knowledge or consent disguised in food or drink (Haw and Stubbs, 2010). The administration of medication covertly to patients with mental capacity is considered unethical, though administration in this way is described in the literature, particularly in relation to patients suffering with schizophrenia where capacity may fluctuate (Whitty and Devitt, 2005). Tablets may be crushed or liquid forms of medication may be used for patients who are either not in a position to give consent or refuse consent because of loss of insight (Kala, 2012). There has been much concern that people with dementia are too frequently given powerful sedative and antipsychotic drugs which make life easier for care staff.

Treolar, Beats and Philpot (2000) and Treolar and Philpot (2001) examined the use of covert medication; at the time of the study, 79% of patients in long-stay care settings for older people had medication administered via deception. This is interesting particularly in light of the possible implications for the lack of transparency and inadequate documentation around this practice within the sector, although this research is now quite dated. In contemporary dementia care, with developments in national law and regulation, there are clear implications for human rights-based approaches. One must be ultimately cognisant of the clinical regulators; in 1996, a senior nurse was suspended from duty and subjected to disciplinary action for obeying the request of her consultant to give a disruptive patient haloperidol disguised in a drink (Ramsay, 2001).

—— Life review and life story ———————————

Health and social care policy and guidance in England are increasingly recommending the use of life story work (LSW) in the care of people with dementia. The National Dementia Strategy for England, for example, refers to the use of life story work as 'an effective vehicle for care home staff to communicate and develop relationships with residents, based on their unique life experiences' (Department of Health, 2009, p.58). Continuity theory (Atchley, 1989, 1999) argues that as people grow older they strive to preserve and maintain continuity in their activities, behaviours, habits, thinking, relationships, values and attitudes. Continuity is a strategy for coping with changes in middle and later life (Atchley, 1989). Typically the older person will attempt to maintain continuity by 'dealing with a new environment in familiar ways…[by] search[ing] for linkages and familiarity' (Atchley, 1989, p.189). Garland and Garland (2001) describe life review as a highly structured form of reminiscence, which allows the participant to ascribe meaning and value to his/her life, and come to terms with uncomfortable issues.

A definition of life review is provided by Woods et al. (2005, p.1): 'Life review typically involves individual sessions, in which the person is guided chronologically through life experiences, encouraged to evaluate them, and may produce a life story book.'

A recent systematic review suggests that individual reminiscence work, using a life review or life story process, shows potential psychosocial benefits for people with dementia (Subramaniam and Woods, 2012). McKeown and colleagues (2006, p.238) defined LSW as 'a term given to biographical approaches in health and social care settings that gives people time to share their memories and talk about their life experiences'. Life Story Books (LSBs) can consist of photographs, written accounts in people's own words and materials relating to a person's life and life history, resulting in the collection of information to form the LSB (Heathcode, 2005). The photographs and memorabilia can be used therapeutically to enhance communication between health professionals, residents, carers and their families. These LSBs can highlight a resident's unique life history and can be used as a basis for individualised care (Wills and Rose Day, 2008).

A life review process, then, helps a person with dementia to recount and evaluate his or her life history in chronological order. The process can be represented in tangible form as a life story book, photo album, scrap book, memory box or memory book (Subramaniam, Woods and Whitaker, 2014). Haight and colleagues (2003) have emphasised the important role of the person with dementia in having editorial control and decision-making power throughout the process of developing the book, with the life review and creation of the book proceeding hand in hand. Transition to care such as a nursing home can present many challenges for older adults as it can create a sharp break with their previous life, resulting in feelings of isolation and anonymity, loss of identity and loneliness (Heliker and Jaquish, 2006).

Heliker (2007) supports the view that a culture of listening and story sharing can promote a caring environment for residents in a continuing care setting. More recently, the use of LSW has been identified as one approach to maintain a person's human rights (McKeown et al., 2015). LSBs further can promote and enhance person-centred care and relationship-centred care (Nolan et al., 2004) (see Chapter 2).

—— Bringing it all together ——————————————

EachStep Blackburn[2] is a new cutting-edge dementia care home, a specialist service providing a range of dementia person-centred care and support, including respite, residential, nursing and end-of-life care. The EachStep approach aims to provide people with tailored support that is delivered by staff who understand residents' life history, have strong values and who are creatively focussed in promoting wellbeing. Part of the Each Step team is a 'Community Circles Connector', who can focus on enabling people to remain connected with their closest and to continue to enjoy the things that are important to them in the community, critical in promoting 'social health'. As a result of a collaborative action of the INTERDEM Social Health Taskforce, the somewhat previously static WHO definition of health has been

2   See https://www.c-i-c.co.uk/eachstep-blackburn-forms-pioneering-partnership-helen-sanderson-associates.

reformulated 'towards a dynamic one based on the ability to physically, mentally and socially adapt and self-manage' (Dröes et al., 2016, p.1). Social health is critical to the wider goal of 'community based rehabilitation' (see Chapter 13).

I first resume discussion of living well and promoting wellbeing in Chapter 7.

——— Essential reading ———

British Psychological Society. 2014. *A Guide to Psychosocial Interventions in Early Stages of Dementia*, London: The British Psychological Society, available at www.bps.org.uk/system/files/user-files/DCP%20Faculty%20for%20the%20Psychology%20of%20Older%20People%20(FPoP)/public/a_guide_to_psychosocial_interventions_in_dementia.pdf (accessed 3 Oct 2016).

Kaiser P, Eley R (eds). 2016. *Life Story Work with People with Dementia: Ordinary Lives, Extraordinary People*, London: Jessica Kingsley Publishers.

——— References ———

Aguirre E, Spector A, Orrell M. 2014. Guidelines for adapting cognitive stimulation therapy to other cultures. Clin Interv Aging, 9, 1003–1007.

Aguirre E, Woods RT, Spector A, Orrell M. 2013. Cognitive stimulation for dementia: a systematic review of the evidence of effectiveness from randomised controlled trials. Ageing Res Rev, 12(1), 253–262.

Atchley RC. 1989. A continuity theory of aging. The Gerontologist, 29, 183–190.

Atchley RC. 1999. *Continuity and Adaptation in Aging*, Baltimore, MD: The Johns Hopkins University Press.

Bahar-Fuchs A, Clare L, Woods B. 2013. Cognitive training and cognitive rehabilitation for mild to moderate Alzheimer's disease and vascular dementia. Cochrane Database Syst Rev, 6, CD003260.

Barrick AL, Sloane PD, Williams CS, Mitchell CM, et al. 2010. Impact of ambient bright light on agitation in dementia. International Journal of Geriatric Psychiatry, 25, 1013–1021.

Basford JR, Malec JF. 2015. Brief overview and assessment of the role and benefits of cognitive rehabilitation. Arch Phys Med Rehabil, 96(6), 977–980.

Bates J, Boote J, Beverley C. 2004. Psychosocial intervention for people with a milder dementing illness: a systematic review. Journal of Advanced Nursing, 45(6), 644–658.

Behrman S, Chouliaras L, Ebmeier KP. 2014. Considering the senses in the diagnosis and management of dementia. Maturitas, 77(4), 305–310.

Belleville S, Clement F, Mellah S, Gilbert B, Fontaine F, Gauthier S. 2011. Training-related brain plasticity in subjects at risk of developing Alzheimer's disease. Brain, 134(6), 1623–1634.

Bouchard R, Rossor MN. 1996. Typical Clinical Features. In S. Gauthier (ed.), *Clinical Diagnosis and Management of Alzheimer's Disease*, London: Martin Dunitz Publishers.

Brandling J, House W. 2009. Social prescribing in general practice: adding meaning to medicine. Br J Gen Pract, 59(563), 454–456.

Breuil V, De Rotrou J, Forette F, Tortrat D, et al. 1994. Cognitive stimulation of patients with dementia: preliminary results. Int J Geriatr Psychiatry, 9, 211–217.

British Psychological Society. 2014. *A Guide to Psychosocial Interventions in Early Stages of Dementia*, London: The British Psychological Society, available at www.bps.org.uk/system/files/user-files/DCP%20Faculty%20for%20the%20Psychology%20of%20Older%20People%20(FPoP)/public/a_guide_to_psychosocial_interventions_in_dementia.pdf (accessed 3 Oct 2016).

Bronfenbrenner U. 2004. *Making Human Beings Human: Bioecological Perspectives on Human Development*, Thousand Oaks, CA: Sage.

Carrion C, Aymerich M, Baillés E, López-Bermejo A. 2013. Cognitive psychosocial intervention in dementia: a systematic review. Dement Geriatr Cogn Disord, 36(5–6), 363–375.

Cassarino M, Setti A. 2015. Environment as 'Brain Training': a review of geographical and physical environmental influences on cognitive ageing. Ageing Res Rev, 23(Pt B), 167–182.

Cheston R, Ivanecka A. 2016. Individual and group psychotherapy with people diagnosed with dementia: a systematic review of the literature. Int J Geriatr Psychiatry, July, doi:10.1002/gps.4529 (e-pub ahead of print).

Chung JC, Lai CK, Chung PM, French HP. 2002. Snoezelen for dementia. The Cochrane Database of Systematic Reviews, 4, CD003152.

Clare L, Jones RS. 2008. Errorless learning in the rehabilitation of memory impairment: a critical review. Neuropsychological Review, 18, 1–23.

Clare L, Woods RT. 2004. Cognitive training and cognitive rehabilitation for people with early-stage Alzheimer's disease: a review. Neuropsychol Rehabil, 14, 385–401.

Clare L, Bayer A, Burns A, Corbett A, et al. 2013. Goal-oriented cognitive rehabilitation in early-stage dementia: study protocol for a multi-centre single-blind randomised controlled trial (GREAT). Trials, 14, 152.

Clare L, Wilson BA, Carter G, Roth I, Hodges JR. 2004. Awareness in early-stage Alzheimer's disease: relationship to outcome of cognitive rehabilitation. J. Clin. Exp. Neuropsychol, 26(2), 215–226.

Clare L, Woods B, Moniz-Cook E, Orrell M, Spector A. 2003. Cognitive rehabilitation and cognitive training for early-stage Alzheimer's disease and vascular dementia. Cochrane Database Syst Rev, 4, CD003260

Cohen D, Eisdorfer C. 1986. *The Loss of Self: A Family Resource for the Care of Alzheimer's Disease and Related Disorders*, New York: WW Norton & Company.

Coleman P. 2005. Uses of reminiscence: functions and benefits. Ageing & Mental Health, 9, 4.

Culley H, Barber R, Hope A, James I. 2013. Therapeutic lying in dementia care. Nursing Standard, 28(1), 35–39.

Day A, James I, Meyer T, Lee D. 2011. Do people with dementia find lies and deception in dementia care acceptable? Ageing and Mental Health, 15(7), 822–829.

Dalton DS, Cruickshanks KJ, Klein BE, Klein R, Wiley TL, Nondahl DM. 2003. The impact of hearing loss on quality of life in older adults. The Gerontologist, 43, 661–668.

De Oliveira TC, Soares FC, De Macedo LD, Diniz DL, et al. 2014. Beneficial effects of multi-sensory and cognitive stimulation on age-related cognitive decline in long-term-care institutions. Clin Interv Aging, 9, 309–320.

Department of Health. 2009. *Living Well with Dementia: A National Dementia Strategy*, London: Department of Health.

Dröes RM, Chattat R, Diaz A, Gove D, et al. 2016. The Interdem Social Health Taskforce. Social health and dementia: a European consensus on the operationalization of the concept and directions for research and practice. Aging Ment Health, Nov 21, 1–14.

Dröes RM, van der Roest HG, van Mierlo L, Meiland FJM. 2011. Memory problems in dementia: adaptation and coping strategies and psychosocial treatment. Expert Reviews, 11, 1769–1782.

Feil N. 1993. *The Validation Breakthrough: Simple Techniques for Communicating with People with Alzheimer's-Type Dementia*, Baltimore, MD: Health Promotion Press.

Garland J, Garland C. 2001. *Life Review in Health and Social Care: A Practitioner's Guide*, Hove: Brunner-Routledge.

General Medical Council. 2013. *Good Medical Practice*, London: GMC, available at www.gmc-uk.org/static/documents/content/GMP_.pdf (accessed 3 Oct 2016).

Gibson F. 2004. *The Past in the Present: Using Reminiscence in Health and Social Care*, Baltimore, MD: Health Professions Press.

Haight BK, Bachman DL, Hendrix S, Wagner MT, Meeka A, Jolene J. 2003. Life review: treating the dyadic family unit with dementia. Clinical Psychology and Psychotherapy, 10, 165–174.

Harris P, Keady J. 2006. Editorial – dementia. The International Journal of Social Research and Practice, 5(1), 5–10.

Haw C, Stubbs J. 2010. Covert administration of medication to older adults: a review of the literature and published studies. J Psychiatr Ment Health Nurs, 17(9), 761–768.

Heathcode J. 2005. Part two: choosing and individual reminiscence approach. Nurse Residential Care, 7, 78–80.

Heiss WD, Kessler J, Slansky I, Mielke R, Szelies B, Herholz K. 1993. Activation PET as an instrument to determine therapeutic efficacy in Alzheimer's disease. Ann N Y Acad Sci, 695, 327–331.

Heliker D. 2007. Story sharing: restoring the reciprocity of caring in long-term care. J Psychosoc Nurs Ment Health Serv, 45, 20–23.

Heliker D, Jaquish A. 2006. Transition of new residents to long-term care: basing practices on residents' perspective. J Gerontol Nurs, 32, 34–42.

Hughes J, Hope T, Reader S, Rice D. 2002. Dementia and ethics: the views of informal carers. Journal of the Royal Society of Medicine, 95, 242–246.

Hulsegge J, Verheul A. 1987. *Snoezelen*, Chesterfield: Rompa.

Iliffe S, Wilcock J, Haworth D. 2006. Delivering psychosocial interventions for people with dementia in primary care: Jobs or skills? Dementia, 5(3), 327–338.

James IA, Powell I, Smith T, Fairbairn A. 2003. Lying to residents: Can the truth sometimes be unhelpful for people with dementia? PSIGE Newsletter, BPS 82, 2628.

Kala AK. 2012. Covert medication; the last option: a case for taking it out of the closet and using it selectively. Indian J Psychiatry, 54(3), 257–265.

Kitwood T. 1997. *Dementia Reconsidered: The Person Comes First*, Buckingham: Open University Press.

Koehler R, Wilhelm E, Shoulson I. 2011. *Cognitive Rehabilitation Therapy for Traumatic Brain Injury. Cognitive Rehabilitation Therapy for Traumatic Brain Injury: Evaluating the Evidence*, Washington, DC: The National Academies Press.

Kovach CR. 2000. Sensoristasis and imbalance in persons with dementia. Journal of Nursing Scholarship, 32, 379–384.

Lawrence V, Fossey J, Ballard C, Moniz-Cook E, Murray J. 2012. Improving quality of life for people with dementia in care homes: making psychosocial interventions work. Br J Psychiatry, 201(5), 344–351.

Lin YC, Dai YT, Hwang SL. 2003. The effect of reminiscence on the elderly population: a systematic review. Public Health Nursing, 20(4), 297–306.

Maci T, Pira FL, Quattrocchi G, Nuovo SD, Perciavalle V, Zappia M. 2012. Physical and cognitive stimulation in Alzheimer Disease. The GAIA Project: a pilot study. Am J Alzheimers Dis Other Demen, 27(2), 107–113.

Malec JF, Basford JS. 1996. Postacute brain injury rehabilitation. Arch Phys Med Rehabil, 77(2), 198–207.

Mapelli D, Di Rosa E, Nocita R, Sava D. 2013. Cognitive stimulation in patients with dementia: randomized controlled trial. Dement Geriatr Cogn Dis Extra, 3(1), 263–271.

McKeown J, Clarke A, Repper J. 2006. Life story work in health and social care: systematic literature review. J Adv Nurs, 55(2), 237–247.

McKeown J, Ryan T, Ingleton C, Clarke A. 2015. 'You have to be mindful of whose story it is': the challenges of undertaking life story work with people with dementia and their family carers. Dementia (London), 14(2), 238–256.

McLellan DL. 1991. Functional Recovery and the Principles of Disability Medicine. In M. Swash and J. Oxbury (eds), *Clinical Neurology*, London: Churchill Livingstone.

Mental Health Foundation. 2014. *Dementia – What is Truth?* Available at www.mentalhealth.org. uk/sites/default/files/Dementia%20truth%20inquiry%20lit%20review%20FINAL%20(3).pdf (accessed 3 Oct 2016).

Miyahara M. 2003. Effects on memory of verbal labeling for hand movements in persons with Alzheimer's disease. American Journal of Alzheimer's Disease and Other Dementias, 18(6), 349–35.

Moebs I, Gee S, Miyahara M, Paton H, Croucher M. 2015. Perceptions of a cognitive rehabilitation group by older people living with cognitive impairment and their caregivers: a qualitative interview study. Dementia (London), October, 1471301215609738 (e-pub ahead of print).

Moniz-Cook E, Agar S, Gibson G, Win T, Wang M. 1998. A preliminary study of the effects of early intervention with people with dementia and their families in a memory clinic. Aging Ment Health, 2, 199–211.

Moniz-Cook E, Vernooij-Dassen M, Woods B, Orrell M. 2011. Psychosocial interventions in dementia care research: the INTERDEM manifesto. Aging Ment Health, 15(3), 283–290.

Moniz-Cook E, Vernooij-Dassen M, Woods R, Verhey F, et al. 2008. A European consensus on outcome measures for psychosocial intervention research in dementia care. Aging Ment Health, 12(1), 14–29.

Neal M, Briggs M. 2000. Validation therapy for dementia. Cochrane Database Syst Rev, 2, CD001394.

NICE. 2012. *Dementia: Supporting People with Dementia and Their Carers in Health and Social Care*, London: National Institute for Health and Clinical Excellence.

Nolan MR, Davies S, Brown J, Keady J, Nolan J. 2004. Beyond person-centred care: a new vision for gerontological nursing. J Clin Nurs, 13(3a), 45–53.

Nursing and Midwifery Council. 2008. *The Code: Standards of Conduct, Performance and Ethics for Nursing and Midwives*, available at www.nmc.org.uk/globalassets/sitedocuments/standards/nmc-old-code-2008.pdf (accessed 3 Oct 2016).

O'Shea E, Devane D, Cooney A, Casey D, et al. 2014. The impact of reminiscence on the quality of life of residents with dementia in long-stay care. Int J Geriatr Psychiatry, 29(10), 1062–1070.

Olazarán J, Reisberg B, Clare L, Cruz I, et al. 2010. Nonpharmacological therapies in Alzheimer's disease: a systematic review of efficacy. Dement Geriatr Cogn Disord, 30(2), 161–178.

Orrell M, Woods B, Spector A. 2012. Should we use cognitive stimulation therapy to improve cognitive function in people with dementia. BMJ, 344, e633.

Papp KV, Walsh SJ, Snyder PJ. 2009. Immediate and delayed effects of cognitive interventions in healthy elderly: a review of current literature and future directions. Alzheimers Dement, 5, 50–60.

Parker J. 2006. 'I remember that…': reminiscence groups with people with dementia. A valuable site for practice learning. Groupwork, 16(1), 7–28.

Prince M, Bryce R, Albanese E, Wimo A, Ribeiro W, Ferri CP. 2013. The global prevalence of dementia: a systematic review and metaanalysis. Alzheimers Dement, 9, 63–75.

Rabipour S, Raz A. 2012. Training the brain: fact and fad in cognitive and behavioral remediation. Brain and Cognition, 79(2), 159–179.

Ramsay S. 2001. UK nurses receive guidance on covert medication of patients. Lancet, 358(9285), 900.

Sachs GA, Carter R, Holtz LR, Smith F, et al. 2011. Cognitive impairment: an independent predictor of excess mortality: a cohort study. Ann Intern Med, 155, 300–308.

Salthouse TA. 2006. Mental exercise and mental aging: evaluating the validity of the 'use it or lose it' hypothesis. Perspectives on Psychological Science, 1, 68–87.

Skills for Care. 2013. Supporting People in the Advanced Stages of Dementia: A Case Study-Based Manager's Guide to Good Practice in Learning and Development for Social Care Workers Supporting People in the Advanced Stages of Dementia.

Spector A, Charlesworth G, King M, Lattimer M, et al. 2015. Cognitive-behavioural therapy for anxiety in dementia: pilot randomised controlled trial. Br J Psychiatry, 206(6), 509–516.

Spector A, Davies S, Woods B, Orrell M. 2000. Reality orientation for dementia: a systematic review of the evidence of effectiveness from randomized controlled trials. Gerontologist, 40(2), 206–212.

Spector A, Gardner C, Orrell M. 2011. The impact of Cognitive Stimulation Therapy groups on people with dementia: views from participants, their carers and group facilitators. Aging Ment Health, 15(8), 945–949.

Spector A, Orrell M, Davies S, Woods B. 2001. Can reality orientation be rehabilitated? Development and piloting of an evidence-based programme of cognition-based therapies for people with dementia. Neuropsychological Rehabilitation.

Spector A, Orrell M, Woods B. 2010. Cognitive Stimulation Therapy (CST): effects on different areas of cognitive function for people with dementia. Int J Geriatr Psychiatry, 25(12), 1253–1258.

Spector A, Thorgrimsen L, Woods B, Orrell M. 2006. *Making a Difference: An Evidence-Based Therapy Programme to Offer Cognitive Stimulation Therapy to People with Dementia*, London: Hawker.

Subramaniam P, Woods B. 2012. The impact of individual reminiscence therapy for people with dementia: systematic review. Expert Review of Neurotherapeutics, 12(5), 545–555.

Subramaniam P, Woods B, Whitaker C. 2014. Life review and life story books for people with mild to moderate dementia: a randomised controlled trial. Aging Ment Health, 18(3), 363–375.

Swaab DF, Lucassen PJ, Salehi A, Scherder EJ, van Someren EJ, Verwer RW. 1998. Reduced neuronal activity and reactivation in Alzheimer's disease. Prog Brain Res, 117, 343–377.

Tardif S, Simard M. 2011. Cognitive stimulation programmes in health elderly: a review. International Journal of Alzheimer's Disease, Article ID 378934.

Taulbee LR, Folsom JC. 1966. Reality orientation for geriatric patients. Hosp Community Psychiatry, 17(5), 133–135.

Treolar A, Philpot M. 2001. Concealing medication in patients' food. Lancet, 357, 62–64.

Treloar A, Beats B, Philpot M. 2000. A pill in the sandwich: covert medication in food and drink. Journal of the Royal Society of Medicine, 93(8), 408–411.

Turner A, Eccles F, Keady J, Simpson J, Elvish R. 2016. The use of the truth and deception in dementia care among general hospital staff. Aging Ment Health, May, 1–8 (e-pub ahead of print).

Valenzuela MJ, Sachdev P. 2009. Can cognitive exercise prevent the onset of dementia? Systematic review of randomized clinical trials with longitudinal follow-up. Am. J. Geriatr. Psychiatry, 17, 179–187.

Van Bogaert P, Van Grinsven R, Tolson D, Wouters K, Engelborghs S, Van der Mussele S. 2013. Effects of SolCos model-based individual reminiscence on older adults with mild to moderate dementia due to Alzheimer disease: a pilot study. J Am Med Dir Assoc, 14(7), 528.e9–13.

Vance DE. 2003. Implications of olfactory stimulation on activities for adults with age-related dementia. Activities, Adaptation & Aging, 27, 17–25.

Wang J. 2007. Group reminiscence therapy for cognitive and affective function of demented elderly in Taiwan. International Journal Geriatric Psychiatry, 22, 1235–1240.

White JM, Cornish F, Kerr S. 2015. Frontline perspectives on 'joined-up' working relationships: a qualitative study of social prescribing in the west of Scotland. Health Soc Care Community, October, doi:10.1111/hsc.12290 (e-pub ahead of print).

Whitty P, Devitt P. 2005. Surreptitious prescribing in psychiatric practice. Psychiatric Services, 56, 481–483.

WHO. 2002. *Active Ageing: A Policy Framework*, Madrid: WHO, available at apps.who.int/iris/bitstream/10665/67215/1/WHO_NMH_NPH_02.8.pdf (accessed 3 Oct 2012).

WHO. 2012. Dementia: A Public Health Priority, available at www.who.int/mental_health/publications/dementia_report_2012/en (accessed 3 Oct 2012).

Wills T, Rose Day M. 2008. Valuing the person's story: use of life story books in a continuing care setting Clin Interv Aging, 3(3), 547–552.

Wilson BA. 1989. Models of Cognitive Rehabilitation. In RL Wood and P Eames (eds), *Models of Brain Injury Rehabilitation*, London: Chapman & Hall.

Wilson BA. 2002. Towards a comprehensive model of cognitive rehabilitation. Neuropsychological Rehabilitation, 12(2), 97–110

Wood-Mitchell A, Mackenzie L, Cunningham J, James I. 2007. Can a lie ever be therapeutic? The debate continues. Journal of Dementia Care, 15(2), 24–28.

Wood-Mitchell A, Waterworth A, Stephenson M, James I. 2006. Lying to people with dementia: sparking the debate. Journal of Dementia Care, 14(6), 30–31.

Woods B. 2002. Editorial: reality orientation: a welcome return? Age & Ageing, 31, 155–156.

Woods B, Aguirre E, Spector AE, Orrell M. 2012. Cognitive stimulation to improve cognitive functioning in people with dementia. Cochrane Database Syst Rev, 2, CD005562.

Woods B, Spector A, Jones C, Orrell M, Davies S. 2005. Reminiscence therapy for dementia. Cochrane Database Syst Rev, 2, CD001120.

Woods B, Thorgrimsen L, Spector A, Royan L, Orrell M. 2006. Improved quality of life and cognitive stimulation therapy in dementia. Aging Ment Health, 10(3), 219–226.

Wu YT, Prina AM, Brayne C. 2015. The association between community environment and cognitive function: a systematic review. Soc Psychiatry Psychiatr Epidemiol, 50(3), 351–362.

Yamagami T, Takayama Y, Maki Y, Yamaguchi H. 2012. A randomized controlled trial of brain activating rehabilitation for elderly participants with dementia in residential care homes. Dement Geriatr Cogn Dis Extra, 2(1), 372–380.

Yates LA, Orrell M, Spector A, Orgeta V. 2015. Service users' involvement in the development of individual Cognitive Stimulation Therapy (iCST) for dementia: a qualitative study. BMC Geriatr, 15, 4.

Zarit SH, Edwards AB. 1996. Family Caregiving: Research and Clinical Intervention. In RT Woods (ed.), *Handbook of the Clinical Psychology of Aging*, Chichester: John Wiley & Sons Ltd.

Chapter 6

ORAL HEALTH AND SWALLOWING

The twentieth century will be remembered chiefly, not as an age of political conflicts and technical inventions, but as an age in which human society dared to think of the health of the whole human race as a practical objective. (Arnold Toynbee, British historian)

Learning objectives

By the end of this chapter, you will:

» be able to outline the critical importance of allied health professionals

» be able to explain the importance of oral health to living better with dementia

» be able to explain which swallowing problems might affect people living with dementia and why they are important

Introduction

Dementia is a team effort in every sense: a person with dementia never receives a diagnosis alone. The success of an approach which attempts to do everything well for a person with dementia, to promote where possible his or her **independence**, depends on key actors who are **interdependent**.

Allied health professionals (AHPs) currently – at the time of writing – make up 6% of the NHS workforce – the third largest professional group – and still more work in social care, housing, local government and the voluntary and private sectors (Oliver, 2015).

The AHPs include 12 professions regulated by the Health and Care Professions Council (HCPC), which collectively make up the third largest workforce in the NHS. They work across a range of sectors including health, social care, education, academia and the voluntary and private sectors across the life course. They include physiotherapists, occupational therapists, podiatrists, dieticians, speech and language therapists, paramedics, radiographers, orthoptists, prosthetists and orthotists, art therapists, music therapists and drama therapists (NHS England/ ahpf (date unclear)).

David Oliver comments on the King's Fund website:

> NHS England's new models of care – especially primary and acute care systems, emergency care networks and improving health care for care home residents – all require input and leadership from skilled AHPs. […] More widely, the push from the Royal College of General Practitioners, the British Geriatrics Society and others to focus more on care planning, care coordination and self-management, and on anticipatory care for older people living with frailty, relies heavily on the role of AHPs. As does the focus on transforming urgent and emergency care services, on improving patient flow and on maintaining performance on the four-hour A&E waiting times target. (Oliver, 2015)

Allied health professionals hold a critical place in delivering the NHS Outcomes Framework (see Figure 6.1).

Domain 1: Preventing people from dying prematurely	Domain 2: Enhancing quality of life for people with long-term conditions	Domain 3: Helping people to recover from episodes of ill-health or following injury	Effectiveness
Domain 4: Ensuring people have a positive experience of care			Experience
Domain 5: Treating and caring for people in a safe environment and protecting them from avoidable harm			Safety

Figure 6.1: NHS Outcomes Framework

The framework is structured around the outcome domains shown below, which set out the high-level national objectives for the NHS. The key focus is around improving health outcomes and reducing health inequalities: **domain 1** – this domain captures how successful the NHS is in reducing the number of avoidable deaths; **domain 2** – this domain captures how successfully the NHS is supporting people with long-term conditions to live as normal a life as possible; **domain 3** – this domain captures how people recover from ill-health or injury and wherever possible how it can be prevented; **domain 4** – this domain looks at the importance of providing a positive experience of care for patients, service users and carers; **domain 5** – this domain explores patient safety and its importance in terms of quality of care to deliver better health outcomes.

There are almost 900 million people aged 60 years and over living worldwide. Rising life expectancy is contributing to rapid increases in this number, and is associated with the increased prevalence of chronic diseases like dementia; between 2015 and 2050, the number of older people living in higher income countries is forecast to increase by just 56%, compared with 138% in upper middle income countries, 185% in lower middle income countries and by 239% (a more than three-fold increase) in low income countries (Alzheimer's Disease International, 2016). The WHO has expressed concern that the oral health of older people is widely neglected. Based on a global survey of older people, the WHO has called for public health action by strengthening health promotion, integrating disease prevention and improving age-friendly primary oral health care. The exclusion of cognitively impaired older adults in the past has led to widespread under-reporting of poor oral health (Foltyn, 2015).

The rationale for including oral health care is based upon it being an essential and integral part of general health with an impact on the quality of life during a person's lifespan. The *World Oral Health Report 2003*, for example, outlines important principles for disease control and oral health promotion in the 21st century, as oral health is a determining factor for quality of life and is strongly associated with general health (WHO, 2003). These principles remain important until the end of life. Yet oral health is often neglected in general health promotion.

Oral health and swallowing difficulties are good examples of where a multidisciplinary approach is ideal.

— Oral health

Survey evidence suggests that oral health problems are common in care homes (e.g. Frenkel et al., 2000) and that institutionalised adults have greater oral health needs than their non-institutionalised peers (Pajukoski et al., 1999). Patients with dementia experience more oral diseases than healthy people (Chalmers, Carter and Spencer, 2003). Furthermore, care home residents who lack the capacity to consent may have greater oral health needs but are usually excluded from studies (Chalmers et al., 2003). As a result, current studies may underestimate the care needs for this group of residents. Currently, effective dental care and maintenance are both needed, but residents' oral health needs are not always adequately addressed (Monaghan and Morgan, 2010). As introduced in Chapter 3, studies show that, as with other developed countries, care home residents in the UK have high levels of dependency, cognitive impairment and multiple morbidity (Gordon et al., 2014). Oral problems are partially a result of barriers to dental services and changed self-perceptions of oral health in the context of multimorbidity, as acknowledged by Fiske and colleagues (2000). The combination of these medical conditions and disabilities increases dental case complexity and can influence dental treatment care particularly when managing dentate patients (Scully, 2010). Both oral disease and case complexity are therefore relevant for dental care and treatment service planning in care homes.

The most significant dental problems of patients with dementia result from a progressive diminution in oral self-care. There is an increasing dependence on the carer to provide oral hygiene, and the dentist has a significant role in ensuring that carers are able to take on these tasks (Moody, 1990). Many people's functions continue to deteriorate until verbal communication is no longer possible; the progressive decline in communicative abilities may hamper pain assessment in people with dementia, especially when it comes to orofacial pain (de Vries et al., 2016).

Not all people with dementia are old, but for the purposes of the discussion here the research is mainly derived from older people in residential settings, the majority of whom live with dementia. Most surveys indicate that the elderly who live in residential care have the worst oral health conditions (Frenkel, Harvey and Newcombe, 2001; Saub and Evans, 2001). Rejnefelt, Andersson and Renvert (2006) point out that people with dementia living in 'special facilities' have more oral health problems than those without dementia. In addition to residents retaining their natural dentition, it is also becoming more evident in the care home population that some individuals have had complex restorative treatment. These restorations require a high level of maintenance, making oral care for residents a much more complex and challenging task than in the past when the majority would have been admitted with dentures (Welsh, Edwards and Hunter, 2012).

The main reasons oral care is important for older people are that poor oral health affects overall health, nutrition, quality of life, communication and appearance; and the number of older people in the population, including dependent older people, continues to rise (NHS Health Scotland, 2013). According to McGrath and Bedi (1999), 72% of elderly people considered oral health important for their quality of life, especially in terms of mastication and comfort. Dental patients present with a spectrum of oral and general health needs which can require a combination of dental care professionals, including general dentists and specialists, to provide care (Morgan et al., 2015). Dental services and professionals worldwide will similarly need to adapt to continue to provide care for dentate older people with a range of complex dental and medical problems.

Many experience oral disease before entering residential care, but once in care this continues to progress. Oral health means more than having good teeth. It is part of (and should not be considered separate from) general health, and it could be argued that a person cannot have a healthy body without having a healthy mouth. The number of teeth with coronal and cervical caries increases with increasing severity of Alzheimer's disease (Ship, 1992). It has been demonstrated that persons with Alzheimer's disease have impaired oral health as a result of poor oral hygiene. For example, patients with Alzheimer's disease have more gingival plaque, bleeding and calculus compared with age-matched, gender-matched adults, and submandibular saliva output is impaired in persons with Alzheimer's disease who are taking medications (Ship et al., 1990).

Caries experience among the institutionalised elderly is associated with disability, and oral care is lacking among the institutionalised elderly in this study. Appropriate preventive measures as well as interventional activities should be undertaken to control oral disease among residential aged care residents (Philip et al., 2012a, b). It is well established that persistent dental plaque (i.e. biofilm) leads to an increased risk of developing dental caries and gingivitis, as well as other infections in the oral cavity. In addition, increasing research evidence indicates a clear relationship between oral infections and general health complications (Preston et al., 1999). Poor oral hygiene and a poor dental status may also result in reduced quality of life and difficulties in maintaining an active social life (Walker and Kiyak, 2007). In a study of 325 residents from nine nursing homes in Islington, almost two-thirds of the sample were dentate (64.5%); 61.3% of dentate and 50.9% of edentate residents reported problems such as dry mouth, sore cracked lips, broken teeth and toothache, and ill-fitting dentures (Porter et al., 2015).

An area which is particularly challenging for care staff is the provision of oral care to residents who resist or reject care, often as a result of dementia. The number of care home residents who have dementia and who also have retained their own teeth is expected to rise significantly in the future (NHS Health Scotland, 2013). Dental treatment planning, oral care and behavioural management for persons with Alzheimer's disease must be designed with consideration for the severity of the disease and must involve family members (Ocasio, Solomowitz and Sher, 2000).

NICE guidance (2016) on oral health in care homes makes particular recommendations for care staff carrying out admissions or assessments.

Dental disease

There are two main types of dental disease – gum (periodontal) disease and tooth decay (dental caries). Both can cause discomfort or pain, and can lead to the development of infection. An increasing number of dentate elderly people have tooth wear, periodontal disease, oral implants and sophisticated tooth- and implant-supported restorations and prostheses. Hence, they are in need of both preventive and curative oral health care continuously (van der Putten et al., 2010).

There is a clear difference between healthy teeth and gums and unhealthy teeth and gums (see Figure 6.2).

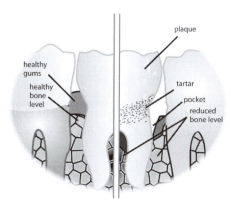

Figure 6.2: Teeth and gums

Gum disease

Gum disease (gingivitis) can cause inflamed and bleeding gums, gum recession, loose teeth and bad breath. It is caused by the accumulation of dental plaque. Good oral hygiene and the use of chlorhexidine tooth gel or mouth rinse can help to control it. Plaque is a combination of food debris and bacteria from the mouth. Everyone has some dental plaque. It leads to gum disease if it is not removed by efficient cleaning as it builds up on the surface of the teeth, particularly at the margin of the gum.

In periodontal disease, the gingivitis has spread below the gum level to involve the bone and the fibres tethering the tooth to the surrounding bone (periodontal membrane). Although this tends to occur in adults, a destructive form may occur in young patients. Although this disease may be treated and its progress checked, its effects are not reversible.

Tooth decay

Recent UK Adult Dental Health Surveys have shown that, similar to most developed countries, more adults are keeping their natural teeth into old age and, whereas 40% of adults aged 75–80 were reported to have 21 or more natural teeth, only 5% had 18 sound and untreated teeth (White et al., 2011). Based on substantial data available in a community-based geriatric dental clinic, dementia does not appear to be associated with tooth loss per se (Chen et al., 2010). The majority of nursing home residents arrive dentate (Dey, 1997). Older adults experience faster plaque production than younger adults because of the dual effects of gingival recession and reduced saliva production (Shay and Ship, 1995).

Tooth decay is caused by the action of dental plaque on the teeth when food and drinks containing sugar are consumed. This may involve the crown of the tooth or, in older patients, the root of the tooth. This involves a softening of the teeth by the removal of calcium by acidic attack from plaque – this is called decalcification.

Essentially, the bacteria in the plaque feed on the sugar, producing acid, which in turn attacks the tooth, causing decay. Dentists recommend restricting the intake of sugar to two or three times a day, preferably at mealtimes, as it is the number of times we eat sugar in a day, rather than the total amount of sugar consumed, which is important in guarding against tooth decay. Gum recession increases the chances of tooth decay occurring at the necks of the teeth unless oral hygiene is excellent and dietary sugar is controlled.

Periodontitis

Poor oral hygiene causes periodontal disease, which in turn creates tooth loss. Chronic periodontitis is a prevalent peripheral infection that is associated with gram-negative anaerobic bacteria and the elevation of serum inflammatory markers including C-reactive protein. The remaining teeth shift, causing the loss of occlusal surfaces and subsequent chewing and swallowing problems; other systemic diseases associated with poor oral hygiene include aspiration pneumonia, diabetes and coronary artery disease (Jablonski et al., 2011a). People with dementia (in some cases Alzheimer's disease specifically) can have significantly poorer gingival health than those without the condition and the increased likelihood of deep periodontal pockets (British Dental Association, 2013). The molecular and cellular mechanisms responsible for the aetiology and pathogenesis of Alzheimer's disease have not been defined; however, inflammation within the brain is thought to play a pivotal role (Kamer et al., 2008). Studies suggest that peripheral infection/inflammation might somehow affect the inflammatory state of the central nervous system.

Based on a six-month observational cohort study of 60 community-dwelling participants with mild-to-moderate Alzheimer's disease, Ide and colleagues (2016) have suggested that periodontitis is associated with an increase in cognitive decline in Alzheimer's disease, independent of baseline cognitive state, which may be mediated through effects on systemic inflammation. It is important to anticipate future oral decline in treatment planning and institute aggressive preventive measures (such as the use of topical fluoride, chlorhexidine or both) and the practice of frequent recall visits and daily oral hygiene (Lapeer, 1998).

Dentures

More people keep their natural teeth into old age. However, a significant number of older people have partial or full dentures. Dentures act like magnets to plaque. If partial dentures are worn, it is important that oral hygiene is well maintained or the increased plaque accumulation will encourage gum disease and tooth decay.

Compared with individuals without dementia, patients with Alzheimer's disease have significantly more gingival plaque, bleeding and calculus and have older and less clean dentures (Ship, 1992). Later on during a dementia, there is the progressive neglect of oral health as a result of forgetting the need, or even how, to brush one's teeth or clean dentures (Kieser et al., 1999). A component of good daily oral hygiene is the removal of dentures overnight to allow the tissues in the mouth to re-oxygenate. The prolonged use of dentures and inadequate cleaning can result in a fungal infection (thrush) forming, resulting in sore red areas under the dentures. Older adults with cognitive impairment have significantly older dentures that are significantly less clean compared with persons who do not have Alzheimer's disease (Ship et al., 1990).

Significantly more persons with Alzheimer's disease do not remove their dentures at night, and persons with dementia are more likely to have poor denture hygiene. Furthermore, the stability and occlusion of dentures are generally less satisfactory as the disorder progresses (British Dental Association, 2013). New dentures may be needed when the person loses all their natural teeth or when existing dentures go missing. In both circumstances the person with dementia may have difficulty coping with their new set of dentures and will need to be encouraged to persevere. A Swiss study of 233 long-term patients revealed that 72% of denture wearers had stomatitis with a clear relationship to poor oral hygiene and the neglect of denture care (Budtz-Jłrgensen et al., 1996). Subjects with dementia can forget to remove prostheses, resulting in the accumulation of food debris and dental biofilm on the remaining teeth (Friedlander et al., 2006). Dentures are also frequently lost or broken. Later deterioration of dental care may lead to the destruction of dentition by caries and periodontal disease. The problems of management may increase because of halitosis and difficulty in eating (Matear and Clarke, 1999).

The study by Fujihara and colleagues (2013) demonstrated that 57 subjects with vascular dementia who demonstrated aggressiveness and those with activity disturbances had significantly lower rates of denture-wearing than those without these two distressed responses. Because subjects with aggressiveness or resistance to receiving nursing care are unlikely to wear dentures by their own will even if they can ask for their carer's assistance, this result was not surprising and suggested that the wearing of dentures should be related to behavioural symptoms, such as aggressiveness and activity disturbances, rather than psychological symptoms.

Edentulism and masticatory function

Economically and socially disadvantaged older adults and the physically impaired are more likely to experience tooth loss (edentulism), untreated dental decay and periodontal diseases (Dolan and Atchison, 1993). Older people tend to have fewer natural teeth, and there are higher rates of edentulism (having no natural teeth) with increasing age (Kelly et al., 2000). The oral health status of older people has been gaining more importance in developing and developed countries in the last decades as the proportion of this group increases because of the increase in life expectancy. The general trend is for a reduction in edentulism and an increase in the retention of natural teeth until later life (Fiske et al., 2000). Patients with dementia can lose teeth, though it is not clear whether the risk, the rate of tooth loss or the prevalence varies for those with dementia compared to those without. There is conflicting data in this area; some data indicate no significant difference between those with dementia and those without, and others indicate that those with dementia have a lower number of teeth (British Dental Association, 2013).

Many people usually lose many teeth with age. The loss of teeth reduces masticatory capacity and subsequently influences the selection of foods and nutritional status. People who have lost many teeth often use dentures to support the impaired masticatory function. The adequate rehabilitation of edentulousness by the wearing of dentures has a beneficial effect on mastication (Shimazaki et al., 2001). One of the most immediate and important functional consequences of oral disorders is a reduction in chewing capacity. The ability to chew influences the types of foods people choose to eat, and this can result in a poor diet (Locker, 2002). Under-nutrition in residents of long-term care facilities has been linked to eating problems (Keller, 1993), and chewing problems can increase the likelihood of weight loss in nursing home residents (Blaum, Fries and Fiatorone, 1995).

The loss of masticatory function is also associated with increased disability and mortality (Shimazaki et al., 2001). Being able to chew properly, therefore, is of utmost importance for elderly persons to maintain a healthy diet and preserve cognition. This is especially the case when they are at risk of, or suffering from, dementia. Unfortunately, many older persons living in nursing homes are completely edentulous (Adam and Preston, 2006), and if they do have teeth remaining, they are often in need of dental care (Wyatt, 2002; Unluer, Gokalp and Dogan, 2007). Offering both oral health care and an improved diet to elderly persons with dementia will most likely improve their health situation and their quality of life (Weijenberg et al., 2013).

Residents in aged care facilities frequently have poor oral health and hygiene with moderate to high levels of oral disease and overall dental neglect. This is reinforced by aged care staff who acknowledge that the demands of feeding, toileting and tackling behavioural issues among residents often take precedence over oral health care regimens (Yi Mohammadi, Franks and Hines, 2015). The current literature shows that there is a general reluctance by aged care staff to prioritise oral care due to limited knowledge as well as existing psychological barriers to working on another person's mouth (Adams, 1996).

Oral lesions

There is conflicting data relating to oral lesions and pathology in people living with dementia. In some cases dementia sufferers (and those without dementia) have no overt signs of soft tissue pathology; in others, denture stomatitis, denture hyperplasia, mucositis denture associated ulceration, general ulceration and angular cheilitis can be seen (British Dental Association, 2013). Furthermore, those with dementia can have an increased prevalence, in some cases significant, of denture-related oral mucosal lesions, angular cheilitis, coated hairy tongue and gingival hyperplasia (British Dental Association, 2013).

General approach

Dental treatment for a patient with dementia is a professional judgement, including the patient's dental pathology as well as the state of cognitive function (British Dental Association, 2013). The effects of different types of intervention on the oral hygiene and health of long-term care residents have been studied, but most interventions have focused on the improvement of the oral condition of healthy or mildly cognitively impaired older people. Only a few studies have revealed the positive effects of residents' education in teeth-brushing techniques or critical self-estimation of one's oral condition (Komulainen et al., 2014).

Currently, the amount of time devoted to oral health care education in basic training for health professionals is limited, to put it diplomatically. The situation is further complicated by high staff turnover and the poor availability of continuing professional development in all disciplines. Education in itself may not be enough, but in combination with other measures such as realistic strategies and oral care procedures, routines and follow-up assessments, it may give positive results (Lindqvist et al., 2013). There has been a real drive to improve oral health by educating care staff (Isaksson et al., 2000). It has been shown that carers' improved knowledge leads to less plaque (Portella et al., 2013) and reduced mucosal (Isaksson et al., 2000) among care dependants.

Over half of all nursing home residents require assistance in all aspects of activities of daily living, including mouth care. One major barrier to the provision of that assistance is care-resistant behaviour (CRB). CRBs are actions 'invoked by a caregiving encounter, defined as the repertoire of behaviors with which persons with dementia withstand or oppose the efforts of a caregiver' (Jablonski et al., 2011b, p.77). A lack of cooperation by residents is a major barrier to the provision of oral health care by nursing home care staff; in particular, residents with dementia may resist care by refusing to open their mouth, turning away their head, verbally assaulting the carer, spitting at or hitting the carer and so forth (Hoben et al., 2016).

Managers who prioritise oral health will have a positive influence on the care practices in their establishments and are encouraged to participate in the training sessions for such (Welsh, Edwards and Hunter, 2012).

NICE (2016) have provided these recommendations recently in a document callhe NICE (2016) guideline 'Oral Health for Adults in Care Homes' (NG48)[1] covers oral health, including dental health and daily mouth care, for adults in care homes. The aim is to maintain and improve their oral health and ensure timely access to dental treatment, and is designed for a number of audiences including care home managers, care staff, health and wellbeing boards, oral health promotion teams or similar services, and dental practitioners.

The complexity of the organisational culture in residential aged care facilities and a lack of knowledge and awareness among carers have compounded the severity of the problem (Chalmers and Pearson, 2005). Restricted access to proper and timely care, difficulties with carers providing care, especially among the cognitively impaired, and the lack of on-site dental care also contribute to the problem (Paley, Slack-Smith and O'Grady, 2009). One way to avoid this is to train nursing staff carefully in how to handle their care recipients, based on mutual respect, in a way that facilitates building psychological bridges (Forsell et al., 2011).

Nonetheless, there are a number of exciting product and service innovations. The use of ultrasonic baths can be a successful means to improve denture hygiene among older people in long-term care with and without dementia. Education for the carer in order to improve oral hygiene, however, seems to be of minor significance and to be more effective for people with dementia (Zenthöfer et al., 2015). The Caring for Smiles guide covers not only core oral health knowledge specific to older people, but also topics such as how to teach, overcoming barriers in providing oral care and overcoming care-resistant behaviour (Welsh et al., 2012). The Mouth Care Without a Battle innovation incorporates person-centred techniques compiled from numerous sources to make care less threatening and thus avoid behaviours that interfere with care (Zimmerman et al., 2014). These strategies are multifaceted and include: choosing the most appropriate time to provide care; having a consistent care provider; making eye contact; having a gentle touch; giving explanations and verbal reassurance; and employing other individualised practices such as the gentle massage of the cheek.

Swallowing difficulties

The prevalence of swallowing difficulties (dysphagia) in patients with dementia ranges from 13% to 57%, depending on subject selection and the method (Rösler

---

1   Available at https://www.nice.org.uk/guidance/ng48 (accessed 28 Oct 2016).

et al., 2008; Alagiakrishnan, Bhanji and Kurian, 2013). The commonly reported symptoms in such patients would include the pocketing of food in the mouth, difficulties with mastication, coughing or choking with food or fluid, and the need for reminders to swallow food (Priefer and Robbins, 1997). Some of the contributing factors to oral phase dysphagia include the inability to recognise food visually, oral-tactile agnosia, and swallowing and feeding apraxia (Logemann, 1998). Because of the almost tenfold risk of aspiration pneumonia in patients with dysphagia, aspiration pneumonia is the leading cause of death in patients with dementia (Rösler et al., 2015). Aspiration pneumonia has further been reported to be a cause of death in patients with dementia (Grasbeck et al., 2003).

Difficulties swallowing are common in patients with advanced dementia and contribute to the mortality-risk factors (Easterling and Robbins, 2008). Dysphagia refers to swallowing difficulties that may occur due to either oropharyngeal or oesophageal problems. Pharyngeal-phase dysphagia leads to aspiration before, during and after swallowing (Finucane, Christmas and Travis, 1999). Unfortunately, the swallowing disorder forms a barrier to food consumption and can lead to weight loss, malnutrition and dehydration (Easterling and Robbins, 2008). Dysphagia may develop in patients with dementia during the course of their disease (Suh, Kim and Na, 2009) and it often complicates the course of illness in these patients. Furthermore, dysphagia has been shown to occur in different types of dementia (Bine, Frank and McDade, 1995). Dysphagia is a growing concern in dementia and can lead to malnutrition, dehydration, weight loss, functional decline and a fear of eating and drinking, as well as a decrease in quality of life.

Alagiakrishnan et al. (2013) conducted a systematic review of the literature to determine the patterns of swallowing deficits in different types of dementia and to look at the usefulness of different diagnostic and management strategies. The prevalence of swallowing difficulties in patients with dementia ranged from 13% to 57%. Dysphagia developed during the late stages of frontotemporal dementia, but it was seen during the early stage of Alzheimer's disease too. Limited evidence was available on the usefulness of diagnostic tests, the effect of postural changes, the modification of fluid and diet consistency, behavioural management and the possible use of medications. One conclusion from this substantial undertaking in research, sadly, is that significant gaps exist regarding the evidence for the evaluation and management of dysphagia in dementia.

According to reported problems pointing to the risk of dysphagia, about 40% of nursing home residents showed symptoms, as was similarly reported in the study of Humbert and Robbins (2008). Clinicians need to recognise the heterogeneity of health determinants and how these factors may influence approaches to dysphagia in different care settings. Current economic restraints are putting pressure on nursing home facilities to identify key issues that are associated with various outcomes, including the burden of respiratory infection resulting from aspiration (Nogueira and Reis, 2013). Depending on the form of dementia, cortical and subcortical lesions can, for example, lead to modifications of tongue movement and hyoid elevation, to upper oesophageal sphincter contraction and to sensory deficits and impaired coordination of movements in the oral, pharyngeal and laryngeal areas. Oropharyngeal dysphagia is the most common cause of aspiration, and pneumonia, presumably from aspiration, is the most common cause of death in persons with dementia (Burns et al., 1990; Chouinard, 2000).

In a systematic review with homogeneity of cohort studies, dysphagia has been found to be strongly associated with aspiration pneumonia in frail older people (van der Maarel-Wierink et al., 2011). Aspiration pneumonia, an inflammatory condition of lung parenchyma usually initiated by the introduction of bacteria into the lung alveoli, is causing high hospitalisation rates, morbidity and often death in frail older people (Welte, Torres and Nathwani, 2012). Therefore, the risk factors of aspiration pneumonia, such as dysphagia, should be prevented in frail older people whenever possible. Dysphagia, or swallowing impairment, has been described as a symptom which refers to difficulty or discomfort during the progression of the alimentary bolus from the oral cavity to the stomach (Rofes et al., 2011).

Essential reading

NHS England/ahpf. No date. *A Strategy to Develop the Capacity, Impact and Profile of Allied Health Professionals in Public Health 2015–2018: Strategy from the Allied Health Professionals Federation supported by Public Health England*, available at www.ahpf.org.uk/files/AHP%20Public%20 Health%20Strategy.pdf (accessed 3 Oct 2016).

References

Adam H, Preston AJ. 2006. The oral health of individuals with dementia in nursing homes. Gerodontology, 23, 99–105.

Adams R. 1996. Qualified nurses lack adequate knowledge related to oral health, resulting in inadequate oral care of patients on medical wards. J Adv Nurs, 24(3), 552–560.

Alagiakrishnan K, Bhanji RA, Kurian M. 2013. Evaluation and management of oropharyngeal dysphagia in different types of dementia: A systematic review. Arch Gerontol Geriatr, 56, 1e9.

Alzheimer's Disease International. 2016. *World Alzheimer Report 2015: The Global Impact of Dementia*, available at www.alz.co.uk/research/world-report-2015 (accessed 3 Oct 2016).

Bine JE, Frank EM, McDade HL. 1995. Dysphagia and dementia in subjects with Parkinson's disease. Dysphagia, 10(3), 160–164.

Blaum C, Fries B, Fiatorone M. 1995. Factors associated with low body mass index and weight loss in nursing home residents. Journal of Gerontology: Medical Sciences, 50A, M162.

British Dental Association. 2013. Dental Problems and their Management in Dementia, available at www.bda.org/dentists/education/sgh/Documents/Dental%20problems%20and%20their%20 management%20in%20patients%20with%20dementia.pdf (accessed 3 Oct 2016).

Budtz-Jĺrgensen E, Mojon P, Banon-Clément JM, Baehni P. 1996. Oral candidosis in long-term hospital care: comparison of edentulous and dentate subjects. Oral Dis, 2(4), 285–290.

Burns A, Jacoby R, Luthert P, Levy R. 1990. Cause of death in Alzheimer's disease. Age Ageing, 19, 341e344.

Chalmers JM, Pearson A. 2005. Oral hygiene care for residents with dementia: a literature review. J Adv Nurs, 52, 410–419.

Chalmers JM, Carter KD, Spencer AJ. 2003. Oral diseases and conditions in community-living older adults with and without dementia. Spec Care Dentist, 23, 7–17.

Chen X, Shuman SK, Hodges JS, Gatewood LC, Xu J. 2010. Patterns of tooth loss in older adults with and without dementia: a retrospective study based on a Minnesota cohort. J Am Geriatr Soc, 58(12), 2300–2307.

Chouinard J. 2000. Dysphagia in Alzheimer disease: a review. J Nutr Health Aging, 4, 214–217.

de Vries MW, Visscher C, Delwel S, van der Steen JT, et al. 2016. Orofacial pain during mastication in people with dementia: reliability testing of the orofacial pain scale for non-verbal individuals. Behav Neurol, 3123402.

Dey AN. 1997. Characteristics of elderly nursing home residents: data from the 1995 National Nursing Home Survey. Adv Data, 2(289), 1–8.

Dolan TA, Atchison KA. 1993. Implications of access, utilization and need for oral health care by the noninstitutionalized and institutionalized elderly on the dental delivery system. J Dent Educ, 57, 876–887.

Easterling CS, Robbins E. 2008. Dementia and dysphagia. Geriatric Nursing, 29(4), 275–285.

Finucane TE, Christmas C, Travis K. 1999. Tube feeding in patients with advanced dementia: a review of the evidence. Journal of the American Medical Association, 282(14), 1365–1370.

Fiske J, Griffiths J, Jamieson R, Mange D. 2000. Guidelines for oral health care for long-stay patients and resident. Gerodontology, 17, 55–64.

Foltyn P. 2015. Ageing, dementia and oral health. Aust Dent J, 60(Suppl 1), 86–94.

Forsell M, Sjögren P, Kullberg E, Johansson O, et al. 2011. Attitudes and perceptions towards oral hygiene tasks among geriatric nursing home staff. Int J Dent Hyg, 9(3), 199–203.

Frenkel H, Harvey I, Newcombe RG. 2000. Oral health care among nursing home residents in Avon. Gerodontology, 17, 33–38.

Frenkel H, Harvey I, Newcombe RG. 2001. Improving oral health in institutionalised elderly people by educating caregivers: a randomised controlled trial. Community Dent Oral Epidemiol, 29(4), 289–297.

Friedlander AH, Norman DC, Mahler ME, Norman KM, Yagiela JA. 2006. Alzheimer's disease: psychopathology, medical management and dental implications. J Am Dent Assoc, 137, 1240–1251.

Fujihara I, Sadamori S, Abekura H, Akagawa Y. 2013. Relationship between behavioral and psychological symptoms of dementia and oral health status in the elderly with vascular dementia. Gerodontology, 30(2), 157–161.

Gordon AL, Franklin M, Bradshaw L, Logan P, Elliott R, Gladman JRF. 2014. Health status of UK care home residents: a cohort study. Age and Ageing, 43, 97–103.

Grasbeck A, Englund E, Horstmann V, Passant U, Gustafson L. 2003. Predictors of mortality in frontotemporal dementia: a retrospective study of the prognostic influence of pre-diagnostic features. International Journal of Geriatric Psychiatry, 18(7), 594–601.

Hoben M, Kent A, Kobagi N, Yoon MN. 2016. Effective strategies to motivate nursing home residents in oral health care and to prevent or reduce responsive behaviours to oral health care: a systematic review protocol. BMJ Open, 6(3), e011159.

Humbert IA, Robbins J. 2008. Dysphagia in the elderly. Phys Med Rehabil Clin N Am, 19(4), 853–866.

Ide M, Harris M, Stevens A, Sussams R, et al. 2016. Periodontitis and Cognitive Decline in Alzheimer's Disease. PLoS One, 11(3), e0151081.

Isaksson R, Paulsson G, Fridlund B, Nederfors T. 2000. Evaluation of an oral health education program for nursing personnel in special housing facilities for the elderly. Part II: clinical aspects. Special Care Dentistry, 20, 109–113.

Jablonski RA, Kolanowski AM, Litaker M. 2011a. Profile of nursing home residents with dementia who require assistance with mouth care. Geriatr Nurs, 32(6), 439–446.

Jablonski RA, Therrien B, Mahoney EK, Kolanowski A, Gabello M, Brock A. 2011b. An intervention to reduce care-resistant behavior in persons with dementia during oral hygiene: a pilot study. Spec Care Dentist, 31(3), 77–87.

Kamer AR, Craig RG, Dasanayake AP, Brys M, Glodzik-Sobanska L, de Leon MJ. 2008. Inflammation and Alzheimer's disease: possible role of periodontal diseases. Alzheimers Dement, 4(4), 242–250.

Keller H. 1993. Malnutrition in institutionalized elderly: how and why? Journal of the American Geriatric Society, 41, 1212.

Kelly M, Steele J, Nuttall N, Bradnock G, et al. 2000. *Adult Dental Health Survey Oral Health in the United Kingdom*, London: The Stationery Office.

Kieser J, Jones G, Borlase G, MacFadyen E. 1999. Dental treatment of patients with neurodegenerative disease. N Z Dent J, 95, 130–134.

Komulainen K, Ylöstalo P, Syrjälä AM, Ruoppi P, et al. 2014. Oral health intervention among community-dwelling older people: A randomised 2-year intervention study. Gerodontology, 34, 19–26.

Lapeer GL. 1998. Dementia's impact on pain sensation: a serious clinical dilemma for dental geriatric caregivers. J Can Dent Assoc, 64, 182–184, 187–192.

Lindqvist L, Seleskog B, Wårdh I, von Bültzingslöwen I. 2013. Oral care perspectives of professionals in nursing homes for the elderly. Int J Dent Hyg, 11(4), 298–305.

Locker D. 2002. Changes in chewing ability with ageing: a 7-year study of older adults. J Oral Rehabil, 29(11), 1021–1029.

Logemann JA. 1998. The evaluation and treatment of swallowing disorders. Current Opinion in Otolaryngology & Head and Neck Surgery, 6, 395–400.

Matear DW, Clarke D. 1999. Considerations for the use of oral sedation in the institutionalized geriatric patient during dental interventions: a review of the literature. Spec Care Dentist, 19, 56–63.

McGrath C, Bedi R. 1999. The importance of oral health to older people's quality of life. Gerodontology, 16, 59–63.

Monaghan N, Morgan MZ. 2010. Oral health policy and access to special care dentistry in care homes. Journal of Disability and Oral Health, 11, 61–68.

Moody GH. 1990. Alzheimer's disease. Br Dent J, 169, 45–47.

Morgan MZ, Johnson IG, Hitchings E, Monaghan NP, Karki AJ. 2015. Dentist skill and setting to address dental treatment needs of care home residents in Wales. Gerodontology, February, doi:10.1111/ger.12185 (e-pub ahead of print).

NHS Health Scotland. 2013. *Caring for Smiles: Guide for Care Homes,* available at www.nes.scot.nhs.uk/media/2603965/caring_for_smiles_guide_for_care_homes.pdf (accessed 3 Oct 2016).

NICE. 2016. Oral Health for Adults in Care Homes, available at www.nice.org.uk/guidance/ng48/resources/oral-health-for-adults-in-care-homes-1837459547845 (accessed 3 Oct 2016).

Nogueira D, Reis E. 2013. Swallowing disorders in nursing home residents: how can the problem be explained? Clin Interv Aging, 8, 221–227.

Ocasio NA, Solomowitz BH, Sher MR. 2000. Dental management of the patient with Alzheimer's disease. N Y State Dent J, 66, 32–35.

Oliver D. 2015. *Allied Health Professionals Are Critical to New Models of Care,* King's Fund blog, 1 December.

Pajukoski H, Meurman J, Snellman-Gröhn S, Sulkava R. 1999. Oral health in hospitalized and non-hospitalized community dwelling elderly patients. Oral Surg. Oral Med. Oral Pathol. Oral Radiol. Endod, 88, 437–443.

Paley GA, Slack-Smith L, O'Grady M. 2009. Oral health care issues in aged care facilities in Western Australia: resident and family caregiver views. Gerodontology, 26, 97–104.

Philip P, Rogers C, Kruger E, Tennant M. 2012a. Caries experience of institutionalized elderly and its association with dementia and functional status. Int J Dent Hyg, 10(2), 122–127.

Philip P, Rogers C, Kruger E, Tennant M. 2012b. Oral hygiene care status of elderly with dementia and in residential aged care facilities. Gerodontology, 29(2), e306–311.

Porter J, Ntouva A, Read A, Murdoch M, Ola D, Tsakos G. 2015. The impact of oral health on the quality of life of nursing home residents. Health Qual Life Outcomes, 13, 102.

Portella FF, Rocha AW, Haddad DC, Fortes CB, et al. 2013. Oral hygiene caregivers' educational programme improves oral health conditions in institutionalised independent and functional elderly. Gerodontology.

Preston AJ, Gosney MA, Noon S, Martin MV. 1999. Oral flora of elderly patients following acute medical admission. Gerontology, 45, 49–52.

Priefer BA, Robbins J. 1997. Eating changes in mild-stage Alzheimer's disease: a pilot study. Dysphagia, 12(4), 212–221.

Rejnefelt I, Andersson P, Renvert S. 2006. Oral health status in individuals with dementia living in special facilities. Int J Dent Hyg, 4, 67–71.

Rofes L, Arreola V, Almirall J, Cabre M, et al. 2011. Diagnosis and management of oropharyngeal dysphagia and its nutritional and respiratory complications in the elderly. Gastroenterol Res Pract, 818979.

Rösler A, Lessmann H, von Renteln-Kruse W, Stansschuss S. 2008. Dysphagia and dementia: disease severity and degree of dysphagia as assessed by fiberoptic endoscopy. Eur J Geriatr, 31, 127–130.

Rösler A, Pfeil S, Lessmann H, Höder J, Befahr A, von Renteln-Kruse W. 2015. Dysphagia in dementia: influence of dementia severity and food texture on the prevalence of aspiration and latency to swallow in hospitalized geriatric patients. J Am Med Dir Assoc, 16(8), 697–701.

Saub R, Evans RW. 2001. Dental needs of elderly hostel residents in inner Melbourne. Aust Dent J, 46, 198–202.

Scully C. 2010. *Medical Problems in Dentistry*, London: Elsevier Health Sciences.

Shay K, Ship JA. 1995. The importance of oral health in the older patient. J Ameriatr Soc, 43(12), 1414–1422.

Shimazaki Y, Soh I, Saito T, Yamashita Y, et al. 2001. Influence of dentition status on physical disability, mental impairment, and mortality in institutionalized elderly people. J Dent Res, 80, 340–345.

Ship JA. 1992. Oral health of patients with Alzheimer's disease. J Am Dent Assoc, 123, 53–58.

Ship JA, DeCarli C, Friedland RP, Baum BJ. 1990. Diminished submandibular salivary flow in dementia of Alzheimer type. J Gerontol Med Sci, 45, 61–66.

Suh MK, Kim H, Na DL. 2009. Dysphagia in patients with dementia: Alzheimer versus vascular. Alzheimer Disease and Associated Disorders, 23(2), 178–184.

Unluer S, Gokalp S, Dogan BG. 2007. Oral health status of the elderly in a residential home in Turkey. Gerodontology, 24, 22–29.

van der Maarel-Wierink CD, Vanobbergen JNO, Bronkhorst EM, Schols JMGA, de Baat C. 2011. Risk factors for aspiration pneumonia in frail older people: a systematic literature review. J. Am. Med. Dir. Assoc, 12, 344–354.

van der Putten GJ, De Visschere L, Schols J, de Baat C, Vanobbergen J. 2010. Supervised versus non-supervised implementation of an oral health care guideline in (residential) care homes: a cluster randomized controlled clinical trial. BMC Oral Health, 10, 17.

Walker RJ, Kiyak HA. 2007. The impact of providing dental services to frail older adults: perceptions of elders in adult day health centers. Spec Care Dent, 27, 139–143.

Weijenberg RA, Lobbezoo F, Knol DL, Tomassen J, Scherder EJ. 2013. Increased masticatory activity and quality of life in elderly persons with dementia – a longitudinal matched cluster randomized single-blind multicenter intervention study. BMC Neurol, 13, 26.

Welsh S, Edwards M, Hunter L. 2012. Caring for smiles – a new educational resource for oral health training in care homes. Gerodontology, 29(2), e1161–1162.

Welte T, Torres A, Nathwani D. 2012. Clinical and economic burden of community-acquired pneumonia among adults in Europe. Thorax, 67, 71–79.

White D, Pitts N, Steele J, Sadler K, Chadwick B. 2011. *Disease and Related Disorders – A Report from the Adult Dental Health Survey 2009*, London: The Health and Social Care Information Centre.

WHO. 2003. World Oral Health Report, available at www.who.int/oral_health/publications/report03/en (accessed 3 Oct 2016).

Wyatt CC. 2002. Elderly Canadians residing in long-term care hospitals. Part II: dental caries status. J Can Dent Assoc, 68, 359–363.

Yi Mohammadi JJ, Franks K, Hines S. 2015. Effectiveness of professional oral health care intervention on the oral health of residents with dementia in residential aged care facilities: a systematic review protocol. JBI Database System Rev Implement Rep, 13(10), 110–122.

Zenthöfer A, Cabrera T, Rammelsberg P, Hassel AJ. 2015. Improving oral health of institutionalized older people with diagnosed dementia. Aging Ment Health, February, 1–6 (e-pub ahead of print).

Zimmerman S, Sloane PD, Cohen LW, Barrick AL. 2014. Changing the culture of mouth care: mouth care without a battle. Gerontologist, 54(Suppl 1), S25–34.

— Chapter 7 ————————————————————

LIVING WELL AND PROMOTING WELLBEING

Learning objectives ————————————————

By the end of this chapter, you will:

- » be able to explain activity theory, and define occupation, activity engagement and continuity

- » understand the importance of promoting wellbeing through diverse channels including: arts, drama and theatre; aromatherapy; dancing; exercise and physical activity; the enjoyment of gardens and horticultural therapy; massage; humour therapy; and music therapy

- » be able to understand how promoting wellbeing might be adapted to suiting an individual's (changing) needs

- » appreciate the importance of physical activity, independence and access to outdoor spaces

—— Introduction ————————————————

Implementing care innovations is not always a matter of course (Burgio et al., 2001a, b). The culture of a care home appears to have a strong influence on the range and quality of activities available. One review of the successful implementation of psychosocial interventions in dementia care pointed out that post-implementation sustainability is given little consideration in implementation studies (Boersma et al., 2014).

But residential settings, as well as care at home, should above all promote wellbeing in accordance with section 1(1) of the Care Act 2014:

1 Promoting individual wellbeing

(1) The general duty of a local authority, in exercising a function under this Part in the case of an individual, is to promote that individual's wellbeing.[1]

A holistic perspective of the person through a multidimensional assessment is now helping to guide rehabilitation and inspire future research. A multidimensional assessment allows for person-centred rehabilitation while considering the individual's activities and participation (Rocha et al., 2013). A need to engage in activity is intrinsic to human beings. People with dementia are no exception, but they often need carers' help to participate (Kitwood, 1997). Everyone has an inbuilt need to participate in activity, and what we do makes us who we are. Engaging in a balance of self-care, work and play activities is essential to our physical and mental wellbeing and quality of life. People with dementia are no exception.

Despite improvements in nursing home policies and programmes regarding quality of care and quality of life over the past 30 years, some of which have been somewhat circular, research continues to show that older adults living in nursing homes spend the majority of their time during the day performing passive activities (e.g. sleeping, doing nothing, fidgeting, waiting, glancing at a television) and exhibiting little emotion (Leedahl, Chapin and Little, 2015). Data from a converging number of studies indicate that residents are frequently unoccupied in these settings. It is not unusual to find residents who are capable of independent activity sitting or lying down for long periods of time (MacRae, Schnelle and Ouslander, 1996). This is incredible. To date, the provision of occupational therapy within UK care homes has been an underdeveloped area of practice but has recently gained more momentum (Wenborn et al., 2013). An increase in occupational therapy provision has previously been recommended, recognising the potential to prevent falls, improve function (Royal College of Physicians, Royal College of Nursing and British Geriatrics Society, 2000) and enhance activity (Mozley et al., 2004). A focus on the human dimension can be lost amid large-scale institutional priorities. Insufficient attention to the psychosocial aspects of service use can threaten identities that have already been compromised by the disease (Lloyd and Stirling, 2015). In long-term care for people with dementia, reaching the best possible quality of life is generally perceived as the primary goal. Health care professionals and researchers alike have placed great value on the idea that activity can be beneficial for persons with dementia (Nolan, Grant and Nolan, 1995).

But it would be amazing to aspire to 'universalise the best', as Nye Bevan once put it.

Andrea Sutcliffe is chief inspector for social care at the Care Quality Commission (CQC). In a blogpost from 2 June 2016 entitled 'The art of being outstanding', she

---

1   See www.legislation.gov.uk/ukpga/2014/23/section/1/enacted (accessed 4 Oct 2016).

has given inspirational examples of the promotion of wellbeing through creativity, quoting from the relevant CQC reports that are all available on the CQC website.

» Peregrine House, Whitby – 'A varied programme of activity: Zumba, Motivation, large drafts or Connect 4, film events, afternoon tea, pampering sessions, and music. The home supported them to run clubs such as poetry, walking, reading, gardening, Scrabble and singing.'

» Prince of Wales House, Ipswich – 'Staff were finding creative ways to support people to live a full life – this included aromatherapy, music therapy, and foot, hand and head massage.'

» Deansfield Residential Care Home, Telford – 'People's individual histories and personalities were valued and made part of their lives, for example, people had a personalised place mat which they had helped make.'

» The Old Hall, Billingborough – 'Reflecting the training they had received… the staff member told us of the importance of music in stimulating memory in people living with dementia… People were supported to attend local groups such as art classes and choirs that they had enjoyed being part of before they moved into the home.'

Sutcliffe further notes: 'A key feature of the outstanding services we see is their person-centred approach which enables people to live full and meaningful lives […] so I was delighted last week to be invited to speak at the 2016 Arts in the Care Home conference.'

—— Meaningful activity and engagement ——

Activity theory has long held that older adults who remain engaged in the world around them experience increased levels of psychological and physical wellbeing as compared to those who are less involved (Havighurst and Albrecht, 1953). This position has been influential in the field of dementia care where the concept of meaningful activity has become ubiquitous. Activities do not need to be structured or complicated. The presence of meaningful activities is a quality indicator for the NHS (Bradshaw, Playford and Riazi, 2012). The scope of 'activity' is diverse, consisting of household chores, recreation, work-related endeavours and social involvement; what makes it meaningful is doing things that matter, the sense of pleasure, connection and the autonomy associated with activity participation, regardless of the level of dependency or cognitive impairment (Roland and Chappell, 2015).

Engaging with meaningful activity can help with coping, and this has been researched in young onset dementia (for a schematic view, see Figure 7.1).

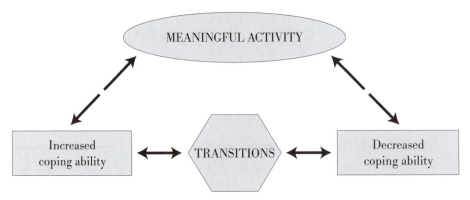

Figure 7.1: The relationship between meaningful activity and transition in early onset dementia

This model illustrates the relationships between the emergent themes and how meaningful activity (with or without the expectation of value from participation in such meaningful activity) can affect a family's coping ability through the transitions experienced in early onset dementia.
Source: from Roach, Drummond and Keady (2016, Fig. 1).

According to a wide range of wellbeing theories, involvement in activities plays an important role in reaching a good quality of life for people in general (Gerritsen et al., 2007). But the focus of the activity at any particular time must be on the person, and not the task.

Table 7.1 provides an overview of 'meaningful' activities.

Table 7.1: Meaningful activities for people with dementia that address fundamental psychological needs according to developmental psychological theory

Meaningful activities for people with dementia	Fundamental psychological needs being addressed
Life review therapy and life story work	Need for life review
Spiritual/religious activities	Need to place continuity of life in context and need for death preparation
Intergenerational activities	Need for intergenerational relationships, particularly understanding of family and friends
Reacquaintance with previously conducted leisure activities	Need for sense of control and to achieve life goals, and for physical activity and exercise
Pursuit of new leisure activities	Need to be creative and pursue wellbeing

SOURCE: ADAPTED FROM NYMAN AND SZYMCZYNSKA (2016, TABLE 1).

People with dementia use professional supports for daytime activities and social company, but available services for such may not be meaningful or valued by individuals with dementia or be matched to individuals' varied interests and abilities (Hancock et al., 2006).

The interaction between residents and others is very important for the development of social capital (see Figure 7.2).

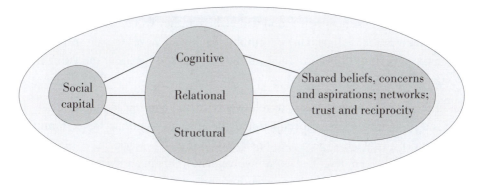

Figure 7.2: Cognitive social capital refers to shared
understandings, values and beliefs

Relational social capital is represented by the characteristics of
relationships such as trust and cooperation. Individuals who trust each
other are more likely to work together in a cooperative manner.
Source: after Dicicco-Bloom et al. (2007, Fig. 1, p.16),
cited in White, Cornish and Kert (2015).

Examples of ways of promoting wellbeing through meaningful activities might include:

» hobbies and crafts: crossword puzzles, painting, gardening, picking berries, visiting a garden centre, knitting or other crafts

» exercise: going for walks, trying yoga or tai chi, or going for a swim

» reminiscing: talking about old times, watching family videos, going through photo albums, making a life story book

» daily tasks and chores: baking together, cleaning up together such as sweeping, wiping the table, folding towels, polishing silverware

» music: listening to favourite music, dancing, singing along.

Engagement in activities is assumed to generate feelings of fulfilment and meaning in life (Westerhof et al., 2010). The question of the meaning of these activities for people with dementia has not been directly addressed. Moreover, most of this research has been conducted in formal care settings with severely impaired individuals, even though the majority of people with dementia live in their own homes (Phinney, Chaudhury and O'Connor, 2007). Indeed, participating in activities may be more important to the psychological wellbeing of people with dementia than the general physical and social environment (Marshall and Hutchinson, 2001).

It is difficult to ignore the impact of activities on general health and wellbeing. One example is a personal view given by Sarah Crockett (2013):

> People may have better continence or better bowel regulation, be more motivated, or calmer, their mood will be better, they will be able to express themselves, they will remain safely mobile for longer, have less pain and have fewer periods of ill health. They will be happier and healthier individuals. (p.23)

Crockett then provides very easy to follow advice on planning activities.

The preventive value of occupational therapy interventions for community-living older people has been demonstrated in the US (Jackson et al., 1998). Occupation has been described as an involvement in life in a way that is personally significant and that engages time, attention and environment (Smit et al., 2015). Occupational therapists define occupations as the activities that we need or choose to do that allow us to live as independently as possible, from self-care to employment, hobbies and interests. A lack of occupation can lead to boredom, apathy, distressed response, a lack of confidence, social exclusion and solitude. Occupation should incorporate meaningful activities; these can be defined as enjoyable activities that engage the resident to the extent that they improve either their emotional wellbeing, cognitive status or their physical function (Morley et al., 2014).

Activity engagement of long-term care residents is not only recognised as an indicator of quality of care, but also through the lens of promoting wellbeing and social interaction. Sometimes it is even assumed that a lack of activity involvement will cause excess disability, meaning more loss of skills and functional capacities than can be explained by the disease on its own (Wells and Dawson, 2000). Activity involvement seems to be beneficial for people with dementia in relation to the care relationship (a resident accepts help, no conflicts with the care staff), positive affect (a resident is relatively content with a positive mood), social networks (has friendly contact with other residents) and having something to do (has things to do without help from others) (Smit et al., 2016). Brooker, Wooley and Lee (2007) have developed a model to stimulate sustainable activities for people with dementia living in long-term care: the Enriched Opportunities Programme. This model is highly impressive and innovative and has been carefully built up by the triangulation of evidence for each element of the programme from the published literature, expert opinion and from feedback from practice (Vernooji-Dassen, 2007).

How wellbeing is promoted in activities is relevant to the mental health of residents (first introduced in Chapter 4). Residents who displayed agitation and/or apathy were more likely to be excluded from activity programmes (Buettner, 1988). Newly admitted nursing home residents with depression were found to have low social engagement, independent of other risk factors (Achterberg et al., 2003). Cognitive impairment and deficits in physical function, as well as visual and hearing deficits, also predicted low engagement (Schroll et al., 1997).

Finally, continuity is vitally important in behaviours promoting wellbeing. Being allowed to carry on with everyday activities for as long as possible will not only help the person hold on to these skills and encourage independence, but will allow him or her to feel able to contribute and know that the help is valued. The challenge of evaluating complex interventions aimed at changing the culture within real-life settings has been discussed previously (Fossey et al., 2006).

Promoting wellbeing

Arts, drama and theatre

The general perception now is that artists and arts organisations are clearly taking a lead in developing creative responses to the challenge posed by dementia. There is the potential for such programmes to improve a broad range of outcomes, such as: wellbeing, quality of life, cognitive function and creative thinking; increases in communication (including non-verbal), facilitating reminiscences and meaningful conversation; regaining a sense of self; increasing self-esteem; and improving the quality of life of carers. This has been suggested by some studies (e.g. Windle et al., 2014).

Article 30 of the UN Convention of the Rights of People with Disabilities invokes participation in cultural life, recreation, leisure and sport.

Article 30(1) states that:

1. States Parties recognise the right of persons with disabilities to take part on an equal basis with others in cultural life, and shall take all appropriate measures to ensure that persons with disabilities:

a) Enjoy access to cultural materials in accessible formats;

b) Enjoy access to television programmes, films, theatre and other cultural activities, in accessible formats;

c) Enjoy access to places for cultural performances or services, such as theatres, museums, cinemas, libraries and tourism services, and, as far as possible, enjoy access to monuments and sites of national cultural importance.

Within dementia care, artistic expressions such as music, pictorial art and dance have been shown to have a positive influence on patients' quality of life (Gjengedal et al., 2014). The arts in their widest sense can touch on so many attributes of excellent care and quality of life: the value of active ageing, choice and control, independence and interdependence, creativity, lifelong learning, identity, confidence, friendship, emotional stimulation, intellectual fulfilment and sensory pleasures. Arts-based activities represent a range of activities, including dance, music, creative writing, visual art and singing (Windle et al., 2014). According to a review of creative therapies for people with dementia (including music, art, drama and dance therapy), many positive effects were found from participation, such as the improvement of interaction skills and people coming to terms and coping better with dementia (Salisbury, Algar and Windle, 2011). The capacity of art to open up for new knowledge is described in a variety of settings, but the use of such performances seems, however, to be less widespread in research related to dementia care (Gjengedal et al., 2014).

Drama is both a method and a subject, seen from an holistic perspective, and integrates thoughts, feelings and actions. It includes, for example, group activity in fictional role-play, where the participants can learn to explore issues, events and relationships (O'Toole and Lepp, 2000). Drama has been used as a method within nursing education and is also suggested to be used in clinical settings. Other results showed that drama can be a means to enhance reflection among staff in residential care for people with dementia (Bolmsjö, Edberg and Andersson, 2014).

Interestingly, crafts are beneficial as memory triggers in reminiscence sessions with older women in residential care who have severe symptoms of dementia and had enjoyed crafting as a leisure activity during their lifetime (Pöllänen and Hirsimäki, 2014). Despite attempts to identify meaningful activities in residential care and find meaningful ways of initiating reminiscence in persons with dementia, little is known about craft-focused reminiscence in residential care settings. There is therefore an identifiable need for more research and practical innovation (e.g. Gitlin et al., 2010).

Finally, a truly great example of the organic growth of a dementia-friendly community, through dementia-friendly performances, is described in Box 7.1 on the West Yorkshire Playhouse.

Box 7.1: Extracts from *West Yorkshire Playhouse Guide to Dementia-Friendly Performances*

In 2014 West Yorkshire Playhouse pioneered the UK/world's first dementia-friendly performance – a mainstream theatre show specifically adapted to meet the needs of people living with dementia and their supporters. All aspects of the production were considered from stage action, technical cues, front of house support and pre-show creative engagement.

INTRODUCTION

The best people to inform dementia-friendly adaptations are people with dementia. They are experts in living with the condition, and we advocate strongly for any theatre considering this approach to consult with people with dementia to ensure decisions are made with them, not for them.

Many people with dementia have spent a lifetime attending theatre, concerts and music halls. A diagnosis of dementia can reduce confidence and increase isolation, leaving people with dementia and their supporters less likely to attempt such trips. As life becomes more mundane, these stimulating, meaningful activities assume greater importance, and present significantly increased potential for enriching lives.

Our aspiration is to increase opportunities for people with dementia to access life-enhancing shows, reconnecting them to their local cultural venues and their communities. We hope theatres across the UK and beyond will find this practical guide an inspiration in advocating for and staging dementia-friendly performances.

MEET AND GREETS

If possible, give your audience the opportunity to meet the company immediately after the show.

This has proved to be a consistent highlight for audience and company members alike. It is a unique chance for people with dementia and their supporters to feel valued and excited, while company members have found, often unexpectedly, a renewed connectedness both with the audience and within the company itself.

Obviously, nothing is compulsory – some company members may have a familial connection with someone living with dementia, and may not wish to engage in the meet and greet. Similarly, some audience members may have transport waiting for them and will be keen to leave immediately.

This variation will facilitate an unhurried, calm emptying of the auditorium, allowing more staff to assist those who are leaving than would be available if everyone exited at the same time.

SOURCE: REPRODUCED FROM TAYLOR (2016) BY KIND PERMISSION.

Engage & Create is a social enterprise dedicated to transforming the quality of life for people with dementia.[2] Ignite Sessions are a tool for engaging people at all stages of dementia, using artworks from gallery and museum collections to spark discussion. These unique sessions offer people with dementia a social experience whatever stage they are at, where the focus is on response, not remembering, and where they can be heard and understood. The versatility of Ignite Sessions means the sessions can be delivered in either a gallery for the more able, as a focus activity in a care home, and even one-to-one at the bedside in hospitals.

---

2   See www.sinc.co.uk/member-directory/engage-create (accessed 4 Oct 2016).

Aromatherapy

Aromatherapy is a non-pharmacological intervention, but it may lie in the grey area between medicine and care along with a number of other complementary therapies (Johannessen, 2013). It is well known that all the five human senses can deteriorate as part of the normal ageing process. However, limited knowledge arguably exists about how the senses change due to dementia, except for olfactory and gustatory dysfunction, which are well documented (Wittmann-Price, 2012). NICE recommends the use of aromatherapy for the behavioural and psychological symptoms of dementia (NICE, 2006), although it has been pointed out that, as olfaction tends to decline in dementia, this may not be an appropriate intervention (Vance, 2003). According to a recent Cochrane review on aromatherapy and dementia, the benefits of aromatherapy for people with dementia are at best 'equivocal' from the seven trials meeting the eligibility criteria (Forrester et al., 2014). It is important to note there were several methodological difficulties with the included studies, such as whether different aromatherapy interventions are comparable and the possibility that outcomes may vary for different types of dementia.

The use of aromatherapy (particularly lavender, rosemary and lemon balm) in dementia is widespread, with much case-based evidence for positive effects in sleep and agitation; however, there is a lack of high-quality trials in the field (Holmes and Ballard, 2004). The oil *Lavendula augustifolia* is one of the most commonly used and cited essential oils, with a number of studies indicating that lavender can decrease stress and pain intensity; it can also assist by reducing insomnia (Lewith, Godfrey and Prescott 2005). Lavender has been postulated to exert a direct action on tryptophan, the precursor of serotonin, which helps put people to sleep (Zeilmann et al., 2003). It has also been reported that the essential oil of lemon affects the antioxidant action of vitamin E and improves the state of blood vessels near the skin (Grassman et al., 2001).

In terms of the functional neuroanatomy of the human brain, the olfactory bulb links to the amygdala, and thus some smells may trigger positive or negative emotional states depending on the person's past experience of the smell (Holmes and Ballard, 2004). With these neural pathways, aromatherapy can mediate our emotional responses by inhalation alone (Snow, Hovanec and Brandt, 2004). This theory may explain why aromatherapy works for people with dementia, who may have an impaired sense of smell.

Dancing

Ravelin and colleagues have defined dance in the following way: *dance is a culturally acquired human resource* (Ravelin, Kylma and Korhonen, 2006; Ravelin, Isola and Kylmä, 2013). It is creative and unique, but also universal. Dance contains bodily expression of the self, emotions and stories in interaction with the self and others. Dance as a method of intervention in nursing can promote understanding of the self as well as social interaction.

Ageing adults, whether living with dementia or not, tend to undergo age-related changes in joint range-of-motion, strength, sensory processing and sensorimotor integration which contribute to balance impairments with increasing age. Residents of nursing homes represent one of the most vulnerable, often functionally impaired, populations of older adults who are at high risk of further decline leading to a complete loss of independence and other related deleterious consequences (Ferrucci et al., 2004). Physical therapists have expressed moderate-to-high agreement that dance could positively impact clients' physiological and psychological states, thus facilitating long-term participation and corresponding health benefits (Abreu and Hartley, 2013). Several studies have explored the effects of dance on mental health, balance, fall risk and function (Hackney and Earhart, 2010). Also, the emotional effects of social dancing have been comprehensively described (Palo-Bengtsson and Ekman, 2000, 2002) (see Figure 7.3).

Dance research has highlighted improvements in physical health and shown increases in social activity among healthy older adults (Bertram and Stickley, 2007; Keogh et al., 2009). In addition to physical and motor skill activities, dance engages cognitive functions, including perception, emotion and memory (Dhami, Moreno and DeSouza, 2014). A longitudinal study has even reported that dancing reduced the risk of developing dementia (Verghese et al., 2003). Anecdotal reports of the benefits of dancing in care homes (Hirsh, 1990), such as the use of line dance (Hayes, 2006), circle dance or ballet (Lehner, 2006), have suggested that the sense of togetherness and socialisation have improved in people with dementia. Dance is therefore currently very promising as an efficient, effective and exhilarating physical therapy intervention, with inherent sources of motivation for long-term neurological and orthopaedic patients in a hospital or community setting (Hecox, Levine and Scott, 1976). It could be beneficial to develop programmes that promote dancing as a form of exercise in ageing adults to increase activity level and exercise compliance, and possibly increase function (Abreu and Hartley, 2013). Their inclusion in the daily life of care homes is therefore much to be welcomed.

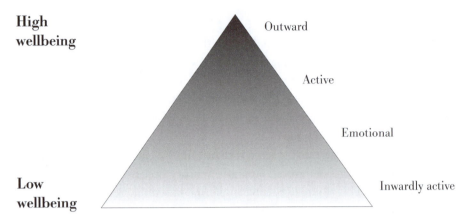

Figure 7.3: Triangle of supportive environments
Source: redrawn from Bengtsson and Grahn (2014, Fig. 1, p.879).

Exercise and physical activity

Exercise and physical activity are complicated.

Physical activity is of special interest. It has been identified as relevant to many health outcomes, including: cardiorespiratory health (coronary heart disease, cardiovascular disease, stroke and hypertension); metabolic health (diabetes and obesity); musculoskeletal health (bone health, osteoporosis); cancer (breast and colon cancer); functional health and the prevention of falls; and depression (WHO, 2010). There has been growing recognition that physical inactivity is reaching global pandemic proportions, with sequelae in morbidity and mortality, requiring collaborative solutions (Ding et al., 2016).

Physical activity should be distinguished from physical exercise which is planned, structured and repetitive and has the objective of improving or maintaining physical fitness (Caspersen, Powell and Christenson, 1985). This is not to say that physical activity interventions need to await further scientific study – there are strong indications of benefits in terms of wellbeing and quality of life, and in terms of physical benefits such as improved balance (preventing falls) and grip strength (supporting independence in activities of daily living) (Bowes et al., 2013). The importance of physical, functional, psychological and social factors in realising a healthy old age is recognised by elderly people, health care professionals and policymakers (Beswick et al., 2008).

Physical activity is often described as 'any bodily movement produced by skeletal muscle that results in energy expenditure' (Saarloos et al., 2008, p.79) and encompasses all activity, such as walking for transport or cleaning the house, whereas exercise is defined as 'a subset of physical activity consisting of planned, structured, repetitive bodily movements with the purpose of improving or maintaining one or more components of physical fitness or health' (Dishman, Heath and Lee, 2013, p.559). There is a vast amount of evidence supporting the role of physical activity in assisting older people to regain or better maintain mobility and functional independence (Burton, Lewin and Boldy, 2015). In addition to reducing the risk of chronic illness, minimising the risk of falls and feeling better mentally (reduced negative moods, higher positive moods, lower anxiety levels) and physically, it is necessary to sustain strength, balance and mobility in one's latter years to live independently without assistance (Gillespie et al., 2012; Robertson et al., 2012).

According to a recent Cochrane review, physical rehabilitation for long-term care residents may be effective, reducing disability with few adverse events, but the effects appear to be quite small and may not be applicable to all residents (Crocker et al., 2013). Moreover, an exercise programme may yield benefits in the management of falls, malnutrition, behavioural disturbances and depression, key problems for people with Alzheimer's disease (Rolland et al., 2007).

Three studies have addressed the effects of the spatial layout of nursing homes on residents' level of physical activity (McAllister and Silverman, 1999; Milke et al., 2009; Zuidema et al., 2010). In the UK, regular exercise therapy is not routinely available to care home residents (Sackley, Gatt and Walker, 2001; Brittle et al., 2009). A controlled study by Alessi et al. (1995) revealed that physical activity helped reduce daytime agitation and night-time restlessness in care home residents with incontinence. A controlled trial of older adults with dementia in a nursing home by Sung and colleagues (2010, 2011) found the forms of movement and music preferred by the patients were beneficial in managing agitation and recommended that these be incorporated into care routines.

Gardens and horticultural therapy

The idea that **gardens** can have calming, restorative and even healing effects is certainly not new to Western medicine. In Victorian Britain, gardens were an important feature of many psychiatric hospitals (Burton, 2014). Public health and urban development strategies have yet to conceive of ways that optimise nature as a health resource for older adults and to realise the full benefits of contact with nature as an upstream health promotion intervention (Maller et al., 2005). The background is that nursing home residents have expressed the loss of freedom, loss of control, feelings of loneliness and a sense of failure at having to stay in nursing homes (Kellett, 1999; Tse, 2007). Moving to and living in a nursing home is a difficult experience for many people. It is likely to be traumatic and depressing for those already struggling with loss of health or ill health, pain, dependency and limited social and material resources (Grek, 2008).

The terms sensory garden and therapeutic garden have slightly different nuances (Gonzalez and Kirkevold, 2014). The label sensory garden refers to the idea that the garden should stimulate the senses, for example sight, vision, hearing, smell and touch. The term therapeutic garden refers to the anticipated benefits of its use, including reducing behaviour problems and improving sleep–wake patterns and muscle strength (e.g. Detweiler et al., 2008), and the effects of therapeutic gardens are truly fascinating. It can be argued that the garden promotes more interaction between staff and residents and also between visitors and residents, and that this is the important factor and not the garden itself. The notion that therapeutic gardens are the environmental change that best promotes the increase in these interactions and are thus pivotal in residents' quality of life can be equally argued (Edwards, McDonnell and Merl, 2013).

Therapeutic landscapes promote physical wellbeing, mental wellbeing and social wellbeing (detailed in Table 7.2).

Table 7.2: Aspects of therapeutic landscapes

Physical wellbeing	Motivated physical activity for both recreation and purposeful exercise. Sense of improved physical health. Daily gardening, in the hope of reducing the incidence of dementia in future years (Simons et al., 2006).
Mental wellbeing	Sense of improved psychological health. Feelings of renewal, restoration and rejuvenation. There has been interest in the therapeutic effects of gardening on mental health in general (Shiue et al., 2016).
Social wellbeing	Essential for social interactions (e.g. planned with family and friends, unplanned with neighbours). Pleasant collective experience of nature (social inclusion; community).

SOURCE: BASED ON FINLAY ET AL. (2015, TABLE 1, P.99).

Horticultural therapy and exposure to gardens have been shown to have positive benefits for the elderly. Indoor gardening has been reported to be effective in improving sleep, agitation and cognition in persons with dementia (Detweiler et al., 2012). Although the theoretical and policy support for the application of horticultural therapy in the holistic care of people with dementia is arguably strong, it remains a relatively overlooked element in dementia care and research, particularly within a community context (Noone et al., 2015). The availability of gardens or outdoor areas at residential homes may offer a range of benefits for people with dementia, including opportunities for active engagement with gardening, walking in an outdoor environment and sitting in soothing surroundings (Whear et al., 2014).

A growing awareness of the importance of access to outdoor environments for people with dementia has developed in recent years, with dementia researchers and care providers acknowledging that contact with the natural world is an essential component of holistic dementia care (Schwarz and Rodiek, 2007). Evidence-based design often takes a salutogenic perspective. Salutogenesis is the study of health development, and thus salutogenic strategies include efforts to create, enhance and improve physical, mental and social wellbeing and to move towards optimal wellbeing (Antonovsky, 1979, 1996). Visiting an outdoor garden has been shown to reduce agitation in nursing home residents who pace (Cohen-Mansfield and Werner, 1998, 1999). The longitudinal study by Mooney and Nicell (1992) also found that the use of exterior environments reduced incidents of aggressive behaviour and contributed significantly to a risk management programme.

Activity theory claims that older people who are active in various occupations and in contact with other people become more satisfied and better adapted in later life than those who are less active (Havighurst, 1968). Leaving some empty space in the garden for high-functioning residents to do their own gardening can help get them actively involved in the garden (Heath, 2004). Previous research on garden environments in health care settings has often focused on specific patient groups or people with particular needs. Such research often aims at describing the experience and use of the outdoors or the perceived benefits of using the outdoors, and the results often need to be reinterpreted to be generally applicable to the process of designing outdoor environments in health care settings (Bengtsson and Grahn, 2014). A health-promoting environment is not only accessible and usable. To optimise health, the environment also has to be interesting, attractive and stimulating (Bengtsson and Carlsson, 2013). Rehabilitation in dementia care is mainly carried out indoors. However, the outdoor environment around a nursing home can be a supplementary environment for treatment, rehabilitation and increasing the quality of life for older persons (Thelander et al., 2008). Exposure to nature (e.g. looking through a window, walking by a park) and actively participating outdoors (e.g. gardening, hiking) promotes both physical and mental health (Pretty, 2004; Maller et al., 2005).

Wendy Brewin (2011) has described the Creative Spaces Project. This innovative initiative used outdoor-related activities and the enhancement of the care home gardens to bring residents and staff closer together with people in the community. It helped raise the quality of life for residents and the quality of working life for staff, and it promoted a better understanding of dementia in the community.

> The outdoor-related activities and use of the garden are now incorporated into people's care plans so that they are a natural part of daily living. Staff are more aware of the support that it provides them; they are finding work less stressful because residents are less stressed as they spend more time outdoors or are involved in an indoor activity that relates to the outdoor environment.

It clearly has a pro-social effect too.

> Strong friendships have been formed as a result; the young people are growing up without fear of dementia and other amenities in the area are now looking at improving their outdoor spaces to help engage with the residents and with others in the community.

Creative Spaces' outdoor activities are helping to re-establish connections between the community and the residents of Trevarna, bringing them together and breaking down social barriers. These have inspired new ideas and triggered memories relating to outdoor environments which have been incorporated into a new garden at the care home. This will not only enhance life quality but will also provide a place where community events and activities can take place.

Current guidelines for dementia recommend that specific attention should be paid to the physical environment where people with dementia live, including the design of and access to gardens, indicating that gardens may be a strong element of future care (NICE, 2006). The NHS is increasingly using social prescribing and community referral schemes to refer patients to a range of local non-clinical services and support in local communities, in the knowledge that much of what determines and supports our health is rooted in social and economic factors. There are an increasing number of community garden schemes – for example, the Lambeth GP Food Co-Op covers 11 practices in South London, where patients with long-term conditions work together to grow food, which is sold to King's College Hospital, enabling one set of patients to provide food for others (Buck, 2016). Results suggest that community gardens were perceived by gardeners as providing numerous health benefits, including improved access to food, improved nutrition, increased physical activity and improved mental health (Wakefield et al., 2007). Community gardens were also seen to promote social health and community cohesion.

Massage

Kitwood has claimed that, in terms of the main psychological needs of people with dementia, love is central, and the five overlapping needs that contribute to this are comfort, attachment, inclusion, occupation and identity (Kitwood, 1997). It can be assumed that closing the distance between the nurse and patient through tactile massage fulfilled the psychological need of attachment (Suzuki et al., 2010). There is a growing body of literature suggesting that complementary and alternative therapies may be effective treatments for reducing stress and inducing comfort in people with dementia. Massage is one such treatment that is thought to be beneficial (Moyle et al., 2014).

Tactile massage, developed by a Swedish nurse named Ardeby and referred to as *taktil massage* in Swedish, is a complementary care method used successfully not only in palliative and geriatric care but also in other health fields to reduce stress (Suzuki et al., 2010). Taylor (1991) defines tactile massage as a series of slow massage strokes applied with firm pressure, mainly using the flat of the hand and fingers. Snyder has shown that hand massage and therapeutic touching did not significantly reduce agitation in elderly patients with dementia in an Alzheimer's care unit during five days of observation, after hand massage and therapeutic touching had been provided once a day in the late afternoon for ten days (Snyder, Egan and Burns, 1995). Massage, in particular, is thought to induce a calming and reassuring sensation, with reduced discomfort and improved mood resulting from the subsequent production of oxytocin (Goldstone, 2000; Uvnās-Moberg, 2004).

A recent Cochrane review found that there was a very limited amount of reliable evidence available in favour of massage and touch interventions for problems associated with dementia. The authors concluded that massage and touch may serve as alternatives or complements to other therapies for the management of behavioural, emotional and perhaps other conditions associated with dementia. More research is needed, however, to provide definitive evidence about the benefits of these interventions (Viggo Hansen, Jørgensen and Ørtenblad, 2006).

In further research, foot massage delivered by a family member or familiar care worker may increase the likelihood of reductions in agitation and aggression (Moyle et al., 2014). A combination of massage, relaxing music and aromatherapy has already been found to be effective in reducing anxiety for emergency nurses (Davis et al., 2005). With massage known to provide relief for patients with chronic pain and already used in this specific population to reduce symptoms associated with dementia and advanced dementia, its use in providing relief of chronic pain for patients with dementia and advanced dementia warrants investigation (Kapoor and Orr, 2015).

Humour therapy

Humour therapy (or laughter therapy, laughter meditation and laughter clubs) has unique implications as group programmes and as self-management techniques. The mechanism by which humour therapy impacts on agitation may be by addressing unmet needs (i.e. for company and meaningful activity) which are thought to be a cause of behavioural disturbance in persons with dementia (Kolanowski et al., 2011).

For practitioners to implement credible programmes and effectively teach self-management techniques, further empirical research on the physical, psychosocial and placebo effects of laughter and humour needs to be conducted (Takeda et al., 2010). Humour can be seen as a specific defence mechanism (see Strotzka, 1956/57), by which positive emotions operate to reduce the undesirable negative emotions involved in a stress situation. The psychological and physiological benefits of humour and laughter are well documented. Although it has been found that humour can decrease fear, stress and anxiety, it can also decrease levels of stress hormones, improve respiration and increase immune function (e.g. Bennett et al., 2003). With this knowledge, researchers and clinicians have tried to implement the use of humour interventions in health care settings (Tan and Schneider, 2009).

Music therapy

The power of music, even in people with pretty advanced dementia, can be striking. The very widely praised film *Alive Inside: A Story of Music and Memory* followed Dan Cohen, a social worker who had decided on a whim to bring iPods to a nursing home.

> Hi, my name is Dan Cohen.
>
> Six years ago I started bringing iPods that were totally personalized to nursing home residents in New York to see what difference it could make in their lives. It was an immediate hit. No matter one's cognitive or physical status, the benefits were clear: ...greater attention and engagement, just a happier state of mind. Families and staff are thrilled when they see their loved ones improve in some way.[3]

The original policy document 'Living Well with Dementia: A National Dementia Strategy' was initially launched in 2009 by the UK Department of Health in order to improve 'the quality of services provided to people with dementia...[and to] promote a greater understanding of the causes and consequences of dementia' (Department of Health, 2009, p.9). The Dementia Strategy focuses both on the individuals and on the community around them, aiming to maximise public awareness of dementia, and ensure high-quality treatment throughout the various stages of the condition (Spiro, Farrant and Pavlicevic, 2015).

Music therapy facilitates intimate emotional-musical communications with those for whom words and language have long ceased to function and works to build flourishing musical communities in residential care homes (Stige et al., 2010).

Music therapy has been defined as 'controlled use of music and its influence on the human being to aid in physiologic, psychologic and emotional integration of the individual during treatment of an illness or disability' (Munro and Mount, 1978, p.1029).

There are two types of music interventions. The first is passive or 'receptive' music therapy, which involves listening only on the part of the recipient (Clark et al., 1998). The second type is active, live or interactive music therapy, which requires individuals to engage in structured sound making (Raglio et al., 2008).

Music in general can have a positive effect on persons with dementia, improving self-esteem, communication, independence, social interaction, participation in meaningful activities, general wellbeing, memory, expression of emotions and alleviation of apathy (van der Vleuten, Visser and Meeuwesen, 2012). Systematic

---

3   See http://icaniwill.alz.co.uk/icaniwill/library/alive-inside-power-music-comes-to-people-with-dementia-via-ipods.html (accessed 4 Oct 2016).

analysis of the role of music in the brain reward circuitry has been explored by many investigators utilising sophisticated neuroimaging tools to dissect specific loci of music activation in the brain (Blum et al., 2016). Music has been shown to influence a broad range of outcomes positively, including alleviating anxiety, promoting relaxation, improving mood, reducing pain, decreasing agitation, improving exercise performance and increasing food intake among various populations (Snyder and Chlan, 1999).

Non-pharmacological interventions such as music therapy, that are person-centred, may be the most effective psychological approach to long-term improvement in the reduction of neuropsychiatric symptoms (Sjogren et al., 2013). A review of the literature by Lou (2001) found that music interventions in six out of seven studies decreased agitation in elderly populations with dementia. Another research study suggests that music decreased patient wandering during treatment sessions (Groene, 1993).

The specific focus of a recent Cochrane review was to assess whether music therapy can diminish behavioural and cognitive problems or improve social and emotional functioning in older people with dementia (Vink et al., 2003). Ten studies have been included in this review which state that music therapy is beneficial for treating older people with dementia. However, the methodological quality of these small, short-term studies was generally poor, as was the presentation of results; no useful conclusions can be drawn.

It is worth noting that concerns exist as to *who* provides music interventions despite the positive, non-invasive aspect of group music interventions. The use of personnel lacking in-depth nursing or musical training conflicts with the nursing paradigm of high-quality, person-centred care and patient safety (Ing-Randolph, Phillips and Williams, 2015). Koger and Brotons (2000) have had similar methodological concerns. No randomised controlled trials, or trials with quantitative data suitable for analysis, were found. The authors concluded that the research into music therapy to date has lacked methodological design rigour.

Following a roundtable discussion in October 2014, the Baring Foundation decided as a first step to undertake a short-term investigation into singing in care homes from the A Choir in Every Care Home project. This would serve a number of aims, including the collation of the existing evidence for the benefits (for staff, family and friends, choir members and residents) of singing/choirs for older people, whether in care homes or in terms of links to the wider community. It would also consider issues of the quality of the artistic experience and the art achieved, with special reference to dementia (Deane, Dawson and Noble, 2015).

—— Essential reading ——

Sutcliffe A. 2016. *The Art of Being Outstanding*, Care Quality Commission blog, 2 June, available at www.cqc.org.uk/content/art-being-outstanding (accessed 3 Oct 2016).

Art, music and creativity

Rahman S. 2015. *Living Better with Dementia*, London: Jessica Kingsley Publishers. Chapter 14, Art, Music and Creativity and Living Better with Dementia, pp.304–320.

Rio R. 2009. *Connecting through Music with People with Dementia: A Guide for Caregivers*, London: Jessica Kingsley Publishers.

General activities

Rahman S. 2014. *Living Well with Dementia*, London: CRC Press. Chapter 10, General Activities that Encourage Wellbeing, pp.161–174.

Leisure activities

Rahman S. 2014. *Living Well with Dementia*, London: CRC Press. Chapter 7, Leisure Activities and Living Well with Dementia, pp.121–132.

Sporting memories

Rahman S. 2015. *Living Better with Dementia*, London: Jessica Kingsley Publishers. Chapter 15, Explaining the Triggering of Sporting Memories in People Living Better with Dementia, pp.304–320.

Other useful books

Baker C. 2014. *Developing Excellent Care for People Living with Dementia in Care Homes*, London: Jessica Kingsley Publishers.

Crockett S. 2013. *Activities for Older People in Care Homes: A Handbook for Successful Activity Planning*, London: Jessica Kingsley Publishers.

Marshall K. 2015. *A Creative Toolkit for Communication in Dementia Care*, London: Jessica Kingsley Publishers.

—— References ——

Abreu M, Hartley G. 2013. The effects of salsa dance on balance, gait, and fall risk in a sedentary patient with Alzheimer's dementia, multiple comorbidities, and recurrent falls. J Geriatr Phys Ther, 36(2), 100–108.

Achterberg W, Pot AM, Kerkstra A, Ooms M, Muller M, Ribbe M. 2003. The effect of depression on social engagement in newly admitted Dutch nursing home residents. Gerontologist, 43(2), 213–218.

Alessi CA, Schnelle JF, MacRae PG, Ouslander JG, et al. 1995. Does physical activity improve sleep in impaired nursing home residents? Journal of the American Geriatrics Society, 43, 1098–1102.

Antonovsky A. 1979. *Health, Stress and Coping*, San Francisco: Jossey-Bass.

Antonovsky A. 1996. The salutogenic model as a theory to guide health promotion. Oxford: Oxford University Press.

Bengtsson A, Carlsson G. 2013. Outdoor environments at three nursing homes: qualitative interviews with residents and next of kin. Urban Forestry and Urban Greening, 12(3), 393–400.

Bengtsson A, Grahn P. 2014. Outdoor environments in health care settings: A quality evaluation tool for use in designing health care gardens. Urban Forestry and Urban Greening, 13, 878–891.

Bennett MP, Zeller JM, Rosenberg L, McCann J. 2003. The effect of mirthful laughter on stress and natural killer cell activity. Altern Ther Health Med, 9(2), 38–45.

Bertram G, Stickley T. 2007. *Young@Heart: An Evaluation of the Young@Heart Dance Project for Older People. Dance 4*, Nottingham: University of Nottingham.

Beswick AD, Rees K, Dieppe P, Ayis S, et al. 2008. Complex interventions to improve physical function and maintain independent living in elderly people: a systematic review and meta-analysis. Lancet, 371(9614), 725–735.

Blum K, Simpatico T, Febo M, Rodriquez C, et al. 2016. Hypothesizing music intervention enhances brain functional connectivity involving dopaminergic recruitment: common neuro-correlates to abusable drugs. Mol Neurobiol, May (e-pub ahead of print).

Boersma P, van Weert JCM, Lakkerveld J, Dröes RM. 2014. The art of successful implementation of psychosocial interventions in residential dementia care: a systematic review of the literature based on the RE-AIM framework. International Psychogeriatrics.

Bolmsjö I, Edberg AK, Andersson PL. 2014. The use of drama to support reflection and understanding of the residents' situation in dementia care: a pilot study. Int J Older People Nurs, 9(3), 183–191.

Bowes A, Dawson A, Jepson R, McCabe L. 2013. Physical activity for people with dementia: a scoping study. BMC Geriatr, 13, 129.

Bradshaw SA, Playford ED, Riazi A. 2012. Living well in care homes: a systematic review of qualitative studies. Age Ageing, 41(4), 429–440.

Brewin W. 2011. *Use Outdoor Spaces Creatively in Residential Homes*, Alzheimer's Disease International (published 22 October).

Brittle N, Patel S, Wright C, Baral S, Versfeld P, Sackley C. 2009. An exploratory cluster randomized controlled trial of group exercise on mobility and depression in care home residents. Clinical Rehabilitation, 23, 146–154.

Brooker DJ, Wooley RJ, Lee D. 2007. Enriching opportunities for people living with dementia in nursing homes: an evaluation of a multi-level activity based model of care. Aging & Mental Health, 11, 361–370.

Buck D. 2016. Gardens and health: implications for policy and practice, London: The King's Fund, available at https://www.kingsfund.org.uk/sites/files/kf/field/field_publication_file/Gardens_and_health.pdf (accessed 29 Nov 2016).

Buettner L. 1988. Utilizing developmental theory and adaptive equipment with regressed geriatric patients in therapeutic recreation. Ther Recreation J, 22(3), 72–79.

Burgio LD, Allen-Burge R, Roth DL, Bourgeois MS, et al. 2001a. Come talk with me: improving communication between nursing assistants and nursing home residents during care routines. Gerontologist, 41(4), 449–460.

Burgio LD, Lichstein KL, Nichols L, Czaja S, et al. 2001b. Judging outcomes in psychosocial interventions for dementia caregivers: the problem of treatment implementation. Gerontologist, 41(4), 481–489.

Burton A. 2014. Gardens that take care of us. Lancet Neurol, 13(5), 447–448.

Burton E, Lewin G, Boldy D. 2015. Physical activity preferences of older home care clients. Int J Older People Nurs, 10(3), 170–178.

Caspersen CJ, Powell KE, Christenson GM. 1985. Physical activity, exercise, and physical fitness: definitions and distinctions for health-related research. Public Health Rep, 100, 126–131.

Clark ME, Lipe AW, Bilbrey M. 1998. Use of music to decrease aggressive behaviors in people with dementia. J. Gerontol. Nurs, 24(7), 10–17.

Cohen-Mansfield J, Werner P. 1998. Visits to an Outdoor Garden: Impact on Behavior and Mood of Nursing Home Residents who Pace. In B Vellas and G Frisoni (eds), *Research and Practice in Alzheimer's Disease*, New York: Springer.

Cohen-Mansfield J, Werner P. 1999. Outdoor wandering parks for persons with dementia: a survey of characteristics and use. Alzheimer Disease & Associated Disorders, 13(2), 109–117.

Crocker T, Forster A, Young J, Brown L, et al. 2013. Physical rehabilitation for older people in long-term care. Cochrane Database of Systematic Reviews, 2, CD004294.

Crockett S. 2013. *Activities for Older People in Care Homes: A Handbook for Successful Activity Planning*, London: Jessica Kingsley Publishers.

Davis C, Cooke M, Holzhauser K, Jones M, Finucane J. 2005. The effect of aromatherapy massage with music on the stress and anxiety levels of emergency nurses. AENJ, 8, 43–50.

Deane K, Dawson E, Noble D. 2015. *A Choir in Every Care Home,* available at achoirineverycarehome. files.wordpress.com/2016/04/wp1-gathering-1-v4.pdf (accessed 3 Oct 2016).

Department of Health. 2009. Living Well with Dementia: A National Dementia Strategy, available at www.gov.uk/government/uploads/system/uploads/attachment_data/file/168220/dh_094051. pdf (accessed 3 Oct 2016).

Detweiler MB, Murphy PF, Myers LC, Kim KY. 2008. Does a wander garden influence inappropriate behaviours in dementia residents? American Journal of Alzheimer's Disease and Other Dementias, 23, 31–45.

Detweiler MB, Sharma T, Detweiler JG, Murphy PF, et al. 2012. What is the evidence to support the use of therapeutic gardens for the elderly? Psychiatry Investig, 9(2), 100–110.

Dhami P, Moreno S, DeSouza JF. 2014. New framework for rehabilitation – Fusion of cognitive and physical rehabilitation: The hope for dancing. Frontiers in Psychology, 5, 1478.

Ding D, Lawson KD, Kolbe-Alexander TL, Finkelstein EA, et al. 2016. The economic burden of physical inactivity: a global analysis of major non-communicable diseases. Lancet, S0140-6736(16)30383-X, doi:10.1016/S0140-6736(16)30383-X (e-pub ahead of print).

Dishman R, Heath G, Lee I. 2013. *Physical Activity Epidemiology*, Champaign, IL: Human Kinetics.

Edwards CA, McDonnell C, Merl H. 2013. An evaluation of a therapeutic garden's influence on the quality of life of aged care residents with dementia. Dementia (London), 12(4), 494–510.

Ferrucci L, Guralnik JM, Studenski S, Fried LP. 2004. Designing randomized, controlled trials aimed at preventing or delaying functional decline and disability in frail, older persons: a consensus report. Journal of American Geriatrics Society, 52, 625–634.

Finlay J, Franke T, McKay H, Sims-Gould J. 2015. Therapeutic landscapes and wellbeing in later life: impacts of blue and green spaces for older adults. Health Place, 34, 97–106.

Forrester LT, Maayan N, Orrell M, Spector AE, Buchan LD, Soares-Weiser K. 2014. Aromatherapy for dementia. Cochrane Database of Systematic Reviews, 2, CD003150.

Fossey J, Ballard C, Juszczak E, James I, Alder N, Jacoby R, Howard R. 2006. Effect of enhanced psychosocial care on antipsychotic use in nursing home residents with severe dementia: cluster randomised trial. Br Med J, 332, 756–758.

Gerritsen D, Ettema TP, Boelens E, Bos J, et al. 2007. Quality of life in dementia: do professional caregivers focus on the significant domains? American Journal of Alzheimer's Disease & Other Dementias, 22(3), 176–183.

Gillespie L, Robertson M, Gillespie W, Sherrington C, et al. 2012. Interventions for preventing falls in older people living in the community. Cochrane report.

Gitlin LN, Hodgson N, Jutkowitz E, Pizzi L. 2010. The cost-effectiveness of a nonpharmacologic intervention for individuals with dementia and family caregivers: the tailored activity program. American Journal of Geriatric Psychiatry, 18(6), 510–519.

Gjengedal E, Lykkeslet E, Sørbø JI, Sæther WH. 2014. 'Brightness in dark places': theatre as an arena for communicating life with dementia. Dementia (London), 13(5), 598–612.

Goldstone LA. 2000. Massage as an orthodox medical treatment past and future. Complementary Therapies in Nursing and Midwifery, 6, 169–175.

Gonzalez MT, Kirkevold M. 2014. Benefits of sensory garden and horticultural activities in dementia care: a modified scoping review. J Clin Nurs, 23(19–20), 2698–2715.

Grassmann J, Schneider D, Weiser D, Elstner EF. 2001. Antioxidative effects of lemon oil and its components on copper induced oxidation of low density lipoprotein. Arzneimittelforschung, 51, 799–805.

Grek A. 2008. Self-harm and suicide in nursing homes. Journal of Affective Disorders, 107, S21–S52.

Groene R. 1993. Effectiveness of music therapy intervention with individuals having senile dementia of the Alzheimer's type. J Music Ther, 30(3), 138–157.

Hackney ME, Earhart GM. 2010. Social partnered dance for people with serious and persistent mental illness: a pilot study. J Nerv Ment Dis, 198(1), 76–78.

Hancock GA, Woods B, Challis D, Orrell M. 2006. The needs of older people with dementia in residential care. Int J Geriatr Psychiatry, 21(1), 43–49.

Havighurst RJB. 1968. Personality and patterns of aging. Gerontologist, 8, 20–23.

Havighurst RJB, Albrecht R. 1953. *Older People*, New York: Longman, Greens.

Hayes L. 2006. Line dancing with dementia. ADQ, 7, 31–34.

Heath Y. 2004. Evaluating the effect of therapeutic gardens. Am J Alzheimers Dis Other Demen, 19(4), 239–242.

Hecox B, Levine E, Scott D. 1976. Dance in physical rehabilitation. Phys Ther, 56(8), 919–924.

Hirsh S. 1990. Dance therapy in the service of dementia. Am J Alzheimer's Care Relat Disord Res, 5, 26–30.

Holmes C, Ballard C. 2004. Aromatherapy in dementia. Advances in Psychiatric Treatment, 10, 296–300.

Ing-Randolph AR, Phillips LR, Williams AB. 2015. Group music interventions for dementia associated anxiety: A systematic review. Int J Nurs Stud, 52(11), 1775–1784.

Jackson J, Carlson M, Mandel D, Zemke R, Clark F. 1998. Occupation in lifestyle redesign: the well elderly study occupational therapy program. Am J Occup Ther, 52(5), 326–336.

Johannessen B. 2013. Nurses experience of aromatherapy use with dementia patients experiencing disturbed sleep patterns. An action research project. Complement Ther Clin Pract, 19(4), 209–213.

Kapoor Y, Orr R. 2015. Effect of therapeutic massage on pain in patients with dementia. Dementia (London), April, 1471301215583391 (e-pub ahead of print).

Kellett U. 1999. Transition in care: family carers' experience of nursing home placement. Journal of Advanced Nursing, 29(Suppl. 6), 1474–1481.

Keogh JWL, Kilding A, Pidgeon P, Ashely L, Gillis D. 2009. Physical benefits of dancing for healthy older adults: a review. JAPA, 17, 479–500.

Kitwood T. 1997. *Dementia Reconsidered: The Person Comes First*, Buckingham: Open University Press.

Koger SM, Brotons M. 2000. Music therapy for dementia symptoms. Cochrane Database Syst Rev, 3, CD001121.

Kolanowski A, Litaker M, Buettner L, Moeller, J, Costa PT Jr. 2011. A randomized clinical trial of theory based activities for the behavioral symptoms of dementia in nursing home residents. J Am Geriatr Soc, 59, 1032–1041.

Leedahl SN, Chapin RK, Little TD. 2015. Multilevel examination of facility characteristics, social integration, and health for older adults living in nursing homes. J Gerontol B Psychol Sci Soc Sci, 70(1), 111–122.

Lehner S. 2006. Benevolent ballet: fall prevention for the elderly. ADQ, 7, 19–22.

Lewith GT, Godfrey AD, Prescott P. 2005. Single-blinded, randomized pilot study evaluating the aroma of Lavandula augustifolia as a treatment for mild insomnia. J Altern Complement, 11(4), 631–637.

Lloyd B, Stirling C. 2015. A tool to support meaningful person-centred activity for clients with dementia – a Delphi study. BMC Nurs, 14, 10.

Lou M. 2001. The use of music to decrease agitated behaviour of the demented elderly: the state of the science. Scandinavian Journal of Caring Sciences, 15(2), 165–173.

MacRae P, Schnelle J, Ouslander J. 1996. Physical activity levels of ambulatory nursing home residents. JAPA, 4, 264–278.

Maller C, Townsend M, Pryor A, Brown P, St Leger L. 2005. Healthy nature healthy people: 'Contact with Nature' as an upstream health promotion intervention for populations. Health Promot. Int, 21(1), 45–54.

Marshall MJ, Hutchinson S. 2001. A critique of research on the use of activities with persons with Alzheimer's disease: a systematic review. Journal of Advanced Nursing, 35, 488–496.

McAllister C, Silverman M. 1999. Community formation and community roles among persons with Alzheimer's disease: a comparative study of experiences in a residential Alzheimer's facility and a traditional nursing home. Qual. Health Res, 9(1), 65–85.

Milke D, Beck C, Danes S, Leask J. 2009. Behavioral mapping of residents' activity in five residential style care centers for elderly persons diagnosed with dementia: small differences in sites can affect behaviors. J. Hous. Elder, 23(4), 335–367.

Mooney P, Nicell PL. 1992. The importance of exterior environment for Alzheimer residents: effective care and risk management. Health Care Management Forum, 5, 23–29.

Morley JE, Philpot CD, Gill D, Berg-Weger M. 2014. Meaningful activities in the nursing homes. J Am Med Dir Assoc, 15(2), 79–81.

Moyle W, Cooke ML, Beattie E, Shum DH, O'Dwyer ST, Barrett S. 2014. Foot massage versus quiet presence on agitation and mood in people with dementia: a randomised controlled trial. Int J Nurs Stud, 51(6), 856–864.

Mozley C, Sutcliffe C, Bagley H, Cordingley L, et al. 2004. Towards quality care: outcomes for older people in care homes. Aldershot: Ashgate in conjunction with Personal Social Service Research Unit (PSSRU).

Munro S, Mount B. 1978. Music therapy in palliative care. Canadian Medical Association Journal, 119, 1029–1034.

National Institute for Health and Clinical Excellence (NICE). 2006. Dementia: Supporting people with dementia and their carers in health and social care. NICE clinical guideline 42. London: National Institute for Health and Clinical Excellence.

Nolan M, Grant G, Nolan J. 1995. Busy doing nothing: activity and interaction levels among differing populations of elderly patients. Journal of Advanced Nursing, 22, 528–538.

Noone S, Innes A, Kelly F, Mayers A. 2015. 'The nourishing soil of the soul': the role of horticultural therapy in promoting wellbeing in community-dwelling people with dementia. Dementia (London), December, 1471301215623889 (e-pub ahead of print).

Nyman SR, Szymczynska P. 2016. Meaningful activities for improving the wellbeing of people with dementia: beyond mere pleasure to meeting fundamental psychological needs. Perspect Public Health, 136(2), 99–107.

O'Toole J, Lepp M. 2000. *Drama for Life: Stories of Adult Learning and Empowerment*, Brisbane: Playlab.

Palo-Bengtsson L, Ekman SL. 2000. Dance events as a caregiver intervention for persons with dementia. Nurs Inquiry, 7(3), 156–165.

Palo-Bengtsson L, Ekman SL. 2002. Emotional response to social dancing and walks in persons with dementia. Am J Alzheimers Dis Other Demen, 17(3), 149–153.

Phinney A, Chaudhury H, O'Connor DL. 2007. Doing as much as I can do: the meaning of activity for people with dementia. Aging Ment Health, 11(4), 384–393.

Pöllänen SH, Hirsimäki RM. 2014. Crafts as memory triggers in reminiscence: a case study of older women with dementia. Occup Ther Health Care, 28(4), 410–430.

Pretty J. 2004. How nature contributes to mental and physical health. Spiritual. Health Int, 5(2), 68–78.

Raglio A, Bellelli G, Traficante D, Gianotti M, et al. 2008. Efficacy of music therapy in the treatment of behavioral and psychiatric symptoms of dementia. Alzheimer Dis. Assoc. Disorders, 22(2), 158–162.

Ravelin T, Isola A, Kylmä J. 2013. Dance performance as a method of intervention as experienced by older persons with dementia. Int J Older People Nurs, 8(1), 10–18.

Ravelin T, Kylma J, Korhonen T. 2006. Dance in mental health nursing: a hybrid concept analysis. Issues in Mental Health Nursing, 27, 307–317.

Roach P, Drummond N, Keady J. 2016. 'Nobody would say that it is Alzheimer's or dementia at this age': family adjustment following a diagnosis of early-onset dementia. J Aging Stud, 36, 26–32.

Robertson R, Robertson A, Jepson R, Maxwell M. 2012. Walking for depression or depressive symptoms: a systematic review. Mental Health and Physical Activity, 5, 66–75.

Rocha V, Marques A, Pinto M, Sousa L, Figueiredo D. 2013. People with dementia in long-term care facilities: an exploratory study of their activities and participation. Disabil Rehabil, 35(18), 1501–1508.

Roland KP, Chappell NL. 2015. Meaningful activity for persons with dementia: family caregiver perspectives. Am J Alzheimers Dis Other Demen, 30(6), 559–568.

Rolland Y, Pillard F, Klapouszczak A, Reynish E, et al. 2007. Exercise programme for nursing home residents with Alzheimer's disease: a 1-year randomized, controlled trial. J Am Geriatr Soc, 55(2), 158–165.

Royal College of Physicians, Royal College of Nursing, British Geriatrics Society. 2000. *Health and Care of Older People in Care Homes: A Comprehensive Interdisciplinary Approach. A Report of a Joint Working Party of the Royal College of Physicians, The Royal College of Nursing and The British Geriatrics Society*. London: Royal College of Physicians.

Saarloos D, Nathan A, Almeida O, Giles-Corti B. 2008. *The Baby Boomers and Beyond Report: Physical Activity Levels of Older Western Australians 2006*. Perth: Western Australian Government.

Sackley CM, Gatt J, Walker M. 2001. The use of rehabilitation services by private nursing homes in Nottingham. Ageing, 30, 532–533.

Salisbury K, Algar K, Windle G. 2011. Arts programmes and quality of life for people with dementia – a review. Journal of Dementia Care, 19, 33–37.

Schroll M, Jonsson PV, Mor V, Berg K, Sherwood S. 1997. An international study of social engagement among nursing home residents. Age Ageing, 26(Suppl 2), 55–59.

Schwarz B, Rodiek S. 2007. Introduction: outdoor environments for people with dementia. Journal of Housing for the Elderly, 21(1–2), 3–11.

Shiue I. 2016. Gardening is beneficial for adult mental health: Scottish Health Survey, 2012–2013. Scand J Occup Ther, 23(4), 320–325.

Simons LA, Simons J, McCallum J, Friedlander Y. 2006. Lifestyle factors and risk of dementia: Dubbo Study of the elderly. Med J Aust, 184(2), 68–70.

Sjögren K, Lindkvist M, Sandman PO, Zingmark K, Edvardsson D. 2013. Person-centredness and its association with resident well-being in dementia care units. J Adv Nurs, 69(10), 2196–2205.

Smit D, de Lange J, Willemse B, Twisk J, Pot AM. 2016. Activity involvement and quality of life of people at different stages of dementia in long-term care facilities. Aging Ment Health, 20(1), 100–109.

Snow AL, Hovanec L, Brandt J. 2004. A controlled trial of aromatherapy for agitation in nursing home patients with dementia. J Altern Complement Med, 10, 431–437.

Snyder M, Chlan L. 1999. Music therapy. Annual Review of Nursing Research 17, 3–25.

Snyder M, Egan EC, Burns KR. 1995. Interventions for decreasing agitation behaviors in persons with dementia. J Gerontol Nurs, 21(7), 34–40.

Spiro N, Farrant C, Pavlicevic M. 2015. Between practice, policy and politics: music therapy and the Dementia Strategy, 2009. Dementia (London), June, 1471301215585465 (e-pub ahead of print).

Stige B, Ansdell G, Elefant C, Pavlicevic M. 2010. *Where Music Helps: Community Music Therapy in Action and Reflection*, Aldershot: Ashgate.

Strotzka H. 1956/57. Versuch über den Humor. Psyche, 10, 97–609.

Sung HC, Chang AM, Lee WL. 2010. A preferred music listening intervention to reduce anxiety in older adults with dementia in nursing homes. J Clin Nurs, 19(7–8), 1056–1064.

Sung HC, Lee WL, Chang SM, Smith GD. 2011. Exploring nursing staff's attitudes and use of music for older people with dementia in long-term care facilities. J Clin Nurs, 20(11–12), 1776–1783.

Suzuki M, Tatsumi A, Otsuka T, Kikuchi K, et al. 2010. Physical and psychological effects of 6-week tactile massage on elderly patients with severe dementia. Am J Alzheimers Dis Other Demen, 25(8), 680–686.

Takeda M, Hashimoto R, Kudo T, Okochi M, et al. 2010. Laughter and humour as complementary and alternative medicines for dementia patients. BMC Complement Altern Med, 10, 28.

Tan T, Schneider MA. 2009. Humor as a coping strategy for adult-child caregivers of individuals with Alzheimer's disease. Geriatr Nurs, 30(6), 397–408.

Taylor A. 1991. *The Principle and Practice of Physical Therapy, 3rd Edition,* Cheltenham and London: Stanley Thamas.

Taylor N. 2016. West Yorkshire Playhouse Guide to Dementia-Friendly Performances.

Thelander VB, Wahlin T-BR, Olofsson L, Heikkilä K, Sonde L. 2008. Gardening activities for nursing home residents with dementia. Advances in Physiotherapy, 10, 53–56.

Tse MYM. 2007. Nursing home placement: perspective of community dwelling older persons. Journal of Clinical Nursing, 16, 911–917.

Uvnås-Moberg K. 2004. *The Oxytocin Factor: Tapping the Hormone of Calm, Love, and Healing,* Cambridge, MA: Da Capo Press.

van der Vleuten M, Visser A, Meeuwesen L. 2012. The contribution of intimate live music performances to the quality of life for persons with dementia. Patient Educ Couns, 89(3), 484–488.

Vance DE. 2003. Implications of olfactory stimulation on activities for adults with age-related dementia. Activities, Adaptation & Aging, 27, 17–25.

Verghese J, Richard B, Lipton RB, Mindy JK, et al. 2003. Leisure activities and the risk of dementia in the elderly. New Engl J Med, 348, 2508–2516.

Vernooij-Dassen M. 2007. Meaningful activities for people with dementia. Aging Ment Health, 11(4), 359–360.

Viggo Hansen N, Jørgensen T, Ørtenblad L. 2006. Massage and touch for dementia. Cochrane Database Syst Rev, 4, CD004989.

Vink AC, Bruinsma MS, Scholten RJPM. 2003. Music therapy for people with dementia. Cochrane Database of Systematic Reviews, 4, CD003477.

Wakefield S, Yeudall F, Taron C, Reynolds J, Skinner A. 2007. Growing urban health: community gardening in South-East Toronto. Health Promot Int, 22(2), 92–101.

Wells DL, Dawson P. 2000. Description of retained abilities in older persons with dementia. Research in Nursing & Health, 23, 158–166.

Wenborn J, Challis D, Head J, Miranda-Castillo C, et al. 2013. Providing activity for people with dementia in care homes: a cluster randomised controlled trial. Int J Geriatr Psychiatry, 28(12), 1296–1304.

Westerhof GJ, Bohlmeijer ET, van Beljouw IMJ, Pot AM. 2010. Improvement in personal meaning mediates the effects of a life review intervention on depressive symptoms in a randomized controlled trial. Gerontologist, 50, 541–549.

Whear R, Coon JT, Bethel A, Abbott R, Stein K, Garside R. 2014. What is the impact of using outdoor spaces such as gardens on the physical and mental wellbeing of those with dementia? A systematic review of quantitative and qualitative evidence. J Am Med Dir Assoc, 15(10), 697–705.

White JM, Cornish F, Kerr S. 2015. Frontline perspectives on 'joined-up' working relationships: a qualitative study of social prescribing in the west of Scotland. Health Soc Care Community, October, doi:10.1111/hsc.12290 (e-pub ahead of print).

Windle G, Gregory S, Newman A, Goulding A, O'Brien D, Parkinson C. 2014. Understanding the impact of visual arts interventions for people living with dementia: a realist review protocol. Syst Rev, 3, 91.

Wittmann-Price RA. 2012. The olfactory sense: a developmental and lifespan perspective. Journal of Clinical Nursing, 21, 2545–2554.

WHO. 2010. *Global Recommendations on Physical Activity for Health,* Geneva: World Health Organization, available at apps.who.int/iris/bitstream/10665/44399/1/9789241599979_eng.pdf (accessed 3 Oct 2016).

Zeilmann CA, Dole EJ, Skipper BJ, McCabe M, et al. 2003. Use of herbal medicine by elderly Hispanic and non-Hispanic white patients. Pharmacotherapy, 23, 526–532.

Zuidema S, Jonghe JD, Verhey F, Koopmans R. 2010. Environmental correlates of neuropsychiatric symptoms in nursing home patients with dementia. Int. J. Geriatr. Psychiatry, 25, 14–22.

— Chapter 8 —

SEXUALITY AND SPIRITUALITY

Learning objectives

By the end of this chapter, you will:

- » be able to briefly discuss the relevance of identity to personhood
- » be able to evaluate critically the importance of religiosity, sexuality and spirituality for living better with dementia, with a particular emphasis on residential care settings

Introduction

Respect for people as people involves giving them space for their unique identity. This is not always easily governed by protocols or operationalised – there needs to be a plurality of views about sensitive topics, such as sexuality, religiosity and spirituality. Professionals can be most uneasy about talking about such matters, yet such things may matter most to people with dementia and their families. **Identity** is a key feature of the Kitwood flower (see Figure 8.1).

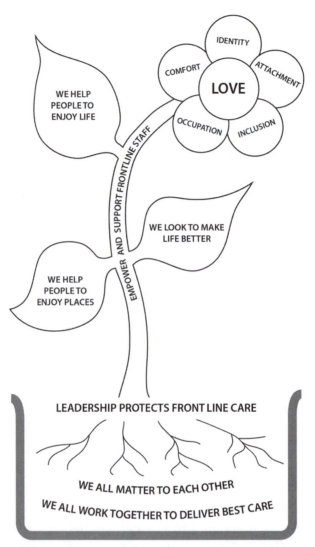

Figure 8.1: The fulfilment of psychological needs depends on a positive care culture – a pictorial representation of how the elements of a positive care culture can support the emotional and psychological wellbeing of people living with dementia in a care setting

Source: inspired by Kitwood (1997a) and reproduced by kind permission from Brooker and Latham (2016, p.35).

Kaufman and Engel (2014) review how Kitwood defines five psychological needs based on clinical observations to establish the main foci for intervention. The need for identity 'involves maintaining a sense of continuity with the past, and some kind of consistency in the present life' (Kitwood, 1997b, p.20).

According to Kitwood and Bredin (1992), a tension exists between medical models of dementia that emphasise loss and deficit on the one hand, and the recognition on the part of primary carers that the intrinsic humanity of people with diseases that lead to dementia symptoms remains intact. Bennett (1980) portrayed the quality of life in long-term care as the satisfaction of basic human needs, whether physiological, social or those to do with safety and security, self-esteem and accomplishment (see Brooker and Latham, 2016, p.35).

I would like to draw attention to how broad the definition of quality of life can be. For example, the Institute of Medicine defined it as a 'subjective or objective judgment concerning all aspects of an individual's existence, including health, economic, political, cultural, environmental, aesthetic, and spiritual aspects' (Institute of Medicine, 2001, p.30, quoted from Gold et al., 1996, p.405). In many post-industrial societies there are increasingly dispersed family networks and complicated family structures. Many countries are increasingly multicultural, with many older people ageing in a second homeland. Moreover, societal views and cultural values about issues such as gender equality and sexual orientation have changed drastically between (and sometimes within) generations (Brooker and Latham, 2016). Providing good transcultural, multicultural and genuinely inclusive care across generational boundaries is not easy.

—— Sexuality ————————————————————————————

How care is provided is a significant influence on residents' adjustment to living in a nursing home, and most nursing home managers will see spiritual care, which includes a range of tasks that are social and emotional in nature, to be an important aspect of the care they provide for residents (Orchard and Clark, 2012). Diseases and disability can reduce the possibility of generally satisfying needs associated with this sphere of life (Laumann et al., 2005; Addis et al., 2006). Staff education should be undertaken, not only in the area of human sexuality, but also in understanding the holistic needs of residents. Holistic nursing targets the physical, mental, social and spiritual needs of people's lives (McSherry, 2006). The most common danger for service providers working with individuals from a different cultural background is to misinterpret culture as something immutable, and then apply it mechanically to all individuals from that background (Elliott et al., 1996).

Sexuality is often misunderstood; social and cultural values place a substantial emphasis on sexual intercourse, reducing sexuality to acts of sexual expression – the observable manifestations of sexual activity and desire. Many younger people have a negative attitude towards sexuality among older people; some even view it as immoral and disgraceful.

Other kinds of sexual behaviour, such as kissing, cuddling and mutual masturbation, are viewed as less significant or non-sexual behaviours. About 25 years ago, Comfort and Dial (1991) stated that older people need, both sexually and medically, what people in general need and that the idea of a decline into a sexless state as acceptable was insulting. Sexuality indeed appears to be an essential part of human existence regardless of one's age (WHO, 2006; Di Napoli, Breland and Allen 2013). In Western countries, despite the increasing 'sexualisation' of popular culture, there is still a certain degree of discomfort and embarrassment in talking about one's own sexuality (Tarzia et al., 2013). Judgement of human behaviour is influenced by our own value system, the society in which we live, our attitude towards sexuality and the policies and controls of the workplace (Alzheimer's Australia, 2010).

Older people themselves have defined sexuality as: looking nice; spending time with the opposite sex; intercourse with a long-time partner; and relieving one's frustrations with a sex worker (Nay, 2004). Sexuality can also refer to: getting dressed up and feeling pampered; looking one's best; enjoying sexually stimulating material; 'talking dirty'; cuddling with a partner in bed; kissing; and masturbating (McAuliffe, Bauer and Nay, 2007). 'Sexuality is with us from the moment of birth to the moment of death' (Zilbergeld, 2004, p.15) and is a fundamental part of being human. However, although there is an increasing emphasis on the application of person-centred approaches to care delivery, many residential aged care service providers still neglect to recognise and address sexuality as a component of wellbeing (Bauer et al., 2014a, b).

Ageism and sexism have been remarkably successful in portraying sexuality as the domain of young people and stereotyping older people as asexual. Older people have colluded in this stereotype by passing themselves off as asexual and generally keeping secret their ongoing interest in, or expression of, sexuality. The label 'deviant' and associated stigma experienced by people who dare to breach societal stereotypes are recognised as tools used by powerful vested interests to maintain and manage the norms and values of society (Nay, McAuliffe and Bauer, 2007). It is argued that many care providers are unaware of the importance of the multiple facets of the care environment that impact on a resident's ability to express their sexuality; they are also unaware of the kind of support that may be required (Bauer et al., 2014a). Some research has indicated that it is inappropriate for older people to have sexual lives (Hsieh, 1995) or that institutions should not allow unmarried older people to have sexual relations and that masturbation will not help older people resolve sexual tensions or impulses (Huang, 1995). Older women are disproportionately affected by dementia primarily because of ageing demographics: women tend to live longer than men and dementia is age-related (Knapp and Prince, 2007). There is an emergent awareness that dementia is a gendered issue, disproportionately affecting women (Bamford, 2011).

Sexuality and sexual needs in older adults remain a neglected area of clinical intervention, particularly so in long-term care settings. Because older adults in medical rehabilitation and long-term care beds present with significant frailties, and often significant neurocognitive disorders, it is difficult for occupational therapists and other staff to evaluate the capacity of an older adult resident to participate in sexual relationships (Lichtenberg, 2014). The way in which they express themselves sexually might, nevertheless, be interfered with by many factors such as age-related health issues, the lack or loss of a partner and perhaps admission to a long-term care facility. Because of various reasons, staying in a long-term care facility might be a barrier to sexual expression (Mahieu and Gastmans, 2015). Research has shown that people still have sexual desires and may remain sexually active well into their 70s and 80s (Delamater, 2012).

A review of the ethics literature reveals the resident's capability to consent as a predominating factor in assessing the moral permissibility of sexual activity. This focus on cognitive capacity does not only tend to disregard the sexual longings of people with dementia (as their ability to make day-to-day decisions might easily be underestimated); it also fails to give an accurate picture of what human sexuality entails, whether one is competent or not (Mahieu, Anckaert and Gastmans, 2014). Esmaill, Esmaill and Munro (2001) pointed to the broad context of human sexuality and psychosexual needs, which comprise five aspects: **sensuality** (awareness of one's own body), **intimacy** (the need for emotional attachment and sexual experience, emotional closeness), **sexual identity** (sexual orientation), **reproduction** (fertility, conceiving a baby and its upbringing) and **sexualisation** (using one's sexuality, keeping one's sex drive under control) (Esmaill et al., 2001). Sexuality is not merely about physical arousal; it is about a particular form of intimacy. That is much more difficult to define, particularly when one presumably wants the intimate relationship between the husband and wife in the scenario above to continue (Bartlett, 2010).

Furthermore, operational definitions for research on sexual interactions are much needed to ensure consistency within the literature (see Table 8.1).

The data from the National Social Life, Health and Aging Project (NSHAP) reveal that sexual activity throughout life is beneficial for health, and may even extend one's lifespan. Research conducted by the NSHAP proved that more than half of people aged 57–85 and about one-third of those aged 75–85 remain sexually active, and their physical health significantly correlates with sexual life (Lindau and Gavrilova, 2010). For older people with dementia living in residential aged care facilities, the issue is more complicated. Staff often struggle to balance residents' rights with their duty of care, and negative attitudes towards older people's sexuality can lead to residents' sexual expression being overlooked, ignored or even discouraged (Tarzia et al., 2013). Nursing staff play a central role in institutionalised elderly care. Their day-to-day contact with residents often develops into a strong relationship based on mutual trust, which eases the sexual expression of the institutionalised elderly (Lyder, 1994).

Table 8.1: Examples of operational definitions in research in sexual behaviour

Concept	Definition
Undoing another's clothes	It was taken to mean undressing another person and taking off his/her clothes, pants or nappies.
Sleeping together and holding each other on the same bed	Referred to two unrelated residents (either by blood or marriage) sleeping together in one bed while they held each other or their genitals touched each other.
Staring at the other's displayed sexuality	Referred to a male patient fixing his eyes on a female's breasts, genitals or bottom, or, in the case of female residents, fixing their eyes on a male's genitals.
Sexual provocation	Referred to using words that implied sexuality or that hinted at sexual desire with the specific objective of flirting with or teasing another person.
Neutral response	Referred to people who saw the sexual behaviour and had a response that was not negative or positive, such as no facial expressions or ignoring the behaviour.

SOURCE: ADAPTED FROM TZENG ET AL. (2009, TABLE 3, P.995).

Denying one's sexuality is seen as having a negative impact on self-image, social relationships and mental wellbeing (Hajjar and Kamel, 2004). There is an increasing body of literature on sexuality and older people, particularly from the US, but it is difficult to locate research that does not suffer from what White (1982, p.12) refers to as 'sample bias' (Archibald, 1998). Particularly when a resident has dementia, staff may be apprehensive, for example, about the abrogation of their duty of care and concerns about unlawful activity, anxiety about potential risks to the resident and even the fear of negative repercussions from a resident's family. This may make many facility managers wary of physically intimate activity among residents (Tarzia, Fetherstonhaugh and Bauer, 2012).

If it is possible to combine expertise from industry, academia and the caring professions at such institutions to probe into this topic, it might contribute to the development of appropriate plans for the sexual care of institutionalised residents with dementia (Tzeng et al., 2009). A study from 198 randomly selected residential aged care facilities (RACFs) in New South Wales, Victoria and Queensland, Australia, provided an overview of the ways in which senior management perceive sexuality to be an issue for RACFs and the state of the current policy and training landscape (Shuttleworth et al., 2010). Formal policies around sexuality-related issues only existed for a relatively small proportion of the facilities. The majority did not have policies that explicitly acknowledged sexuality as part of residents' lives but only dealt with such issues in an informal and ad hoc way. However, the sexual behaviours and desires of older adults do not cease upon nursing home admission. In fact, Bretschneider and McCoy (1988) found that 70% of male and

50% of female nursing home residents had thoughts about being close or intimate (to the present author's knowledge, more recent estimates are not available). Hubbard, Tester and Downs (2003) reported that institutional care residents often engage in intimate touching, kissing, sexual talk, flirting and teasing. The study by Lester and colleagues (2016) proposed that nursing homes should have a clear policy addressing resident sexual activity. It would be beneficial for such a policy to be communicated to residents and their families as part of an admission package instead of waiting for sexual interest to be noticed. This would enable residents to engage in sexual activity with understanding and support, rather than hiding it.

A more open approach to sexuality may encourage a more imaginative and experimental approach to sexual expression and activity, and may enable people with Alzheimer's disease to achieve pleasure and intimacy in diverse and unique ways (Dourado et al., 2010). Staying in a long-term care facility might be a barrier to sexual expression. Research has shown that the overall lack of physical privacy and privacy of information, negative staff attitudes, the absence of a sexual partner and the focus on safety and physical care needs often prevailing in long-term care facilities might impede residents' sexual expression (Elias and Ryan, 2011; Makimoto et al., 2015). Relationships between the staff in a care home and residents' family members may be positive but may also be subject to mutual misunderstanding in that the way family members behave towards staff may affect the level and type of care provided (Wiskerke and Manthorpe, 2016).

Ehrenfeld and colleagues (1999, p.146) have placed sexual behaviour into three groups:

» **love and caring** ('strong affection, a feeling of attraction or desire for someone, longing and sensuality')

» **romance** ('an emotional and mental experience of love in which one tends to idealize the object of one's affection')

» **eroticism** ('sexual excitement or desire').

It is at best doubtful whether, in such a fundamental area of personal life as sexuality, such attitudes should be permitted to determine the permissibility of behaviour. However, at the same time, this may be a practical reality: the administration of the balancing process would presumably rest with the institutional staff of the care home (Bartlett, 2010). However, aggression and agitation are common problems seen in the geriatric population with moderate-to-severe stages of impaired cognition, and especially in long-term care patients with dementia. The prevalence of physically aggressive behaviour increases with the progression of dementia, and it often heralds a poor prognosis (Alagiakrishnan et al., 2005). The prevalence of 'inappropriate sexual behaviour' (ISB) exhibited by people with a dementia varies between 1.8% and 17.5% (Johnson, Knight and Alderman, 2006), although this is likely to be an underestimate as the literature is scarce and definitions obscure.

Resident-to-resident sexual aggression (RRSA) is defined as sexual interactions between long-term care residents that, in a community setting, at least one of the recipients would be likely to construe as unwelcome and that have the high potential to cause physical or psychological distress in one or both of the residents involved. Although RRSA may be common, the physical and psychological consequences for victims may be significant (Rosen, Lachs and Pillemer, 2010).

An extensive review of ISB (Johnson et al., 2006) revealed a multitude of definitions, including sexual advances, hypersexuality, propositioning and inappropriate comments. Following their review, ISB has been defined as 'a verbal or physical act of an explicit, or perceived, sexual nature, which is unacceptable within the social context in which it is carried out' (Johnson et al., 2006, p.688). A recent study explored staff experiences of ISB exhibited by older adults with a dementia (Hayward, Robertson and Knight, 2013). Shock, embarrassment and incomprehension were prominent when ISB was initially encountered. Nurses can often feel ashamed, powerless, angry or even disgusted when they encounter sexual incidents.

—— Religiosity and spirituality ——

The religious and spiritual needs and interests of individuals with dementia have been neglected in research and health care (Doherty, 2006). All good care should have a strong spiritual dimension at its heart, depending on patients' perspectives. It is important to distinguish between spirituality and religion. A working definition could be that religious care is given in the context of shared beliefs, values and liturgies, while spiritual care is usually given in a one-to-one relationship and is person-centred. Religion not only structures how people worship; it also provides the tools for worship, including songs, sacred texts and prayer. Spirituality, which may or may not be linked to a particular religion, is more focused on a search for meaning in life. Being spiritual means being connected in some way to a divine or transcendent sense of purpose.

In Schnell's (2011) study, four main sources related to creating meaning were highlighted:

» Self-transcendence:

- Vertical self-transcendence: orientating towards an immaterial, supernatural power such as faith in God

- Horizontal self-transcendence: taking responsibility for (worldly) affairs beyond one's immediate concerns, such as self-knowledge or unison with nature.

» Self-actualisation: employing, challenging and fostering one's capacities, such as experiences of freedom, creativity and power.

» Order: holding on to values, practicality, decency and the tried and tested, which can be linked to morals and traditions.

» Wellbeing and relatedness: cultivating and enjoying life's pleasures in private and in company, such as experiences of harmony, comfort, love, fun and community.

As revealed by Bonelli and Koenig (2013), religion and spirituality have been increasingly examined in medical research during the past two decades. In nursing, there are accepted nursing diagnoses of spiritual distress or the risk of spiritual distress (Ralph and Taylor, 2008). Interestingly, Finlay (2015) argues that a potentially useful parallel is found when comparing the experience of dementia to the experience of cancer. Dame Cicely Saunders, founder of the modern hospice movement, developed the concept of total pain, the idea that the pain a person experiences can be a combination of physical, emotional, social and spiritual components (Baines, 1990). It is possible to view dementia through a similar lens in that it affects every aspect of a person's life and that the best care will take these varied aspects into account.

When people face situations over which they have little control, they may use spiritual or religious beliefs to manage feelings of helplessness and give meaning and order to the events of their lives (Katsuno, 2003). It is not uncommon when faced with a crisis to ask, 'Why me?' or 'Why is this happening?' Rabbi Harold Kushner's acclaimed book *When Bad Things Happen to Good People* has long been an illuminating text for many people of different faiths seeking to understand the meaning behind tragedy and loss (Snyder, 2003).

However, there are common themes across the various dimensions of religiosity and spirituality (Stuckey and Gwyther, 2003). Religion most often refers to a particular doctrinal framework that guides a system of belief that is sanctioned by a broader faith community. Carers in a study more than a decade ago reported that their religiosity, spirituality and ethnicity impacted their lives and caring efforts (Nightingale, 2003). From the standpoint of practice, health professionals can assist these carers by recognising their belief systems within the care plan. Spirituality is generally described as more inclusive than religiosity and is the overall concept of which religiosity is a subset (Koenig, 2008; Vachon, Fillion and Achille, 2009).

Religion involves specific practices and beliefs that may be associated with an organised group. Spirituality is 'a person's search for or expression of his or her connection to a greater and meaningful context' (Barnum, 2003, p.1). Although religiosity or religion may provide spiritual expression with intellectual, behavioural and social form, the common assessment of spirituality has been limited to its degree or intensity or the frequency of religious involvement (Song and Hanson, 2009). Carers often use religiosity to cope with illness and stressors in their lives. In some samples, the majority have reported that they pray nearly every day and perceive religion as important (Herbert, Dang and Schulz, 2007).

Nagpal and colleagues (2015), based on 107 individuals with mild-to-moderate dementia and their family carers, found that the religiosity of both the carer and the individuals with dementia affected the perception of the quality of life of individuals living with dementia. Religiosity is considered to have three dimensions: organisational, non-organisational and subjective. Organisational religiosity addresses formal religious involvement, such as attending services or events at a place of worship. Non-organisational religiosity addresses private practices, including prayer or reading religious texts. Navaie-Waliser et al. (2001) completed a large study in New York City using phone interviews comparing white, African-American and Hispanic carers. They determined that African-American carers developed increased religiosity after becoming carers and used their religious beliefs as coping mechanisms more often than the white informants.

Puchalski and Romer (2000) define spirituality as 'that which allows a person to experience transcendent meaning in life. This is often expressed as a relationship with God, but it can also be about nature, art, music, family, or community – whatever beliefs and values give a person a sense of meaning and purpose in life' (p.129). Once the word 'spiritual' is used, there has been a slight tendency for care staff to opt out and defer to those from the church. If spiritual care is an important part of holistic care, it is not then the exclusive domain of the church, but the concern of all involved in care. When a person has dementia, the task of offering spiritual care is made even more difficult (Goodall, 2009). For many people, spirituality is synonymous with religion, and not long ago it would have been unusual to hear the word other than in a religious context (Airey et al., 2002). But it could be concluded that spiritual care is that which gives meaning to life and is not necessarily religious, while religious care should always be spiritual (Levison, 2005). Trevitt and MacKinlay (2004) asked whether people with more advanced memory problems could still engage with and talk about spirituality. Their participants talked fully about their early religious activities and how these had changed across their lives.

Spiritual care is generally based on meeting humans' expressions of spirituality and spiritual needs (Narayanasamy, 2004), but people with dementia do not always express their spiritual needs clearly due to their cognitive decline, which makes caring for the spiritual dimensions in their lives challenging (Sabat, 2006; Swinton, 2014). Many clinicians find it challenging to initiate discussions with patients about their spirituality. Some may feel uncomfortable because they do not see it as within their role or scope; others may think that patients will find such discussions too intimate or intrusive; yet others may not have personal spiritual or religious beliefs or practices (Richardson, 2014).

Daaleman and colleagues (2008) conducted a study on the importance of spiritual care in long-term care settings. They found that spiritual care and support are associated with better overall care at the end of life for long-term care residents, and that the best target for interventions to improve this is interaction between residents and facility staff. Spiritual needs are particularly important in crisis-like periods and at the end of life (Molzahn, 2007). Too often individuals visiting health care facilities are seen as a 'disease that needs to be fixed' quickly and cheaply rather than as human beings with complex needs, including those of a spiritual nature (Puchalski et al., 2014). Although nurses claim that they work from a holistic nursing perspective, they admit to a general lack of knowledge about how to meet residents' spiritual needs (Ødbehr et al., 2014). Another challenge nurses face when providing spiritual care is related to the abstract nature of descriptions of spirituality, which blur the understanding of spiritual care (Ramezani et al., 2014). Sawatzky and Pesut (2005) highlight the significance of altruistic care, which implies that nurses show attitudes such as cheerfulness, compassion and kindness, love, joy and peace in their encounters with residents.

However, there have also been a few studies that have described spiritual needs from the residents' perspective. Their findings revealed that residents identified spiritual needs as experiences of meaning in different ways. The sense of meaning could be provided by relationships with family members, friends or through communication (Trevitt and MacKinlay, 2004).

A recent study revealed that residents with dementia do not differ greatly from cognitively healthy people in terms of the spiritual needs of belonging, self-esteem and security (Ødbehr et al., 2014).

Spirituality is, of course, of particular significance in end-of-life care (see Table 8.2).

Table 8.2: Potential predictors of the provision of spiritual
end-of-life care through previous work

Quality of care	Long-term care facility type/physician presence Urbanisation level Staffing Evaluation of quality of care, e.g. communication
A more individualised or more person-centred approach of care; religious backgrounds	Philosophy of care related to individualised approach (individualised person-centred approach: home-like, small-scale living might involve a more individualised approach) Religious affiliation Religious backgrounds and concordance between care provider/patient Importance of faith or spirituality in life and concordance between care provider/patient Religious activities involvement Quality of family–physician relationship
Palliative care	Palliative care explicitly provided at location Palliation as the care goal that takes priority Anticipating death Recognising terminality (recognising dementia as a terminal disease may be a basis for the provision of palliative care)
Other factors or unclear expectations with regard to the direction of a possible association	Facility size and type Demographics Dementia severity Closeness of relationship

FOR MUCH FULLER DETAILS, PLEASE REFER TO VAN DER STEEN ET AL. (2014, TABLE 1, PP.3–7).

Namaste Care

The case for research into spiritual approaches for people with dementia across all levels of capacity is very strong. There are many ethical considerations to do with persons with advanced dementia participating in research, such as how they can consent to take part in a study if they do not realise they have the condition (Higgins, 2013). But there are other important issues too (see, for example, Higgins, 2013). The Namaste Care programme developed by Simard (2007) focuses on the evident need for gentle touch for people with end-stage dementia; namaste is an Indian word with much cultural and spiritual significance. Reaching out to others is part of this. The Namaste Care programme initiates a 'therapeutic relationship' which assists the person to engage with their immediate environment and promotes an environment that is as comfortable and home-like as possible (Nicholls et al., 2013).

In therapeutic relationships, 'understanding the service recipient's perspective on the therapeutic relationship is vital if appropriate interventions are to be developed and implemented' (Shattell, Starr and Thomas, 2007, p.276). The study by Fullarton and Volicer (2013) raised the possibility that involvement in Namaste Care might achieve antipsychotic reduction and discontinuation in residents in a nursing home. A Namaste carer can become very knowledgeable about each resident's history by reading up on their social history and activity interest assessment and by talking to care staff and the resident's family (Simard and Volicer, 2010).

But consent issues in such research are also very interesting. In a study of the effects of Namaste Care on behavioural symptoms in care home residents with advanced dementia, Stacpoole and colleagues (2015, p.704) have remarked on their own methodology:

> An assessment was made of each resident's mental capacity to give informed consent. Where residents lacked this capacity, the decision whether they should participate was made on the basis of their best interests, taking into account the views of family members invited to represent them; or, in the absence of a family member, a professional, not directly involved in the research, was nominated to do so as laid out in legislation (Mental Capacity Act, 2007). Process consent was negotiated on a day to day basis.

But note also Jan Dewing's excellent critique in her own seminal paper (Dewing, 2007, p.23):

> In the situation where the older person with dementia has very little capacity for expressing their consent through facial, behavioural and bodily communication, the need for the researcher to be open and transparent with decision-making is further heightened in order to avoid transgressing boundaries of trust. Having an independent researcher or skilled practitioner to analyse decision-making trials would be one way of achieving openness and transparency. The researcher always has the options of excluding the person or trying to keep the person included, if others known to the person can provide evidence to show that either exclusion or inclusion in the research would most likely have been what the person would have wished for themselves.

Essential reading

Baker C. 2014. *Developing Excellent Care for People Living with Dementia in Care Homes*, London: Jessica Kingsley Publishers.

Jewell A. 2011. *Spirituality and Personhood in Dementia*, London: Jessica Kingsley Publishers.

MacKinley E, Trevitt C. 2015. *Facilitating Spiritual Reminiscence for People with Dementia: A Learning Guide*, London: Jessica Kingsley Publishers.

References

Addis IB, Van Den Eeden SK, Wassel-Fyr CL, Vittinghoff E, Brown JS, Thom DH. 2006. Reproductive risk factors for incontinence study at Kaiser study group: sexual activity and function in middle-aged and older women. Obstet Gynecol, 107(4), 755–764.

Airey J, Hammond G, Kent P, Moffitt L. 2002. *Frequently Asked Questions on Spirituality and Religion*, Derby: Christian Council on Ageing.

Alagiakrishnan K, Lim D, Brahim A, Wong A, et al. 2005. Sexually inappropriate behaviour in demented elderly people. Postgrad Med J, 81(957), 463–466.

Alzheimer's Australia. 2010. *Quality Dementia Care Series: Understanding Dementia Care and Sexuality in Residential Facilities*, Kingston: Alzheimer's Australia.

Archibald C. 1998. Sexuality, dementia and residential care: managers report and response. Health Soc Care Community, 6(2), 95–101.

Baines M. 1990. Tackling total pain. In C Saunders (ed.), *Hospice and palliative care: An interdisciplinary approach*, London: Edward Arnold.

Bamford S. 2011. *Women and Dementia – Not Forgotten*, London: ILC-UK, available at www.ilcuk. org.uk/index.php/publications/publication_details/women_and_dementia_not_forgotten (accessed 3 Oct 2016).

Barnum B. 2003. *Spirituality in Nursing: From Traditional to New Age*, New York: Springer Publishing Company.

Bartlett P. 2010. Sex, dementia, capacity and care homes. Liverpool Law Review, 31(2), 137–154.

Bauer M, Fetherstonhaugh D, Tarzia L, Nay R, Beattie E. 2014a. Supporting residents' expression of sexuality: the initial construction of a sexuality assessment tool for residential aged care facilities. BMC Geriatr, 14, 82.

Bauer M, Nay R, Tarzia L, Fetherstonhaugh D, Wellman D, Beattie E. 2014b. 'We need to know what's going on': views of family members towards the sexual expression of people with dementia in residential aged care. Dementia (London), 13(5), 571–585.

Bennett C. 1980. *Nursing home life: What it is and what it could be*, New York: Tiresias Press.

Bonelli RM, Koenig HG. 2013. Mental disorders, religion and spirituality 1990 to 2010: a systematic evidence-based review. J Relig Health, 52(2), 657–673.

Bretschneider JG, McCoy NL. 1998. Sexual interest and behavior in healthy 80–102 year olds. Archives of Sexual Behavior, 17, 109–129.

Brooker D, Latham I. 2016. *Person-Centred Dementia Care Making Services Better with the VIPS Framework,* London: Jessica Kingsley Publishers.

Comfort A, Dial LK. 1991. Sexuality and ageing: an overview. Clinics in Geriatric Medicine, 7, 1–7.

Daaleman TP, Williams CS, Hamilton VL, Zimmerman S. 2008. Spiritual care at the end of life in long- term care. Med Care, 46, 85–91.

Delamater J. 2012. Sexual expression in later life: a review and synthesis. J. Sex Res, 49(2–3), 125–141.

Dewing J. 2007. Participatory research. A method for process consent with persons who have dementia. Dementia, 6(1), 11–25.

Di Napoli EA, Breland GL, Allen RS. 2013. Staff knowledge and perceptions of sexuality and dementia of older adults in nursing homes. J Aging Health, 25(7), 1087–1105.

Doherty D. 2006. Spirituality and dementia. Spirituality and Health International, 7, 203– 210.

Dourado M, Finamore C, Barroso MF, Santos R, Laks J. 2010. Sexual satisfaction in dementia: perspectives of patients and spouses. Sex Disabil, 28, 195.

Ehrenfeld M, Bronner G, Tabak N, Alpert R, Bergman R. 1999. Sexuality among institutionalized elderly patients with dementia. Nursing Ethics, 6(2), 144–149.

Elias J, Ryan A. 2011. A review and commentary on the factors that influence expressions of sexuality by older people in care homes. J Clin Nurs, 20(11–12), 1668–1676.

Elliott KS, Di Minno M, Lam D, Tu AM. 1996. Working with Chinese families in the context of dementia. In G Yeo, D. Gallagher-Thompson (eds), *Ethnicity and the dementias*, Washington, DC: Taylor & Francis.

Esmaill S, Esmaill Y, Munro B. 2001. Sexuality and disability: the role of health care professionals in providing options and alternatives for couples. Sexuality and Disability, 19, 267–287.

Finlay MR. 2015. Righteousness in the land of forgetfulness. J Relig Health, 54(1), 279–286.

Fullarton J, Volicer L. 2013. Reductions of antipsychotic and hypnotic medications in Namaste Care. J Am Med Dir Assoc, 14(9), 708–709.

Gold MR, Siegel JE, Russell LB, Weinstein MC (eds). 1996. *Cost-Effectiveness in Health and Medicine*, New York: Oxford University Press.

Goodall MA. 2009. The evaluation of spiritual care in a dementia care setting. Dementia, 8(2), 167–183.

Hajjar RR, Kamel HK. 2004. Sexuality in the nursing home, part 1: attitudes and barriers to sexual expression. Journal of the American Medical Directors' Association, 5, S43–S47.

Hayward LE, Robertson N, Knight C. 2013. Inappropriate sexual behaviour and dementia: an exploration of staff experiences. Dementia (London), 12(4), 463–480.

Herbert RS, Dang Q, Schulz R. 2007. Religious beliefs and practices are associated with better mental health in family caregivers of patients with dementia: findings from the REACH study. American Journal of Geriatric Psychiatry, 15, 292–300.

Higgins P. 2013. Involving people with dementia in research. Nursing Times, 109(28), 20–23.

Hsieh YH. 1995. Sexual problems of the aged. Formosan Journal of Sexology, 1, 99–103.

Huang TM. 1995. Sexual knowledge and attitude towards elderly in Chinese people. Formosan Journal of Sexology, 1, 104–113.

Hubbard G, Tester S, Downs MG. 2003. Meaningful social interactions between older people in institutional care settings. Ageing and Society, 23, 99–114.

Institute of Medicine (US) Committee on Improving Quality in Long-Term Care. 2001. *Improving the Quality of Long-Term Care*, Washington, DC: National Academies Press, available at www.ncbi.nlm.nih.gov/books/NBK224500/pdf/Bookshelf_NBK224500.pdf (accessed 3 Oct 2016).

Johnson C, Knight C, Alderman N. 2006. Challenges associated with the definition and assessment of inappropriate sexual behaviour among individuals with an acquired neurological impairment. Brain Injury, 20, 687–693.

Katsuno T. 2003. Personal spirituality of persons with earlystage dementia: is it related to perceived quality of life. Dementia, 2, 315–335.

Kaufmann EG, Engel SA. 2014. Dementia and wellbeing: a conceptual framework based on Tom Kitwood's model of needs. Dementia (London), June, 1471301214539690 (e-pub ahead of print).

Kitwood T. 1997a. *Dementia Reconsidered: The Person Comes First*. Buckingham: Open University Press.

Kitwood T. 1997b. The experience of dementia. Aging & Mental Health, 1, 13–22.

Kitwood T, Bredin K. 1992. Towards a theory of dementia care: personhood and wellbeing. Ageing and Society, 12(3), 269–287.

Knapp M, Prince M. 2007. *Dementia UK: A Report to the Alzheimer's Society*, London: Alzheimer's Society, available at www.alzheimers.org.uk/site/scripts/download_info.php?fileID=2 (accessed 3 Oct 2016).

Koenig HG. 2008. Concerns about measuring 'spirituality' in research. Journal of Nervous and Mental Disease, 196, 349–355.

Laumann EO, Nicolosi A, Glasser DB, Paik A, Gingell C, Moreira E. 2005. Sexual problems among women and men aged 40–80: prevalence and correlates identified in the Global Study of Sexual Attitudes and Behaviors. International Journal of Impotence Research, 17, 39–57.

Lester PE, Kohen I, Stefanacci RG, Feuerman M. 2016. Sex in nursing homes: a survey of nursing home policies governing resident sexual activity. J Am Med Dir Assoc, 17(1), 71–74.

Levison C. 2005. Partners in care. Nursing Management, 12(6), 8–21.

Lichtenberg PA. 2014. Sexuality and physical intimacy in long-term care. Occup Ther Health Care, 28(1), 42–50.

Lindau ST, Gavrilova N. 2010. Sex, health, and years of sexually active life gained due to good health: Evidence from two US population based cross sectional surveys of ageing. British Medical Journal, 340.

Lyder CH. 1994. The role of the nurse practitioner in promoting sexuality in the institutionalized elderly. Journal of the American Academy of Nurse Practitioners, 6(2), 61–63.

Mahieu L, Anckaert L, Gastmans C. 2014. Intimacy and sexuality in institutionalized dementia care: clinical-ethical considerations. Health Care Anal, October (e-pub ahead of print).

Mahieu L, Gastmans C. 2015. Older residents' perspectives on aged sexuality in institutionalized elderly care: a systematic literature review. Int J Nurs Stud, 52(12), 1891–1905.

Makimoto K, Kang HS, Yamakawa M, Konno R. 2015. An integrated literature review on sexuality of elderly nursing home residents with dementia. Int J Nurs Pract, 21(Suppl 2), 80–90.

McAuliffe L, Bauer M, Nay R. 2007. Barriers to the expression of sexuality in the older person: the role of the health professional. Int J Older People Nurs, 2(1), 69–75.

McSherry W. 2006. *Making Sense of Spirituality in Nursing and Health Care Practice: An Interactive Approach*, London: Jessica Kingsley Publishers.

Molzahn AE. 2007. Spirituality in later life: effect on quality of life. J Gerontol Nurs, 33(1), 32–39.

Nagpal N, Heid AR, Zarit SH, Whitlatch CJ. 2015. Religiosity and quality of life: a dyadic perspective of individuals with dementia and their caregivers. Aging Ment Health, 19(6), 500–506.

Narayanasamy A. 2004. Spiritual care. The puzzle of spirituality for nursing: A guide to practical assessment. British Journal of Nursing, 13(19), 1140–1144.

Navaie-Waliser M, Feldman P, Gould D, Levine C, Kuerbis A, Donelan K. 2001. The experiences and challenges of informal caregivers: common themes and differences among whites, blacks, and Hispanics. The Gerontologist, 41(6), 733–741.

Nay R. 2004. Sexuality and Older People. In R Nay and S Garratt (eds), *Nursing Older People: Issues and Innovations*, Marrickville: Elsevier.

Nay R, McAuliffe L, Bauer M. 2007. Sexuality: from stigma, stereotypes and secrecy to coming out, communication and choice. Int J Older People Nurs, 2(1), 76–80.

Nicholls D, Chang E, Johnson A, Edenborough M. 2013. Touch, the essence of caring for people with end-stage dementia: a mental health perspective in Namaste Care. Aging Ment Health, 17(5), 571–578.

Nightingale, MC. 2003. Religion, spirituality, and ethnicity What it means for caregivers of persons with Alzheimer's disease and related disorders, Dementia, 2(3), 379–391.

Ødbehr L, Kvigne K, Hauge S, Danbolt LJ. 2014. Nurses' and care workers' experiences of spiritual needs in residents with dementia in nursing homes: a qualitative study. BMC Nurs, 13, 12.

Orchard H, Clark D. 2012. Tending the soul as well as the body: Spiritual care in nursing and residential homes. International Journal of Palliative Nursing, 7(11), 541–546.

Puchalski CM, Romer AL. 2000. Taking a spiritual history allows clinicians to understand patients more fully. J Palliat Med, 3, 129–137.

Puchalski CM, Vitillo R, Hull SK, Reller N. 2014. Improving the spiritual dimension of whole person care: reaching national and international consensus. J Palliat Med, 17(6), 642–656.

Ralph S, Taylor C. 2008. *Nursing Diagnosis Reference Manual*, Philadelphia: Lippincott Williams & Wilkins.

Ramezani M, Ahmadi F, Mohammadi E, Kazemnejad A. 2014. Spiritual care in nursing: a concept analysis. Intern Nurs Review, 61(2), 211–219.

Richardson P. 2014. Spirituality, religion and palliative care. Ann Palliat Med, 3(3), 150–159.

Rosen T, Lachs MS, Pillemer K. 2010. Sexual aggression between residents in nursing homes: literature synthesis of an under recognized problem. J Am Geriatr Soc, 58(10), 1970–1979.

Sabat SR. 2006. Implicit memory and people with Alzheimer's disease: implications for caregiving. American Journal of Alzheimer's Disease and Other Dementias, 21(1), 11–14.

Sawatzky R, Pesut B. 2005. Attributes of spiritual care in nursing practice. J of Hol Nurs, 23(1), 19–33.

Schnell T. 2011. Individual differences in meaning-making: considering the variety of sources of meaning, their density and diversity. Pers Indiv Differ, 51(5), 667–673.

Shattell MM, Starr SS, Thomas SP. 2007. 'Take my hand, help me out': mental health service recipients' experience of the therapeutic relationship. Int J Ment Health Nurs, 16(4), 274–284.

Shuttleworth R, Russell C, Weerakoon P, Dune T 2010. Sexuality in Residential Aged Care: A Survey of Perceptions and Policies in Australian Nursing Homes. Sex Disabil, 28, 187–194.

Simard J. 2007. *The End-of-Life Namaste Care Program for People with Dementia*, Baltimore, MD: Health Professions Press.

Simard J, Volicer L. 2010. Effects of Namaste Care on residents who do not benefit from usual activities. Am J Alzheimers Dis Other Demen, 25(1), 46–50.

Snyder L. 2003. Satisfactions and challenges in spiritual faith and practice for persons with dementia. Dementia, 2(3), 299–313.

Song MK, Hanson LC. 2009. Relationships between psychosocial-spiritual well-being and end of-life preferences and values in African American dialysis patients. J Pain Symptom Manage, 38(3), 372–380.

Stacpoole M, Hockley J, Thompsell A, Simard J, Volicer L. 2015. The Namaste Care programme can reduce behavioural symptoms in care home residents with advanced dementia. Int J Geriatr Psychiatry, 30(7), 702–709.

Stuckey JC, Gwyther LP. 2003. Dementia, religion, and spirituality. Dementia, 2, 291.

Swinton J. 2014. What the body remembers: theological reflections on dementia. Journal of Religion, Spirituality & Aging, 26(2–3), 160–172.

Tarzia L, Bauer M, Fetherstonhaugh D, Nay R. 2013. Interviewing older people in residential aged care about sexuality: difficulties and challenges. Sex Disabil, 31, 361.

Tarzia L, Fetherstonhaugh D, Bauer M. 2012. Dementia, sexuality and consent in residential aged care facilities. J Med Ethics, 38(10), 609–613.

Trevitt C, MacKinlay E. 2004. 'Just because I can't remember. . .' Religiousness in older people with dementia. Journal of Religion, Spirituality and Aging, 16, 109–121.

Tzeng YL, Lin LC, Shyr YI, Wen JK. 2009. Sexual behaviour of institutionalised residents with dementia – a qualitative study. J Clin Nurs, 18(7), 991–1001.

Vachon M, Fillion L, Achille M. 2009. A conceptual analysis of spirituality at the end of life. Journal of Palliative Medicine, 12, 53–59.

van der Steen JT, Gijsberts MJ, Hertogh CM, Deliens L. 2014. Predictors of spiritual care provision for pa tients with dementia at the end of life as perceived by physicians: a prospective study. BMC Palliat Care, 13(1), 61.

White C. 1982. Sexual interest, attitudes, knowledge and sexual history in relation to sexual behaviour in the institutionalised aged. Archives of Sexual Behaviour, 11(1), 11–21.

WHO. 2006. *Defining Sexual Health: Report of a Technical Consultation on Sexual Health*, Geneva: WHO, available at www.who.int/reproductivehealth/publications/sexual_health/defining_sexual_health.pdf (accessed 3 Oct 2016).

Wiskerke E, Manthorpe J. 2016. Intimacy between care home residents with dementia: findings from a review of the literature. Dementia (London), July, 1471301216659771 (e-pub ahead of print).

Zilbergeld B. 2004. *Better Than Ever*, Trowbridge, UK: Crown House Publishing, Cromwell Press.

Chapter 9

REGULATION, RESEARCH AND STAFF

By the end of this chapter, you will be able to:

» define and recognise abuse, neglect and mistreatment

» explain principles of safeguarding

» explain barriers to research, particularly in relation to novel drug development

» evaluate critically evidence concerning staff engagement and performance, and staff culture especially with regard to staff turnover, person-centred care, barriers to care, staff culture and staffing, particularly in relation to residential settings

» identify with key issues in leadership

—— Introduction ——————————————————————

Three central levers for improving dementia care, health and wellbeing are further research, regulation and staff performance. No one component offers a full solution. For example, in viewing the importance of regulation, some believe an obsession with measuring the dimensions of a pig can divert attention from nourishing the pig adequately in the first place. But such arguments should not be allowed to engender a general ethos of nihilism in improving the quality of dementia care. Although formidable barriers exist, for example staff morale or developing new drugs for dementia, lessons can be learned if one aspires not to make the same mistakes again.

—— Five key questions ——————————————

The regulator, the Care Quality Commission (CQC), has developed five key questions (see Figure 9.1).

Is this service safe?

Is this service effective?

Is this service caring?

Is this service responsive to people's needs?

Is this service well led?

Figure 9.1: The key five questions

Source: Care Quality Commission (no date, pp.11–12). The CQC intends
to ensure that person-centred care is at the heart of the questions we
ask of adult social care services and how CQC rates services.

The CQC feels that answers to these questions can improve care in five key ways:[1]

» **Safe:** you are protected from abuse and avoidable harm.

» **Effective:** your care, treatment and support achieves good outcomes, helps you to maintain quality of life and is based on the best available evidence.

» **Caring:** staff involve and treat you with compassion, kindness, dignity and respect.

» **Responsive:** services are organised so that they meet your needs.

» **Well led:** the leadership, management and governance of the organisation ensure the provision of high-quality care that is based on patients' individual needs, the encouragement of learning and innovation, and the promotion of an open and fair culture.

—— Abuse and neglect ——————————————

Abuse and neglect can occur anywhere: in your own home or a public place, while you are in hospital or attending a day centre, or in a college or care home. You may be living alone or with others. The person causing the harm may be a stranger to you, but more often than not the person is known, and

---

1   See www.cqc.org.uk/content/five-key-questions-we-ask (accessed 4 Oct 2016).

it can be the case that you usually feel safe with them. They are usually in a position of trust and power, such as a health and care professional, relative or neighbour. (NHS Choices, 2015)

Abuse and neglect are two concrete examples of where it is necessary to have a clear idea about locally enforceable regulations and international frameworks.

Since the publication of Goffman's classic *Asylums* in 1968, a large body of scientific literature has underscored the organisational and institutional limits faced by residential care facilities, which can rapidly become restrictive, debilitating and even abusive (Lindbloom et al., 2007). Despite cultural differences in how abuse is conceptualised (Phelan, 2009), the central concern should be working to promote equality, dignity and human rights (Phelan, 2008). *No Secrets* (Department of Health, 2000), the government guidance for protecting vulnerable adults from abuse in England, stated that abuse can occur in different forms including physical, sexual, psychological and financial abuses, discrimination and neglect.

Elder abuse of all types can have profoundly negative consequences and there is evidence of increased mortality rates among older adults who have suffered mistreatment (Lachs et al., 1998). It is widely suggested that people with dementia face particular risks arising from their vulnerabilities and vulnerable situations, although some of these are faced by older people more generally (e.g. Manthorpe, 2015).

The caring relationship between the carer and the care recipient in the overall caring culture is pivotal to the emergence of neglect and abuse (see Figure 9.2).

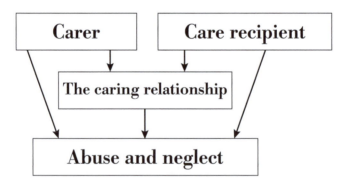

Figure 9.2: Theoretical model for risk of elder
mistreatment by dementia caregivers
Source: Wiglesworth et al. (2010, Fig. 1, p.495).

Neglect implies withholding expected levels of comfort, for example withholding food or medications. *Medical neglect* is another form (Anetzberger, 2005) and refers to postponing medical needs and services by failing to give medicines on time or provide regular medical follow-up (Collins, 2006).

Elder **abuse** has been defined by the WHO as a single or repeated act, or the lack of an appropriate action, occurring within any relationship where there is an expectation of trust and where harm or distress is caused to an older person. It may take several forms.[2]

Physical abuse encompasses a wide range of forms of abuse, including striking, pushing, shoving, choking, burning the skin and other forms of physical injury. It can include being assaulted, hit, slapped, pushed, restrained, denied food or water or not being helped to go to the bathroom. It can also include the misuse of medication.

Psychological or emotional abuse may be subtle but includes withholding funds, food and medication, isolation, belittling or ignoring, and other forms of non-physical abuse. This includes emotional abuse, threats of hurting someone or threats of abandonment, stopping someone from seeing people, and humiliating, blaming, controlling, intimidating or harassing someone. It also includes verbal abuse, cyberbullying and isolation, or the unreasonable and unjustified withdrawal of services or support networks.

Financial abuse is fairly frequent – family members and others may restrict access to much-needed funding. Money or valuables may be stolen, or someone appointed to look after patients' money may spend it inappropriately or coerce patients into spending it in ways they do not want. In addition, pensions, annuity funds, social security cheques or personal savings may be confiscated. Some institutions and private families are guilty of practising and perpetuating these various forms of elder abuse and neglect. Internet scams and doorstep crime are becoming increasingly common forms of financial abuse.

Discriminatory abuse includes forms of harassment, slurs or similar unfair treatment relating to race, gender and gender identity, age, disability, sexual orientation or religion.

There are many definitional issues in the study of elder mistreatment (Dixon et al., 2009) that have become increasingly inclusive in terms of setting, identity or intent (Johnson, 2011).

However, a broad definition may suffice, such as the one used in the US National Research Council Panel on Elder Mistreatment (Bonnie and Wallace, 2003). Elder abuse may be defined as outlined below:

> Intentional actions that cause harm or create a serious risk of harm (whether or not harm is intended) to a vulnerable elder by a caregiver or other person who stands in a trust relationship to the elder; failure by a caregiver to

---

2   A fuller definition is provided by the Office of the Inspector General of the Department of Health and Human Services which has identified seven different types of elder abuse of nursing home residents: physical abuse, misuse of restraints, verbal/emotional abuse, physical neglect, medical neglect, verbal/emotional neglect and personal property abuse (material goods) (Hirst, 2002).

satisfy the elder's basic needs or to protect the elder from harm. (Bonnie and Wallace, 2003, p.40)

Mistreatment conveys two ideas: that some injury, deprivation or dangerous condition has occurred to the elder person and that someone else bears responsibility for causing this or failing to prevent it.

Elder neglect is part of a wider phenomenon of mistreatment by some family members and carers. Abuse has been widely researched, but neglect has received very little attention (Fulmer et al., 2004).

Lachs and Pillemer (2004) have reviewed the elder abuse literature, focusing mainly on community settings. They have cited evidence for a set of risk factors which increases the risk of mistreatment: shared living situations (e.g. living with adult children); having dementia; social isolation; psychological problems or substance abuse of perpetrators; and dependence of perpetrators on the older people they mistreat. All of these factors also suggest the importance of the dynamics between older people and family carers or paid care workers in explaining mistreatment. Kelly (2010) concludes that it is through a lack of recognition of and support for the three kinds of self that practices emerge that may underpin mistreatment in long-term care settings.

Such **malignant positioning** and attacks on selfhood do not necessarily qualify as mistreatment, although they may certainly be seen as a 'permissor' of mistreatment – a pattern of behaviour and practice that makes more serious episodes of mistreatment less unacceptable.

Also noteworthy is aggression which can occur between residents, known as Resident to Resident Aggression (RRA). RRA has been defined as:

negative and aggressive physical, sexual or verbal interactions between long-term care residents that in a community setting would likely be construed as unwelcome and have high potential to cause physical or psychological distress in the recipient. (Rosen et al., 2008, p.78)

I will return to malignant positioning in Chapter 14.

Although more research has been done on both elder abuse perpetrated by family members in community settings (Baker, 2007) and by staff in nursing homes, much less is known about RRA in nursing homes (Shinoda-Tagawa et al., 2004).

Care home regulation and principles of safeguarding

The general remit of the Care Quality Commission is crucial in the regulation of care homes (see Box 9.1).

Box 9.1: Cracks in the Pathway

Overall, the Care Quality Commission in their very helpful report[3] found more good care than poor in the care homes and hospitals we visited, but the quality of care for people with dementia varies greatly and it is likely that they will experience poor care at some point along their care pathway. They reported that clear guidance has been available for years, but improvements in care are still needed and overdue.

ASSESSMENT OF CARE NEEDS

In 29% of care homes and 56% of hospitals, the Care Quality Commission found aspects of variable or poor care regarding how a person's needs were assessed.

PROVIDERS WORKING TOGETHER

In 27% of care homes and 22% of hospitals, the Care Quality Commission found aspects of variable or poor care regarding the arrangements for how they shared information when people moved between services.

INVOLVEMENT

In 33% of care homes and 61% of hospitals, the Care Quality Commission found aspects of variable or poor care regarding people or their families and carers not being involved in decisions about their care and choices about how to spend their time.

PLANNING AND DELIVERY OF CARE

In 42% of hospitals, the Care Quality Commission found aspects of variable or poor care regarding how the care met people's physical and mental health and emotional and social needs.

STAFFING

In 27% of care homes and 56% of hospitals, the Care Quality Commission found aspects of variable or poor care regarding staff's understanding and knowledge of dementia care.

MONITORING THE QUALITY OF CARE

In 37% of care homes and 28% of hospitals, the Care Quality Commission found aspects of variable or poor practice in the way providers monitored the quality of dementia care.

---

3   Available at www.cqc.org.uk/sites/default/files/20141009_cracks_in_the_pathway_final_0.pdf (accessed 4 Oct 2016).

Adult safeguarding is the process of protecting adults with care and support needs from abuse or neglect. It is an important part of what many public services do, but the key responsibility is with local authorities in partnership with the police and the NHS.

It is argued that poor care standards and rigid institutional regimes contribute to a poor quality of life among care home residents (Ronch, 2004). Social workers and care providers need to work closely with residents to ensure that the individual is enabled to make choices, even if those choices appear unwise and include an element of risk (SCIE, 2012). Safeguarding has been described by the Care Quality Commission (CQC) in their document Our *Safeguarding Protocol* (CQC, 2013).

The term safeguarding describes a range of activities that organisations should have in place to protect both children and adults, unless stated otherwise, whose circumstances make them particularly vulnerable to abuse, neglect or harm. CQC recognises that a person's ability to keep themselves safe is partly determined by their individual circumstances and that this may change at different stages in a person's life.

Three important aspects of safeguarding from the CQC are:

» acting promptly on safeguarding issues

» speaking with people using services, and their carers and families

» holding providers to account by taking regulatory action.

The Care Act 2014 puts adult safeguarding on a legal footing. From April 2015 each local authority must:

» make enquiries, or ensure others do so, if it believes an adult is subject to, or at risk of, abuse or neglect; an enquiry should establish whether any action needs to be taken to stop or prevent abuse or neglect, and if so, by whom

» set up a Safeguarding Adults Board (SAB) with core membership from the local authority, the police and the NHS (specifically the local Clinical Commissioning Group/s) and the power to include other relevant bodies

» arrange, where appropriate, for an independent advocate to represent and support an adult who is the subject of a safeguarding enquiry or Safeguarding Adult Review (SAR) where the adult has 'substantial difficulty' in being involved in the process and where there is no other appropriate adult to help them

» cooperate with each of its relevant partners in order to protect adults experiencing or at risk of abuse or neglect.

People who may need safeguarding are defined under section 42 of the Care Act 2014 as adults: who have care and support needs; who are experiencing, or are at risk of, abuse or neglect; and who, because of their care and support needs, cannot protect themselves against actual or potential abuse or neglect.

The statutory guidance enshrines the six principles of safeguarding, as described in Age UK (2015):

» **empowerment** – presumption of person-led decisions and informed consent

» **prevention** – it is better to take action before harm occurs

» **proportionality** – proportionate and least intrusive response appropriate to the risk presented

» **protection** – support and representation for those in greatest need

» **partnerships** – local solutions through services working with their communities

» **accountability** – accountability and transparency in delivering safeguarding.

The Care Act 2014 also recognises the key role of carers in safeguarding. For example, a carer may: witness or report abuse or neglect; experience intentional or unintentional harm from the adult they are trying to support; or unintentionally or intentionally harm or neglect the adult they support.

The overall context of the Adult Social Care Outcomes Framework (ASCOF) is pivotal (see Figure 9.3).

Domain 1: Ensuring quality of life for people with care and support needs

Domain 2: Delaying and reducing the need for care and support

Domain 3: Ensuring that people have a positive experience of care and support

Domain 4: Safeguarding adults whose circumstances make them vulnerable and protecting them from avoidable harm

Figure 9.3: The Adult Social Care Outcomes Framework 2015/16
Source: Department of Health (2014).

—— Barriers to research ——————————————

There are different reasons why qualitative and quantitative research become compromised; research to find 'a new cure' for dementia will also hit different obstacles compared to research into the quality of care in care homes.

Arguably, there is an urgent need to find interventions that will prevent, delay the onset, slow the progression or improve the symptoms of Alzheimer's disease, but the difficulty of advancing the treatment agenda for Alzheimer's is shown by the absence of any new approved therapies since 2004 (Appleby et al., 2013). The scientific pathway towards a cure is uncertain, and the research and development required will take considerable time and financial resources. The World Dementia Council and other organisations have called for the development of a cure or disease-modifying therapy by the year 2025, and efforts are being undertaken globally to lower the barriers to progress.

In Long (2015, p.3), this cautionary warning is given:

> Dementia research and development is at a crossroads. The past decade has seen very little in the way of progress in drug development, and the disease has suffered from a lack of funding in innovation, research and development. Part of the problem is the high failure rate of candidate drugs, predominantly in the early stages of development, which is symptomatic of the gaps in the biology. However, in order to confront this problem we need understand the wider culture of breakdown in the development of dementia drugs. Gaps in knowledge around the disease biology and how conducive it is to the regulatory science, scant openness with data-sharing, and the need for better understanding of regulatory challenges all lead to slow and inefficient translation of research into successful clinical results that can pave the way.

Psychosocial interventions can improve behaviour and mood in people with dementia, but it is unclear how to maximise their effectiveness or acceptability in residential settings. Lawrence and colleagues (2012) found that the successful implementation of such interventions rested on the active engagement of staff and family and the continuing provision of tailored interventions and support.

Clinical research is best done when aligned with clinical care – that is, when the patient can be identified, recruited and, in many instances, researched in parallel with the delivery of clinical service. However, to achieve this effectively requires identifying the additional cost to the NHS clinical support services and the development of an appropriately skilled workforce. The National Institute for Health Research in England funded the Dementias and Neurodegenerative Diseases Research Network (DeNDRoN), and its success thus far has been formidable (Kotting et al., 2012). Building research capacity, collaborating on an international action plan and facilitating research recruitment are all fundamental to the work that DeNDRoN does.

There are known issues about barriers to research in drug development.

The literature is massively biased towards Alzheimer's disease, or dementia of the Alzheimer's type. This skews the discussion to suit Big Pharma, but is Big Pharma able to 'call the shots' as it holds the purse strings?

Trial design

It has been proposed by Fillit and colleagues (2002) that better clinical trial designs to increase the efficiency of the process are needed. The length of trial has to reconcile what is ethical with the progressive nature of disease (Karlawish and Whitehouse, 1998; Kawas et al., 1999). Clinical trial methodologies should be scrutinised to ensure that the design behind each phase tests the intended hypothesis for that phase (Long, 2015).

Therapeutic targets

Despite decades of research, there remains a lack of validated therapeutic targets, presumably stemming from our incomplete understanding of the pathogenesis of the disease (Selkoe, 1991).

Business risk and financial risk

Barriers to the discovery and development of drugs for Alzheimer's at the major pharmaceutical companies comprise concerns about the business risks associated with developing drugs for the disease. In order to manage financial risks and use limited resources efficiently, clinical programmes are designed to allow for an early verification of the therapeutic hypothesis through iterative processes in translational studies.

Regulatory authorities

Regulatory agencies are a key, independent partner for innovators in drug development for Alzheimer's disease in that they govern the approval and provision of drugs. The unique needs of the disease, persistent knowledge gaps and failure in the delivery of disease-modifying drugs have shaped regulatory processes and governance models for product development in this sector. Another issue that affects the pharmaceutical and biotechnology industries is the lack of international harmonisation of clinical trial and regulatory requirements (Spiegel and Irwin, 1996).

Academic infrastructure

Academic drug discovery and development programmes are typically underfunded and lack infrastructure, in terms of staff and equipment, especially at the preclinical level. In addition, there is a general lack of interaction and collaboration between teams of researchers (Fillit et al., 2002).

Better understanding of the disease process

There is a critical need to better understand the complex aetiology of dementia. The lack of success, despite significant investment, may indicate that the gaps in the research science still need to be addressed and agreed on (Long, 2015).

There is also currently a huge effort to improve research into quality of care, including care homes.

In the UK, care homes continue to be one of the main providers of long-term care for older people with dementia. Despite the recent increase in care home research, residents with dementia are often excluded from studies. Care home research networks have been recommended by the Ministerial Advisory Group on Dementia Research as a way of increasing research opportunities for residents with dementia; the Ministerial Advisory Group on Dementia Research was established in February 2010 to consider ways to increase the volume and impact of high-quality dementia research. The feasibility and early impact of an initiative to increase care home participation in research have, in particular, been closely scrutinised (e.g. Davies et al., 2014).

As discussed in Chapter 3, older people in residential settings often experience a range of symptoms which can impact or confound all aspects of the research process, including participant recruitment, and data collection, quality and analysis (Uman and Urman, 1990). While the importance of informed consent is widely acknowledged, the practical aspects of conducting research in this environment can present a unique set of challenges (Hall, Longhurst and Higginson, 2009). I gave one example of this in my discussion of Namaste Care in Chapter 8.

—— Staff engagement and performance ——

Mistry, Levack and Johnson (2015), from inpatient ward research, discovered that patients valued staff who worked together as a cohesive team, treated them as individuals, practised in a collaborative way and used enabling approaches to support their recovery. The dynamics of this relationship depend on how well staff feel nurtured, engaged and supported; this was not just an issue for hospitals, but also for all care settings, even care at home, which I discuss in Chapter 13.

Staff turnover

Turnover of licensed nursing staff in long-term care (LTC) settings (e.g. nursing homes) is a mounting concern and is associated with poor quality of care and low staff morale. Retention and turnover research in LTC has focused primarily on direct care workers (i.e. nurse aides), leaving the issues largely unexplored for licensed nursing staff (i.e. registered nurses and licensed practical nurses). High turnover rates of nursing staff in LTC are detrimental to staff. They have been linked to: lower job satisfaction, increased overtime, role conflict on the unit and increasing the workload for the remaining staff (Chu, Wodchis and McGilton, 2014). Staff turnover also weakens the standard of resident care, as it has been empirically shown to increase catheter use, restraint use, disruptions in the continuity of care, the probability of medical errors, the risk of developing contractures and pressure ulcers, and a prolonged length of stay for residents in LTC (Chu et al., 2014).

Registered nurses have been leaving the aged care sector in large numbers in some jurisdictions, leading to substantial changes in workloads, roles and responsibilities for nurses. Reasons for this include retirement, job dissatisfaction and an unsupportive work environment (Cameron and Brownie, 2010). In a systematic review of international research, organisational commitment, job satisfaction, leadership practices and the working environment were found to influence licensed nursing staff's intentions to stay in all types of health care settings (Cowden, Cummings and Profetto-McGrath, 2011). For example, without a change in workforce trends, high-quality care for older Americans cannot be guaranteed (Lerner et al., 2014). This is reflected in many other developed economies. It is frequently observed that changing demographics and an ageing population are increasing the demand for social care while traditional pools of social care staff are shrinking (Hussein, Ismail and Manthorpe, 2016).

Person-centred care

The increasing prevalence of dementia has challenged residential aged care facilities to recognise the need to go beyond medical care and towards the concept of person-centred care as a key approach to creating a more positive psychosocial environment for residents with dementia (Barbosa et al., 2014). Tom Kitwood propelled this approach in dementia care and inspired many leaders of today in the process. I briefly introduced this in Chapter 2.

Kitwood (1997) argued that the behaviours of people with dementia who are distressed are not just the result of changes in the brain but a consequence of a complex interaction between neuropathology and the person's psychosocial environment. Within this essential reframing, many of the difficulties people with dementia experience are not just a consequence of the disease itself but are the result of threats to one's personhood, brought about by negative interactions with others. Kitwood termed this 'malignant social psychology'.

Promoting a positive and supportive psychosocial climate and a work environment where staff experience a balance between demands from and control over their work, to enable person-centred care practice, seems to have important implications for managers and leaders in residential aged care (Sjögren et al., 2015).

Barriers to care

Many studies indicate that job satisfaction is a core indicator for staff wellbeing and mental health. Job satisfaction has a strong moderating effect on the relationships between work exposure, nurses' attitudes and behavioural outcomes (such as an 'intention to leave'), and job turnover. For example, one aspect of nursing job satisfaction is the satisfaction with the quality of care (Schmidt et al., 2014).

Occupational and resident characteristics affect levels of staff stress and satisfaction in nursing homes, and levels of staff turnover are high. The demand/control model of job strain is widely used in studies of the relationship between work characteristics and health outcomes (Karasek and Theorell, 1990).

Staff culture

The heterogeneous nature of dementia has many implications for the workforce and service providers (Elliott et al., 2015). The culture of the members of staff themselves is intimately associated with their values from recruitment to current employment conditions. Resilience can be defined as an ability to rebound from adversity and overcome difficult circumstances in one's life. This is an attribute that can assist staff to adapt successfully to the demanding physical, mental and emotional nature of their profession (McAllister and McKinnon, 2008), as well as persons with dementia and carers being able to cope with living with the condition themselves.

Culture is paramount for quality of care (see Figure 9.4). For example, researchers have also found that nurses working in contexts with a more positive culture, leadership and evaluation reported more research utilisation, staff development and lower rates of adverse events for patients and staff (Cummings et al., 2007). Nursing managers and leaders must consider that work culture is crucial for improving the quality of care in nursing homes (André et al., 2014). If job satisfaction can be increased through employee empowerment, by extension it seems reasonable to expect that career planning will also be nurtured by an empowering organisational environment that promotes vocational development (Coogle, Parham and Rachel, 2011).

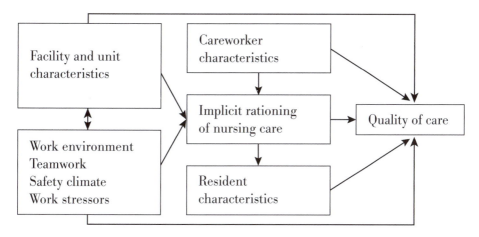

Figure 9.4: Factors related to quality of care
Source: redrawn from Zúñiga et al. (2015, Fig. 1).

Burnout is one syndrome linked to the emotional strains experienced at work. It is a very well-known subject within dementia care. Tom Kitwood provides a brilliant synopsis of the issue in *Dementia Reconsidered* (1997, p.107):

> A considerable body of research on this topic, however, comes strongly to the conclusion that the main causes lie in the way organisations function, particularly inadequacies in the design of jobs, the lack of support structures, and in the workload itself.

The most widely accepted conceptualisation originates from the work of Maslach and Jackson (1986). They consider burnout as an ongoing emotional state, typically characterised by the three dimensions of emotional exhaustion, depersonalisation and reduced personal accomplishment. Reduced personal accomplishment refers to a decline in feelings of competence and personal achievement (Duffy, Oyebode and Allen, 2009). The causes of burnout are indeed multifactorial, involving both the individual struggling to cope with the demands and stresses of work, and the organisation failing to regulate the demands placed on workers or support their workforce adequately. Lazarus and colleagues have developed a process model of stress and coping (e.g. Lazarus, 1993).

Staffing

Staffing has emerged as a key focus of quality of care in various residential long-term care settings. Nursing homes are faced with the challenge of providing 'acceptable' levels of quality at reasonable costs. Jurisdictions attempt to influence this trade-off between cost and quality by regulating the level of nurse staffing a nursing home must have per resident. Indeed, in the US, minimum direct care staffing requirements change the staffing levels and the skills mix, thereby improving certain aspects of quality, but this can also lead to the use of care practices associated with lower quality (Bowblis, 2011). The quest for the ideal staff-to-resident ratio has led to several recommendations. There is general agreement that turnover of direct care workers, registered nurses or managerial professionals (directors of nursing, facility social workers, administrators/directors) disrupts the function and quality of care delivered in residential settings (Zhang et al., 2006). Quality of care can be considered as an outcome determined by structure and process factors, such as organisational, personnel and resident characteristics, as well as the work environment, work stressors and the necessity of rationing care. The relationships between staffing level, turnover or staff mix with quality of care have been broadly researched in nursing homes, with a tendency for better quality of care to be associated with better staffing factors, but results are still inconclusive (Zúñiga et al., 2015).

Many staffing models exist, but which model is associated with the best outcomes for residents of aged care facilities is not well established. A Cochrane review entitled 'Effectiveness of Staffing Models in Residential, Subacute, Extended Aged Care Settings on Patient and Staff Outcomes' found no conclusive research to suggest that any nursing model or skills-mix model would be effective at improving patient or staff wellbeing (Hodgkinson et al., 2011). Backhaus and colleagues (2014) looked at the relationship between nurse staffing and the quality of care in nursing homes. The evidence for this relationship, however, is currently weak because most studies employ a cross-sectional design. No consistent relationship was found between nurse staffing and quality of care. Higher staffing levels were associated with higher as well as lower indicators of quality of care.

Although a growing body of literature examines the relationships between nurse staffing levels in nursing homes and quality of care, this predominantly focuses on US nursing facilities. The studies present a wide range and varied mass of findings that use disparate methods to define and measure quality of care and nurse staffing. Karen Spilsbury and colleagues (2011) concluded that focusing on actual numbers of nurses fails to address the influence of other staffing factors (e.g. turnover, agency staff use), the training and experience of staff, and care organisation and management. 'Quality' is a difficult concept to capture directly, and the measures used focus mainly on the clinical outcomes for residents.

—— Other issues

Leadership

Head nurses and nursing directors can help frontline nurses face this challenge through empowerment and role modelling. The same applies to professionals and practitioners.

Strong leadership can lead to adequate staffing, involvement in policymaking and better collaboration with physicians. It can also improve clinical and practitioner outcomes for patients and users, organisations (e.g. efficiency, innovation and quality) and personnel (e.g. job satisfaction, less absenteeism) (van Oostveen, Mathijssen and Vermeulen, 2015). Aiken, Smith and Lake (1994) attributed the better outcomes in high-performance organisations to professional nursing work systems in particular, where nurses experienced more autonomy and control. Researchers have also found that nurses working in contexts with a more positive culture, leadership and evaluation reported more research utilisation, staff development and lower rates of adverse events for patients and staff (Cummings et al., 2007).

Leadership is also very much about establishing and developing a work culture, where care is given in line with the patients' and their families' individual beliefs, concerns and expectations. A leader must trust his or her staff members to deliver care in line with legislation, professional principles and the institution's set of values, and that this is reciprocated (Jakobsen and Sørlie, 2015).

Staff education and culture change

There are international policy concerns about improving the qualifications of nursing home staff and retaining an adequately educated and skilled workforce in nursing homes (OECD, 2005). More staff (**quantity**) – that is, the number of staff hours per resident day – does not necessarily equate to better care (**quality**). With care provision, quality of life (QoL) may be used as a benchmark for caring. Understanding QoL from the perspective of the person with dementia can help to enhance respect for the individual and improve care provision (Moyle et al., 2015). Competence is important, since it improves opportunities to control situations at work (Josefsson, Sonde and Wahlin, 2007). Joy, Carter and Smith (2000) have emphasised the importance of a multidisciplinary approach to meet the care needs of older persons and the facilitation of teamwork.

There have been mixed findings from studies evaluating the effectiveness of staff training programmes. Most have utilised uncontrolled research methodologies, and often small samples from only one or two facilities. Training programmes that provide staff with information-based sessions and additional support to help facilitate change appear to be more likely to promote continued improvement in skills (Davison et al., 2007).

Settings

Residential aged care facilities

The ability of staff at residential aged care facilities and GPs to identify and respond to dementia is of critical importance. Training programmes in dementia care for staff at such facilities are relatively common and have been systematically reviewed (Kuske et al., 2007). Programmes that seek to move care staff away from focusing on the physical deficits associated with dementia (i.e. the biomedical model), and more towards a greater appreciation of the person's abilities and their maintained sense of personhood, can positively influence attitudes and knowledge levels, and possibly improve job satisfaction and staff morale (Moyle et al., 2011). Home residents have a 'right to health' (see the Preface and Chapter 1).

A positive attitude towards people with dementia and stronger intentions to implement person-centred care strategies predicted a greater sense of competence to provide care, whereas knowledge and training did not predict this outcome (Mullan and Sullivan, 2015). Findings suggest that a comprehensive multifaceted intervention designed for instructing nursing homes on prescribing antipsychotics might improve knowledge of the medication risks of antipsychotics, change beliefs about the appropriateness and effectiveness of their use in behaviour management, and impart strategies and approaches for non-pharmacological behaviour management (Lemay et al., 2013).

The care home workforce is rather overlooked compared to their NHS counterparts, with a lack of career structure and training opportunities. However, a radical new vision called the Care Home Innovation Centre in the UK incorporates the core components of a teaching nursing home with training opportunities for care home staff in the region, in addition to helping undergraduate and postgraduate students in medicine, nursing and the allied health professions to change the culture and image of care homes (Hockley et al., 2016).

Acute hospitals

There has to be greater scrutiny of how transferable research findings are between different care settings, jurisdictions, 'pressures' and means of validation of outcome scores. There is a recent powerful example of the problems inherent to the meaningfulness of the traditional approach here. For some time now in the UK, staff working in acute hospitals have tended to report a lack of knowledge, skills and confidence in caring for people with dementia. A recent study aimed to evaluate the efficacy of a specialist training programme for acute hospital staff in terms of improving attitudes, satisfaction and feelings of caring efficacy when providing care to people with dementia (Surr et al., 2016). The training programme produced a significant positive change on all three outcomes following intermediate training compared to baseline.

This type of research requires careful execution for conclusions to be extrapolated reliably. For example, it is somewhat unclear from the study by Surr and colleagues (2016) what precisely the training background of the study participants is. There are wider concerns also – for example, how valid the study tools are in 'measuring' person-centred care across different settings. One has also to be very cautious about the extent to which person-centred care might be compromised by much wider issues in the 'health economy' such as rota gaps in staff provision. These concerns would have to be addressed adequately for this research to be of stronger impact.

—— Essential reading ————————————————————

Baker C. 2014. *Developing Excellent Care for People Living with Dementia in Care Homes*, London: Jessica Kingsley Publishers.

—— References ————————————————————————

Age UK. 2015. Factsheet FS78: Safeguarding Older People from Abuse and Neglect, available at www.ageuk.org.uk/Documents/EN-GB/Factsheets/FS78_Safeguarding_older_people_from_abuse_fcs.pdf?epslanguage=en-GB?dtrk=true (accessed 3 Oct 2016).

Aiken LH, Smith HL, Lake ET. 1994. Lower medicare mortality among a set of hospitals known for good nursing care. Med. Care, 32(8), 771–787.

André B, Sjøvold E, Rannestad T, Ringdal GI. 2014. The impact of work culture on quality of care in nursing homes--a review study. Scand J Caring Sci, 28(3), 449–457.

Anetzberger GJ. 2005. The Reality of Elder Abuse. In GJ Anetzberger (ed.), *The Clinical Management of Elder Abuse*, New York: Haworth Press.

Appleby BS, Nacopoulos D, Milano N, Zhong K, Cummings JL. 2013. A review: treatment of Alzheimer's disease discovered in repurposed agents. Dement Geriatr Cogn Disord, 35(1–2), 1–22.

Backhaus R, Verbeek H, van Rossum E, Capezuti E, Hamers JP. 2014. Nurse staffing impact on quality of care in nursing homes: a systematic review of longitudinal studies. J Am Med Dir Assoc, 15(6), 383–393.

Baker MW. 2007. Elder mistreatment: risk, vulnerability and early mortality. Journal of the American Psychiatric Nurses Association, 12(6), 313–321.

Barbosa A, Sousa L, Nolan M, Figueiredo D. 2014. Effects of person-centred care approaches to dementia care on staff: a systematic review. Am J Alzheimers Dis Other Demen, January (e-pub ahead of print).

Bonnie RJ, Wallace RB. 2003. *Elder Mistreatment: Abuse, Neglect and Exploitation in an Aging America*, Washington, DC: National Research Council, available at www.nap.edu/openbook.php?record_id=10406&page=1 (accessed 3 Oct 2016).

Bowblis JR. 2011. Staffing ratios and quality: an analysis of minimum direct care staffing requirements for nursing homes. Health Serv Res, 46(5), 1495–1516.

Cameron F, Brownie S. 2010. Enhancing resilience in registered aged care nurses. Australas J Ageing, 29(2), 66–71.

Care Quality Commission. 2013. *Our Safeguarding Protocol: The Care Quality Commission's Responsibility and Commitment to Safeguarding*, available at www.cqc.org.uk/sites/default/files/documents/20130123_800693_v2_00_cqc_safeguarding_protocol.pdf (accessed 3 Oct 2016).

Care Quality Commission. No date. A Fresh Start for the Regulation and Inspection of Adult Social Care: Working Together to Change How We Inspect and Regulate Adult Social Care Services.

Chu CH, Wodchis WP, McGilton KS. 2014. Turnover of regulated nurses in long-term care facilities. J Nurs Manag, 22(5), 553–562.

Collins KA. 2006. Elder maltreatment: a review. Archives of Pathology and Laboratory Medicine, 130, 1290–1296.

Coogle CL, Parham IA, Rachel CA. 2011. Job satisfaction and career commitment among Alzheimer's care providers: addressing turnover and improving staff empowerment. Am J Alzheimers Dis Other Demen, 26(7), 521–527.

Cowden T, Cummings G, Profetto-McGrath J. 2011. Leadership practices and staff nurses' intent to stay: a systematic review. Journal of Nursing Management, 19(4), 461–477.

Cummings GG, Estabrooks CA, Midodzi WK, Wallin L, Hayduk L. 2007. Influence of organizational characteristics and context on research utilization. Nurs Res, 56, S24–39.

Davies SL, Goodman C, Manthorpe J, Smith A, Carrick N, Iliffe S. 2014. Enabling research in care homes: an evaluation of a national network of research ready care homes. BMC Med Res Methodol, 14, 47.

Davison TE, McCabe MP, Visser S, Hudgson C, Buchanan G, George K. 2007. Controlled trial of dementia training with a peer support group for aged care staff. Int J Geriatr Psychiatry, 22(9), 868–873.

Department of Health. 2000. *No Secrets: Guidance on Developing and Implementing Multi-Agency Policies and Procedures to Protect Vulnerable Adults from Abuse*, London: Department of Health, available at www.gov.uk/government/uploads/system/uploads/attachment_data/file/194272/No_secrets__guidance_on_developing_and_implementing_multi-agency_policies_and_procedures_to_protect_vulnerable_adults_from_abuse.pdf (accessed 3 Oct 2016).

Department of Health. 2014. *The Adult Social Care Outcomes Framework 2015/16*, London: Department of Health.

Dixon J, Biggs S, Tinker A, Stevens M, Lee L. 2009. *Abuse, Neglect and Loss of Dignity in the Institutional Care of Older People*, London: NatCen.

Duffy B, Oyebode JR, Allen J. 2009. Burnout among care staff for older adults with dementia: the role of reciprocity, self-efficacy and organizational factors. Dementia, 8(4), 515–541.

Elliott KJ, Stirling CM, Martin AJ, Robinson AL, Scott JL. 2015. We are not all coping: a cross-sectional investigation of resilience in the dementia care workforce. Health Expect, October, doi:10.1111/hex.12419 (e-pub ahead of print).

Fillit HM, O'Connell AW, Brown WM, Altstiel LD, et al. 2002. Barriers to drug discovery and development for Alzheimer disease. Alzheimer Dis Assoc Disord, 16(Suppl 1), S1–8.

Fulmer T, Faan R, Guadagno L, Dyer CB, Connoll, MT. 2004. Progress in elder abuse screening and assessment instruments. Journal of American Geriatric Society, 52(2), 297–304.

Hall S, Longhurst S, Higginson IJ. 2009. Challenges to conducting research with older people living in nursing homes. BMC Geriatr, 9, 38.

Hirst SP. 2002. Defining resident abuse within the culture of long-term care institutions. Clin Nurs Res, 11, 267–284.

Hockley J, Harrison JK, Watson J, Randall M, Murray S. 2016. Fixing the broken image of care homes, could a 'care home innovation centre' be the answer? Age Ageing, September (e-pub ahead of print).

Hodgkinson B, Haesler EJ, Nay R, O'Donnell MH, McAuliffe LP. 2011. Effectiveness of staffing models in residential, subacute, extended aged care settings on patient and staff outcomes. Cochrane Database of Systematic Reviews, 6, CD006563.

Hussein S, Manthorpe J. 2011. *Longitudinal Changes in Care Worker Turnover and Vacancy Rates and Reasons for Job Leaving In England (2008–2010). Longitudinal Analysis of the National Minimum Data Set for Social Care (NMDS-SC), Analysis Report 1. Social Care Workforce Research Unit*, London: King's College.

Hussein S, Ismail M, Manthorpe J. 2016. Changes in turnover and vacancy rates of care workers in England from 2008 to 2010: panel analysis of national workforce data. Health Soc Care Community, 24(5), 547–556.

Jakobsen R, Sørlie V. 2015. Ethical challenges: trust and leadership in dementia care. Nurs Ethics, May, 0969733015580810 (e-pub ahead of print).

Johnson F. 2011. Problems with the term and concept of 'abuse': critical reflections on the Scottish adult support and protection study. British Journal of Social Work.

Josefsson K, Sonde L, Wahlin TB. 2007. Registered nurses' education and their views on competence development in municipal elderly care in Sweden: a questionnaire survey. Int J Nurs Stud, 44(2), 245–258.

Joy JP, Carter DE, Smith LN. 2000. The evolving educational needs of nurses caring for the older adult: a literature review. Journal of Advanced Nursing, 31(5), 1039–1046.

Karasek R, Theorell T. 1990. Healthy Work. Stress, Productivity, and the Reconstruction of Working Life, New York: Basic Books.

Karlawish JH, Whitehouse PJ. 1998. Is the placebo control obsolete in a world after donepezil and vitamin E? Arch Neurol, 55, 1420–1424.

Kawas CH, Clark CM, Farlow MR, Knopman DS, et al. 1999. Clinical trials in Alzheimer disease: debate on the use of placebo controls. Alzheimer Dis Assoc Disord, 13(3), 124–129.

Kelly F. 2010. Abusive interactions: research in locked wards for people with dementia. Social Policy and Society, 9(2), 267–277.

Kitwood T. 1997. Dementia Reconsidered: The Person Comes First, Buckingham: Open University Press.

Kotting P, Beicher K, McKeith IG, Rossor MN. 2012. Supporting clinical research in the NHS in England: the National Institute for Health Research Dementias and Neurodegenerative Diseases Research Network. Alzheimers Res Ther, 4(4), 23.

Kuske B, Hanns S, Luck T, Angermeyer MC, Behrens J, Riedel-Heller SG. 2007. Nursing home staff training in dementia care: a systematic review of evaluated programs. International psychogeriatrics/IPA, 19(5), 818–841.

Lachs MS, Pillemer K. 2004. Elder abuse. Lancet, 364(9441), 1263–1272.

Lachs MS, Williams CS, O'Brien S, Pillemer KA, Charison ME. 1998. The mortality of elder mistreatment. Journal of the American Medical Association, 280(5), 428–432.

Lawrence V, Fossey J, Ballard C, Moniz-Cook E, Murray J. 2012. Improving quality of life for people with dementia in care homes: making psychosocial interventions work. Br J Psychiatry, 201(5), 344–351.

Lazarus RS. 1993. Coping theory and research: past, present and future. Psychosomatic Medicine, 55, 234–247.

Lemay CA, Mazor KM, Field TS, Donovan J, et al. 2013. Knowledge of and perceived need for evidence-based education about antipsychotic medications among nursing home leadership and staff. J Am Med Dir Assoc, 14(12), 895–900.

Lerner NB, Johantgen M, Trinkoff AM, Storr CL, Han K. 2014. Are nursing home survey deficiencies higher in facilities with greater staff turnover. J Am Med Dir Assoc, 15(2), 102–107.

Lindbloom EJ, Brandt J, Hough LD, Meadows SE. 2007. Elder mistreatment in the nursing home: a systematic review. Journal of the American Medical Directors' Association, 8(9), 610–616.

Long R. 2015. Finding a Path for the Cure for Dementia: An Independent Report into an Integrated Approach to Dementia Research, London: Department of Health.

Manthorpe J. 2015. The abuse, neglect and mistreatment of older people with dementia in care homes and hospitals in England: the potential for secondary data analysis: innovative practice. Dementia (London), 14(2), 273–279.

Maslach C, Jackson SE. 1986. Maslach Burnout Inventory Manual (2nd ed.), Palo Alto, CA: Consulting Psychologists Press.

McAllister M, McKinnon J. 2008. Resilience and the Health Professionals: A Critical Review of the Literature, Queensland: University of the Sunshine Coast.

Mistry H, Levack WM, Johnson S. 2015. Enabling people, not completing tasks: patient perspectives on relationships and staff morale in mental health wards in England. BMC Psychiatry, 15(1), 307.

Moyle W, Fetherstonhaugh D, Greben M, Beattie E; AusQoL Group. 2015. Influencers on quality of life as reported by people living with dementia in long-term care: a descriptive exploratory approach. BMC Geriatr, 15, 50.

Moyle W, Murfield JE, Griffiths SG, Venturato L. 2011. Care staff attitudes and experiences of working with older people with dementia. Australas J Ageing, 30(4), 186–190.

Mullan MA, Sullivan KA. 2015. Positive attitudes and person-centred care predict of sense of competence in dementia care staff. Aging Ment Health, March, 1–8 (e-pub ahead of print).

NHS Choices. 2015. Abuse and Neglect of Vulnerable Adults, available at www.nhs.uk/conditions/social-care-and-support-guide/pages/vulnerable-people-abuse-safeguarding.aspx (accessed 3 Oct 2016).

Organisation for Economic Co-operation and Development. 2005. Ensuring quality long-term care for older people OECD, Paris, available at https://www.oecd.org/els/health-systems/Ensuring-quality-long-term-care-for-older-people.pdf (accessed 29 Nov 2016).

Phelan A. 2008. Elder abuse, ageism, human rights and citizenship: implications for nursing discourse. Nursing Inquiry, 15, 320–329.

Phelan A. 2009. Elder abuse and neglect: the nurse's responsibility in care of the older person. International Journal of Older People Nursing, 4, 115–119.

Ronch JL. 2004. Changing institutional culture: can we re-value the nursing home? Journal of Gerontological Social Work, 43(1), 61–82.

Rosen T, Lachs MS, Bharucha AJ, Stevens SM, et al. 2008. Resident-to-resident aggression in long-term care facilities: insights from focus groups of nursing home residents and staff. Journal of the American Geriatrics Society, 56(8), 1398–1408.

Schmidt SG, Dichter MN, Bartholomeyczik S, Hasselhorn HM. 2014. The satisfaction with the quality of dementia care and the health, burnout and work ability of nurses: a longitudinal analysis of 50 German nursing homes. Geriatr Nurs, 35(1), 42–46.

SCIE. 2012. Safeguarding and Quality in Commissioning Care Homes, available at www.scie.org.uk/publications/guides/guide45 (accessed 3 Oct 2016).

Selkoe DJ. 1991. The molecular pathology of Alzheimer's disease. Neuron, 6, 487–498.

Shinoda-Tagawa T, Leonard R, Pontikas J, John E, et al. 2004. Resident-to-resident violent incidents in nursing homes. Journal of the American Medical Association, 291(5), 591–598.

Sjögren K, Lindkvist M, Sandman PO, Zingmark K, Edvardsson D. 2015. To what extent is the work environment of staff related to person-centred care? A cross-sectional study of residential aged care. J Clin Nurs, 24(9–10), 1310–1319.

Spiegel R, Irwin P. 1996. Designing dementia treatment studies: diagnosis, efficacy criteria, and duration. Eur Psychiatry, 11, 149–154.

Spilsbury K, Hewitt C, Stirk L, Bowman C. 2011. The relationship between nurse staffing and quality of care in nursing homes: a systematic review. Int J Nurs Stud, 48(6), 732–750.

Surr CA, Smith SJ, Crossland J, Robins J. 2016. Impact of a person-centred dementia care training programme on hospital staff attitudes, role efficacy and perceptions of caring for people with dementia: a repeated measures study. Int J Nurs Stud, 53, 144–151.

Uman GC, Urman HN. 1990. The challenges of conducting clinical nursing research with elderly populations. Association of Perioperative Registered Nurses Journal, 52, 400–406.

van Oostveen CJ, Mathijssen E, Vermeulen H. 2015. Nurse staffing issues are just the tip of the iceberg: a qualitative study about nurses' perceptions of nurse staffing. Int J Nurs Stud, 52(8), 1300–1309.

Wiglesworth A, Mosqueda L, Mulnard R, Liao S, Gibbs L, Fitzgerald W. 2010. Screening for abuse and neglect of people with dementia. J Am Geriatr Soc, 58(3), 493–500.

Zhang NJ, Unruh L, Liu R, Wan TT. 2006. Minimum nurse staffing ratios for nursing homes. Nursing Economics, 24(2), 78–85.

Zúñiga F, Ausserhofer D, Hamers JP, Engberg S, Simon M, Schwendimann R. 2015. Are staffing, work environment, work stressors, and rationing of care related to care workers' perception of quality of care? A cross-sectional study. J Am Med Dir Assoc, 16(10), 860–866.

Chapter 10

CARE HOMES AND INTEGRATED CARE

Learning objectives

By the end of this chapter, you will be able to:

» understand the impact of inpatient services on persons with dementia and carers

» discuss wider issues in the health economy which might impact on the performance of dementia care as a whole, including avoidable emergency hospital admissions, hospital admissions and hospital readmissions, care transitions, case management, proactive discharge planning, delayed discharges and delayed transfers of care

» explain the critical importance of clinical specialist nurses, such as Admiral nurses, in promoting the health, care and wellbeing of people with dementia and their carers

Introduction

A care home or nursing home should promote a resident's health and wellbeing. If such needs are not fully met, it may be essential for persons to go to other places of care. However, the current workload of acute hospitals in the NHS is enormous (see Box 10.1), and this chapter will give an account of the health and social care system, focused on a person entering and leaving hospital in a timely fashion.

Box 10.1: Hospitals at a glance

HOW MANY BEDS ARE THERE IN ACUTE HOSPITALS?

Some 107,444 hospital beds are provided for general and acute services in England each year (April 2011–March 2012). The number of general and acute beds has decreased by one-third in the past 25 years.

HOW MANY PEOPLE GET ADMITTED TO HOSPITAL?

In 2010–11, 3.6 million people who attended A&E were then admitted to hospital.

There has been a 37% increase in emergency hospital admissions in the past ten years.

Emergency hospital admissions account for over one-third (35%) of all hospital admissions, costing an estimated £11 billion per year.

There are more than two million unplanned hospital admissions for people over 65.

Mortality rates for emergency admissions after 30 days of discharge is 3.6%, compared with 0.7% for elective admissions.

WHO IS IN HOSPITAL?

Nearly two-thirds (65%) of people admitted to hospital are over 65 years old. People over 65 occupy more than 51,000 acute care beds at any one time.

People over 85 years old account for 25% of bed days – this has increased from 22% over the past ten years.

HOW LONG DO PEOPLE STAY IN HOSPITAL?

The average length of stay for acute care in UK hospitals in 2010 was 7.7 days, higher than the OECD average of 7.1 days and significantly in excess of averages in Australia (5.1), the Netherlands (5.8) and the US (4.9).

SOURCE: ADAPTED FROM DATA FROM THE ROYAL COLLEGE OF PHYSICIANS (2012, P.7).

With the patient, each professional will co-create a different narrative; when providers come together as an interprofessional team, these different stories must be recognised as such and effectively integrated into an overall assessment and care plan that incorporates many clinical voices (Clark, 2015). New discharge and home care practices such as case/care management and coordination, multidisciplinary team work, discharge, integrated care and educational programmes have been developed to address shortcomings and cut or restrain the costs of health and social care. The ageing population and the increased prevalence of chronic diseases require a strong reorientation away from the current emphasis on acute and episodic care towards prevention, self-care, more consistent standards of primary care and care that is well coordinated and integrated (Naylor et al., 2015). People benefit from care that is **person-centred, integrated and coordinated** within health care settings, across mental and physical health and across health and social care.

Integrated care may be defined as service development that achieves any of the following outcomes either individually or in combination through integration. Integrated care:

» enhances the patient experience

» avoids clinically inappropriate or unnecessary hospital-based activity

» enables more sustainable and better value solutions for clinically appropriate hospital-based activity.

For care to be integrated, organisations and care professionals need to bring together all the elements of care that a person needs. Integrated care is essential to meet the needs of the whole population, transforming the way care is provided for people with long-term conditions, and enabling people with complex needs to live healthy, fulfilling and independent lives (Naylor et al., 2015). A core part of the vision laid out in the NHS Five Year Forward View involves acute hospitals becoming more closely integrated with other forms of care. If the health and social care system is to respond to the changing needs of the population, and address the financial challenges it faces, acute hospitals will need to play a fundamentally different role within local health economies (Naylor, Alderwick and Honeyman, 2015). The robust integration of health and social care services and the voluntary sector may lead to better outcomes for the health and wellbeing of older individuals.

—— Avoidable emergency hospital admissions ——

Avoiding emergency hospital admissions is a major concern for the NHS, not only because of the high and rising unit costs of emergency admission compared with other forms of care, but also because of the disruption it causes to elective health care – most notably inpatient waiting lists – and to the individuals admitted themselves (Audit Commission, 2009).

Intermediate care was originally launched in the National Service Framework of Older People in 2001 and was conceived of as a platform for integration between providers and health and social care professionals (NHS Benchmarking Network, 2015). There would ideally be a major expansion of both community health and social care services (Stevenson and Spencer, 2002). Intermediate care needs are not always clear when people are referred to social services and, more significantly, people diagnosed with a mental illness, specifically older people, often do not meet the services' criteria for rehabilitation (Manzano-Santaella and Goode, 2011).

Admissions can be identified as 'avoidable' based on the reasons for the admission being avoidable (see Table 10.1).

Table 10.1: Categorisation of avoidable admissions

Theme	Definition
Alternatives to admission	An alternative to admission could have been used and would have been as or more appropriate at the time of admission
Intermediate care	There was a need for intermediate care (nursing, social, physiotherapy, occupational therapy and/or medical) that could be provided in the community
More timely referral	An earlier referral to specialist services would likely have prevented decline and avoided a hospital admission
Better hospital care	Better management by the hospital during a previous admission (or planned follow-up) could have avoided the admission
Better primary care	Better management in primary care could have prevented the admission
More responsive social care	The patient's primary needs were a rapid increase in social support, which could not be provided in a timely fashion, resulting in admission
Palliative care	Patient admitted with a terminal diagnosis, where appropriate planning and/or access to community palliative care could have facilitated more appropriate management in the community

SOURCE: BASED ON MYTTON ET AL. (2012, TABLE 1).

Ambulance services are working hard to ensure that fewer patients need to be taken to A&E and that more patients are treated in their own home (Ambulance Service Network, NHS Confederation, 2010). It is reported that emergency crews frequently encounter older people with dementia, and it can be difficult to take their history, assess their pain and access suitable alternatives to A&E, especially out of hours (Buswell et al., 2016).

Many referrals to the emergency department are potentially preventable, but this would require enhancements to be made to the package of care available within the NHS (Briggs et al., 2013). Many risk stratification instruments focus on measures of disease severity and fail to measure the patient factors that modify subsequent health care utilisation behaviour (Hutchinson et al., 2015). Furthermore, the identification of individuals with advanced disease who may benefit from advance care planning or more palliative approaches to disease management is reportedly poor.

Cognitive impairment and dementia are often significantly associated with admission for pneumonia and urinary tract infections. These are ambulatory care-sensitive conditions (see Box 10.2) for which admissions are thought to be avoidable or manageable with prompt access to medical care; that is, those that could have been prevented or treated in the community (Sampson et al., 2009). Rudolph and colleagues (2010) have attempted to identify the specific causes for emergency department visits for older adults with an increased risk of hospitalisation, including individuals with dementia. Some of the most commonly seen conditions or complications include physical health problems, such as urinary tract infections, delirium, pressure ulcers, falls, fractures, seizures, infections and pneumonia, which are highly associated with hospital admissions (Rudolph et al., 2010; Toot et al., 2013). Psychiatric factors, particularly behavioural problems, are also a key risk factor for hospital admissions, and many people admitted to hospital with dementia enter institutional care on discharge, rather than returning to their own homes (for a review see Toot et al., 2013).

Box 10.2: Ambulatory care-sensitive conditions

Ambulatory care-sensitive conditions (ACSCs) are conditions for which effective management and treatment should prevent admission to hospital. They can be classified as: chronic conditions, where effective care can prevent flare-ups; acute conditions, where early intervention can prevent more serious progression; and preventable conditions, where immunisation and other interventions can prevent illness (Ham, Imison and Jennings, 2010). The 19 ACSCs are listed below (NHS Institute for Innovation and Improvement, no date).

THE 19 AMBULATORY CARE-SENSITIVE CONDITIONS

Vaccine-preventable

1. Influenza and pneumonia

2. Other vaccine-preventable conditions

Chronic

3. Asthma

4. Congestive heart failure

5. Diabetes complications

6. Chronic obstructive pulmonary disease (COPD)

7. Angina

8. Iron-deficiency anaemia

9. Hypertension

10. Nutritional deficiencies

Acute

11. Dehydration and gastroenteritis

12. Pyelonephritis

13. Perforated/bleeding ulcer

14. Cellulitis

15. Pelvic inflammatory disease

16. Ear, nose and throat infections

17. Dental conditions

18. Convulsions and epilepsy

19. Gangrene

WHY LOOK AT EMERGENCY HOSPITAL ADMISSIONS FOR ACSCs?

High levels of admissions for ACSCs often indicate poor coordination between the different elements of the health care system, in particular between primary and secondary care. An emergency admission for an ACSC is a sign of the poor overall quality of care, even if the ACSC episode itself is managed well. The wide variation in emergency hospital admissions for ACSCs implies that they, and the associated costs for commissioners, can be reduced.

SOURCE: THE KING'S FUND (NO DATE, PP.2–3). REPRODUCED BY KIND PERMISSION OF THE KING'S FUND.

Based on observational studies examining reasons for the hospitalisation of persons with dementia, future intervention studies should test approaches to managing chronic conditions and preventing injuries in persons living in the community with dementia. Current work in the area of dementia and multiple chronic conditions may help shape this understanding (Phelan et al., 2015). Research shows that geriatric evaluation and management improve outcomes and save money (Bernabei et al., 1998). Geriatricians working together with coordinated multidisciplinary teams are well placed to manage the care needs of care home residents with multiple morbidity (Lisk et al., 2012). Increasing rates of hospital admission have not necessarily been related to improved outcomes for very elderly people (Wasson et al., 1998). More recently, a number of authors have described the impact of the input of a geriatrician to supplement and support the work of primary care practitioners. These interventions have been reported to have led to reductions in hospital admissions and an increase in the number of residents with an advance care plan in place, with a consequent increase in the number of residents dying in their preferred place of care (in the care home) (e.g. Burns and Nair, 2014).

Avoidable admissions are a prime consideration in the new models of care. The Gateshead Care Home Project new model of care will build on a well-established proactive service based on 'ward-rounds' that sees GP practices and community nursing teams aligned to care homes across the borough.[1] Personalised care delivery and multidisciplinary working are starting to successfully reduce avoidable hospital admissions, as well as an improvement in the quality of care delivered. The next steps through vanguard acceleration will focus on cementing these principles for a wider cohort of patients and families who currently access home services (e.g. intermediate care).

Pain and acute medicine

Arguably, little attention has been given to pain in people with dementia in general hospitals, despite the fact that dementia is common in older hospital inpatients, with a prevalence on medical wards of around 40% (Sampson et al., 2015). Managing acute pain in people with cognitive impairment can be challenging for emergency nurses operating within an often chaotic and fast-paced setting. Studies have demonstrated that older people with cognitive impairment experience analgesic delay in emergency departments (Fry et al., 2011, 2014). There is also evidence that cognitive impairment is a significant risk factor for analgesic delay (Fry et al., 2014). The delivery of appropriate pain management for older people with cognitive impairment and acute pain poses specific challenges for emergency clinicians. Yet nurses are well positioned to contribute to compassionate care through the timely delivery of analgesia (Fry, Chenoweth and Arendts, 2016).

There are particular challenges for clinical staff when caring for patients in acute settings who have dementia; for example, they may not be able to report their pain experiences verbally and are therefore at increased risk of having their pain inadequately assessed and managed (Sampson et al., 2015). A number of studies have highlighted particular issues faced by clinical staff when assessing and managing pain in older adults and those with dementia; communication with patients may be problematic if they are unable to express their pain experiences clearly, organisational issues may impact when older adults receive pain relief, and trying to balance effectively treating pain while minimising the side effects of analgesics have been reported as challenging (e.g. Coker et al., 2010; Manias, 2012).

---

1   See www.england.nhs.uk/ourwork/futurenhs/new-care-models/care-homes-sites (accessed 4 Oct 2016).

Hospital in the home and hospital in the nursing home

Hospital in the home (HiTH) services may offer one means of reducing demand for emergency departments. They may also facilitate more efficient use of inpatient beds, providing an alternative to in-hospital admission and enabling patients to be transferred home earlier, thereby increasing inpatient bed availability (Varney, Weiland and Jelinek, 2014). This definition nonetheless includes services that substitute acute care for home-based management (admission avoidance) and those that support discharge with community-based post-acute care and rehabilitation (discharge support) (Wilson and Parker, 2005). These are special services that have been developed to provide people with hospital care in their homes. Typically, these people would require treatment in an acute care hospital for a period. Instead, a team of health care professionals, such as doctors, nurses and physiotherapists, provide them with treatment at home.

HiTH has been extended in some areas to include a Hospital in the Nursing Home (HiNH) model of admission-avoidance service delivery. However, like HiTH, research related to HiNH has been limited and derived from various health care systems internationally (Crilly et al., 2011). Based in the hospital, the HiNH programme acts as an outreach service to deliver acute care services for Academic Fellowship Clinician (ACF) residents and provide advice and education to ACF staff and GPs. Initially, the programme operated from 08:00 to 16:30, Monday to Friday. Outside these hours, ACF residents were either admitted to a hospital ward for care continuation or admitted to an observation unit for HiNH referral the next day (Crilly, Chaboyer and Wallis, 2012). (Observation units are designated areas often adjacent to the emergency department for emergency department patients who may benefit from an extended observation period.)

Hospital admissions and readmissions

An emergency admission to hospital is a disruptive and unsettling experience, particularly for older people, exposing them to new clinical and psychological risks and increasing their dependency (Glasby, 2003). A hospital readmission is the hospitalisation of a patient that occurs within a specific period after a previous hospital admission referred to as 'the index'. Most studies refer to the concept of hospital readmission within 30 days of discharge as an indicator of the activity and quality of health care (Matesanz-Fernández et al., 2015). There are studies that have identified some factors associated with hospital readmissions and with multiple hospital admissions: male sex, previous hospital admissions, comorbidity, chronic disease, functional state, vascular diseases, adverse events during the index hospitalisation, etc. (Matesanz-Fernández et al., 2015). Who is to blame for older people's readmissions, however? Cuts to social care funding have left even people with substantial needs unsupported (Oliver, 2015).

Acute hospitals can often be confusing environments for a person with dementia, and pre-existing cognitive deficiencies can be exacerbated by the hospital environment and an underlying physical health problem. A policy guidance document has reported that 40% of people in general hospitals in the UK have dementia (Department of Health, 2010). The literature identifies that older people who commonly present with more urgent conditions more frequently require hospital admission from the emergency department and experience a longer length of stay than younger adults (Aminzadeh and Dalziel, 2002; Lutze, Fry and Gallagher, 2015). Older patients with dementia are more likely to require treatment in a general hospital for comorbid health issues and are at greater risk of requiring treatment for falls, dehydration, malnutrition and infection than elderly patients without the diagnosis (Van Doorn et al., 2003; Natalwala et al., 2008).

Older people with cognitive impairment are high users of emergency department services and often present with a complaint of pain. Researchers have identified that between 50% and 80% of patients presenting to emergency departments present with a complaint of pain (Holdcroft and Power, 2003). There is a large body of evidence which indicates that the way hospitals are run can influence the number of admissions and patients' length of stay. According to Grober and colleagues (2011), individuals with dementia are also more likely to present to an emergency department with various other comorbidities. Park and colleagues (2004) identified a number of potential explanations for the extended length of stay for those with dementia in acute settings, including the presence of multiple interdependent comorbidities, the predisposition of older patients with dementia to hospital-acquired infections and complications in treatment, and difficulties in arranging placement or community services.

The pressures on the acute service in England are relentless and intense. These include:

» increasing clinical demand

» changing patients, changing needs

» fractured care (a lack of continuity of care)

» out-of-hours care breakdown especially at weekends

» looming workforce crisis in the medical workforce.

(Royal College of Physicians, 2012)

John's Campaign, with the aim of giving carers of those living with dementia the right to stay with them in hospital, has now been adopted in the Commissioning for Quality and Innovation (CQUIN) payment framework from NHS England for 2016–17. A different initiative called 'the Butterfly Scheme'[2] has been devised by a carer whose mother had lived with dementia following two years of consultation with hundreds of people with dementia and their carers. When a patient or carer opts into the scheme, a discreet butterfly symbol will be placed next to the patient's name. This prompts all staff to follow a special response plan known as REACH. It has now been successfully adopted by over a hundred hospitals in the UK.

Care home residents have traditionally been regarded as a cohort with a poor prognosis. Care home residents were certainly unwell on admission, with background functional impairment. However, the majority can survive to discharge, and their short-term outcomes can be no different from those of the matched controls (Quinn, 2011). It is feasible to develop tools for monitoring admissions to hospital from care homes. Continuous monitoring allows for a process for alerting when admission numbers are unusually high; signals need to be interpreted carefully and followed up appropriately (Sherlaw-Johnson, Smith and Bardsley, 2016).

In 2016, the British Geriatrics Society issued a press release on the provision of GP services in care homes:

> We must ensure that care home residents can continue to access the health care services they need. We call on the BMA and GPs to ensure that, in protecting the future sustainability of their services, they do not classify care home residents as anything less than full members of society, with the same health care entitlements as the rest of us.

According to the Royal College of Physicians' Future Hospital Commission (2013):

> Geriatricians and their specialist teams also have an important role in providing skills to the staff who work in care homes; pilot projects suggest that this may reduce the need for acute admissions. (Royal College of Physicians, 2013, p.59)

Hospital admission increases the risk for people with dementia of institutionalisation on discharge, accelerated morbidity and mortality, and they often die with inadequate pain control or without the benefits of hospice care (de Vries, Drury-Ruddlesden and Gaul, 2016). When people are taken to hospital as an emergency, they want prompt, safe and effective treatment that alleviates their symptoms and addresses the underlying causes of their illness. In short, they want care aiming at

---

2   Available at butterflyscheme.org.uk (accessed 28 Oct 2016).

getting them better, quickly and safely. Improving the experience of those with dementia in acute hospitals will likely lead to cost savings for the health service; however, it will require a number of measures including earlier diagnosis, training for medical professionals and improvements in the built environment (Connolly and O'Shea, 2015).

The admission, person-centred care and family carer

Many people with dementia are admitted to general hospitals, yet doctors feel ill-prepared to manage them. Problems are often multiple and complex. In many cases, dementia is complicated by delirium (Harwood, 2012). Transfers to emergency departments among the nursing home population are: (a) recognised as often placing residents at significant risk for poor health outcomes and decline; (b) often prompted by weak evidence and poor decision-making; (c) plagued by operational inefficiencies that are reinforced by health system fragmentation; and (d) extremely costly to the health care system (Robinson et al., 2012). The transition of nursing home residents to and from hospitals can be problematic, particularly when communication between facilities is inadequate and vital information about residents is not communicated across settings (McCloskey, 2011).

The goal of person-centred approaches to care is to respect personhood despite cognitive impairment (Skaalvik, Normann and Henriksen, 2010). Where the personhood of the individual is recognised and valued, the person with dementia is awarded standing and status as a respected and valued social being (Clissett et al., 2013). Hospital admission of a person with dementia can have a significant impact on the family carer, who temporarily relinquishes caring to health professionals (Bloomer et al., 2014). Adjusting to the change in the carer's role can be challenging and result in feelings of helplessness, loneliness, loss of control and being undervalued. Family members and carers of people with dementia are frequently dissatisfied with their experience of hospital care, including staff not recognising or understanding dementia, a lack of activity and social interaction, inadequate involvement in decision-making and a perceived lack of dignity and respect (Alzheimer's Society, 2009). Understanding the perspective of the family carer, and recognising elements of the 'cycle of discontent', could help ward staff anticipate carer needs and enable relationship building to pre-empt or avoid dissatisfaction or conflict (Jurgens et al., 2012).

Care transitions

Care transitions, or 'transitions between health care settings', can be burdensome for patients with life-threatening illnesses and their families, particularly if they occur at the end of life and involve admissions to acute care settings (Teno et al., 2013). Major gaps exist in our understanding of transitions in care for older persons living in nursing homes. Robinson and colleagues (2012) identified key elements that influence the success of transitions experienced by nursing home residents when they required transfer to a hospital emergency department. These included: knowing the resident; critical geriatric knowledge and skilled assessment; positive relationships; effective communication; and timeliness. When one or more of the elements was absent or compromised, the success of the transition was also compromised. There is consistent evidence that people prefer to die in their own home or home-replacing environment, and that being moved between settings increases the risk of fragmented care from multiple carers and medical errors that impede the provision of high-quality palliative care (van den Block et al., 2015).

Persons with dementia may be particularly at risk of experiencing preventable transitions in care because of the large number of their care transitions, comorbid medical conditions and the severity of cognitive impairment (Callahan et al., 2015). Poorly executed, non-standardised transitions result in a multitude of adverse effects with wide-ranging consequences for both patients and their carers (Coleman, 2003).

The ongoing change in long-term care from institutional care to housing services causes major challenges to the continuity of end-of-life care. To guarantee good-quality care during the last days of life for people with dementia, the underlying reasons behind transitions at the end of life should be investigated more thoroughly (Aaltonen et al., 2014). Freeman and Hughes (2010) offer a useful distinction between two different aspects of continuity: (a) continuity of relationship, which refers to continuous therapeutic relationships with one or more clinicians; and (b) continuity of management, which refers to the continuity and consistency of clinical management, including the provision and sharing of information and communication about care planning, along with coordination of the care required by the patient.

Case management

Case management is an established tool in integrating services around the needs of individuals with long-term conditions. It is a targeted, community-based and proactive approach to care that involves case-finding, assessment, care planning and care coordination.

Many countries reorganising their public policy for individuals with cognitive disorders are hoping that case management will improve care. As with many complex interventions, case management also targets more than one recipient: people with dementia and/or their carers (Köpke and McCleery, 2015; see Box 10.3).

Box 10.3: Case management

For those seeking to commission or deliver case management, the evidence suggests that the following factors are most likely to achieve successful outcomes:

* assigned accountability

* role and remit

* skills and support

* case-finding

* targeting

* caseloads

* a single point of access

* a joint care plan (can support clarity and consistency in the delivery of services)

* continuity of care

* self-care

* communication

* integration and collaboration

* aligned financial incentives

* access to community-based services

* part of a programme approach.

SOURCE: ADAPTED FROM ROSS, CURRY AND GOODWIN (2011, P.26).

The following factors are linked to the achievement of successful outcomes:

» clarity about the role of the case managers and support to ensure they have the right clinical and managerial competencies

» a single point of access for assessment and a joint care plan

» continuity of care to reduce the risk of an unplanned admission to hospital

» self-care, to empower patients to manage their own condition

» joined-up health and social care services with professionals working together

» information systems that support communication, and data that are used proactively to drive quality improvements

(Ross et al., 2011)

International research has revealed the potential benefits of a collaborative case management approach to the assessment and care of people with dementia (Waugh et al., 2013). There is some evidence from the Cochrane review 'Case Management Approaches to Home Support for People with Dementia' that case management is beneficial in improving some outcomes at certain time points, both in the person with dementia and in their carer (Reilly et al., 2015). There was not enough evidence to clearly assess whether case management could delay institutionalisation in care homes.

Despite the intuitive appeal of case management to all stakeholders, there are multiple barriers to implementation in primary care in England. These include: difficulties in embedding case managers within existing well-established community networks; the challenges of keeping time for case management; and case managers' inability to identify and act on emerging patient and carer needs (an essential, but previously unrecognised, training need) (Bamford et al., 2014). In light of these barriers, it is unclear whether primary care is the most appropriate setting for case management in England (Bamford et al., 2014). Innovative service delivery methods may also facilitate the prescribing of anti-cholinesterase drugs (Callahan et al., 2006) in countries where prescribing rates are low, possibly due to restrictions on primary care prescribing (O'Brien, 2008; Robinson et al., 2010).

—— Proactive discharge planning ——

It is well known that discharges can often go wrong (see Box 10.4), but discharges can be planned even from the point of admission.

Box 10.4: The reasons why things go wrong

The core reasons why people feel their departure was not handled properly:

* people are experiencing delays and a lack of coordination between different services

* people are feeling left without the services and support they need after discharge

* people feel stigmatised and discriminated against and that they are not treated with appropriate respect because of their conditions and circumstances

* people feel they are not involved in decisions about their care, or given the information they need people feel that their full range of needs is not considered.

SOURCE: HEALTHWATCH ENGLAND (2015, P.9).

Delivering integrated care is essential to improve outcomes for people who use health and social care services. Reducing gaps and inefficiencies in care should also be able to offer some opportunities for financial savings. Inpatient flow and bed management are a growing problem for acute hospitals as health care treatments improve year on year and patient demand increases. Discharge from hospital is a process and not an isolated event. The importance of the identification, assessment and support of carers as expert partners in hospital discharges is well recognised (ADASS, 2010).

Proactive discharge planning involves thinking about how to move people on from services safely and appropriately as early as possible in the care pathway. This involves working to prioritise discharge planning within organisations, but also improving the communication and coordination between services such as hospital and community care (Bryan, 2010). It may also involve assigning staff especially to concentrate on discharge processes or having nurses rather than doctors undertake the majority of discharge work. Special 'discharge rounds', rapid discharge units or other proactive approaches may also be used (e.g. Dutton et al., 2003). In England, the Community Care (Delayed Discharge) Act 2003 and subsequent policy initiatives have aimed to address delayed discharges, such as through investment in intermediate care services to promote independence among older people after hospital admission, and joint working between health and social services (Bryan, 2010).

As a consequence of delayed discharge, some frail patients deteriorated while others were transferred to other parts of the hospital (Health Foundation, 2013, 2014). These transfers sometimes resulted in vital information being lost, resulting in further deterioration, rework and delay. On average, patients spent four times longer in hospital than was initially estimated by geriatric medicine consultants involved in their care.

—— Delayed discharges and delayed transfers of care

Studies conducted in various countries show that a significant proportion of patients experience delayed discharge because they cannot be transferred to rehabilitation/

residential facilities or moved back home (Lenzi et al., 2014). As is increasingly clear, however, this is often totally inaccurate, as it is the system itself which causes many such blockages, not the individual patient (who often wishes to return home as soon as possible).

As Christina Victor (1991, p.123) explains:

> The whole notion of bed blocking seems to imply that older people enter hospital and then wilfully continue to occupy a bed which, in the views of staff, they no longer require. Older people (or indeed patients of any age) do not become bed blockers of their own intent. Rather where such cases do occur it is because the health and social care system cannot provide the type of care they need.

Delayed transfers of care, where patients are ready to return home or transfer to another form of care but still occupy a hospital bed, are a hot topic of discussion right now – whether because of money, the impact on patient experience or hospital flow (Thompson, 2015).

Delays can occur when patients are being discharged home or to a supported care facility such as a residential or nursing home, or if they require further, less intensive care and are awaiting transfer to a community hospital or hospice. A delayed transfer of care from acute or non-acute (including community and mental health) care occurs when a patient is ready to depart from such care and is still occupying a bed (NHS England, 2013). NHS England, the body responsible for monitoring delayed transfers of care nationally, defines a patient as being ready for transfer when: a clinical decision has been made that the patient is ready for transfer, and a multidisciplinary team has decided that the patient is ready for transfer and the patient is safe to discharge/transfer.

Efficient access to social care is a key aspect of improving discharges from acute psychiatric beds, but it is not the only one. Resources identified as fundamental include 'total dependency psychiatric care, day hospitals, inpatient observation facilities and continuing care wards' (Glasby and Lester, 2004). Discharge planning is the development of an individualised discharge plan for the patient prior to leaving hospital, with the aim of containing costs and improving patient outcomes. Discharge planning should ensure that patients are discharged from hospital at an appropriate time in their care and that, with adequate notice, the provision of other services will be organised.

Reducing delayed transfers of care is at the heart of the challenge of delivering integrated services, especially continuity of care for older people in hospitals. Official figures show the number of delayed transfers for older people – that is, where a patient remains in hospital after the clinicians and professionals involved in their care decide they are ready to leave – increased by 31% to 1.15 million bed days between 2013 and 2015 (House of Commons Committee of Public Accounts,

2016). As was clearly signposted back in 2008 in the report by the Alzheimer's Society (2009), *Counting the Cost*, if a patient has dementia, that length of stay will almost invariably be longer and involve far greater costs for the health system. When these patients are finally released from hospital, it is often without adequate discharge planning to ensure follow-up care. A significant percentage of them will undergo adverse events and unplanned readmissions (Chenoweth, Kable and Pond, 2015). Shepherd and colleagues (2013) investigated discharge planning from hospital to home for a Cochrane review. Their review found that a structured discharge plan tailored to the individual patient probably brings about a reduction in hospital length of stay and readmission rates and an increase in patient satisfaction. The impact on health outcomes is uncertain.

Reasons for delay are monitored in a number of categories, which identify the agency (either the NHS or social services) responsible for this situation (Manzano-Santaella and Goode, 2011). These include:

» awaiting completion of assessment

» awaiting public funding

» delays due to waits for NHS non-acute care

» awaiting care home placements

» awaiting a domiciliary care package

» waiting for equipment and adaptations

» delays caused by patient/family choice

» delays caused between agencies

» homelessness.

The fragility of the adult social care provider market is clearly exacerbating the difficulties in discharging older patients from hospital. NHS England believes the increasing pressure on adult social services will prevent significant progress being made in reducing the number of delayed discharges over the next five years. Local authority spending on adult social services has fallen by 10% in real terms between 2009–10 and 2014–15 (House of Commons Public Accounts Committee, 2016).

Discharge planning of older people with dementia can pose difficult ethical dilemmas to the general hospital clinician. These difficulties may be particularly pronounced for those who are moderately severely affected and for whom hazards are anticipated on discharge home. In many cases, the wishes of the individual to return home may differ markedly from those of health care professionals, carers or relatives (Brindle and Holmes, 2005). At the point of discharge they often express a desire to return home (even though their concept of home may relate to a time in the past, without the dangers they have encountered in more recent times). Alternatively, health and social care professionals, along with relatives, may express concerns that home no longer represents the most suitable environment for the person's future wellbeing, with discharge into long-term residential care proposed as the 'safer' and more appropriate discharge option (Emmett et al., 2013). Care systems also have a responsibility to protect impaired older people from risks in the event of deterioration in both decision-making capacities and functional abilities. This tension between autonomy and protection can be particularly marked in the case of older people with dementia when planning discharge from general hospital settings (Brindle and Holmes, 2005).

Clinical nursing specialists

The need for clinical nursing specialists in dementia can in fact be understood from the first and only (thus far) English dementia strategy document, *Living Well with Dementia*, from the Department of Health (2009). Priorities then included raising awareness of dementia among staff in the acute general hospital (objective 1) and providing good-quality information for people with dementia and their carers (objective 3). Furthermore, such a role has a focus on improving care for patients with the condition and, where appropriate, facilitating optimum end-of-life care for them (objectives 8 and 12) (Elliot and Adams, 2011). Priorities invariably include expert guidance for other members of staff, and promoting choice and control in care. The strategy concerning the clinical nursing specialist in dementia fundamentally adopts the person-centred approach (Griffiths et al., 2015).

Central to understanding carer outcomes is carer coping: this holds the key for the NHS and social care to manage the demand on services in the future, and this has clear resource ramifications. The approach requires investment to safeguard the future of dementia care in England against funding threats. Coping strategies predict carer outcomes such as anxiety, depression and quality of life, and they can ultimately influence the move for the person with dementia to enter a residential care setting (Roche, McCann and Croot, 2016). The benefits of clinical specialist nurses are outlined in Box 10.5.

Box 10.5: Benefits of clinical specialist nurses

* Care at reduced cost and increased efficiency

* System leadership and service redesign

* Bringing care closer to home and reducing the burden of long-term conditions

* Seamless, integrated, multidisciplinary care

* Treating the person, not the condition

* Excellent patient care and experience

SOURCE: HSJ (2015, P.3).

Palliative care intends to improve the quality of life for patients with dementia, and awareness and evidence are growing that an early palliative care approach would benefit people with any type of chronic, life-limiting illness (Beernaert et al., 2015). The **Mental Capacity Act 2005** has the potential for supporting the safeguarding and empowerment role of community nurses. However, nurse specialists providing support to carers and people with dementia may need a greater familiarity with legal provisions. This may assist them in providing general information, making timely referrals to sources of specialist legal advice and in using the Act to reduce anxiety, conflict and disputes (Samsi et al., 2012). Excellent dementia care is highly reliant on exceptional communication skills, and there is nothing more important for involving patients in decisions than communication.

It is becoming increasingly acknowledged that Admiral nurses from Dementia UK are pivotal to promoting health, care and wellbeing for people living with dementia and their carers (see Box 10.6).

Box 10.6: The Admiral nurses' service approach

First, focus on the needs of the family carer, including psychological support, to help family carers understand and deal with their thoughts, feelings and behaviour and to adapt to the changing situation.

Second, use a range of specialist interventions that help people live well with the condition and develop skills to improve communication and maintain relationships.

Third, work with families as an invaluable source of contact and support at particular points of difficulty in the dementia journey, including diagnosis, when the condition progresses, or when tough decisions need to be made such as moving a family member into residential care. Anticipated problems are misdiagnosis, delayed diagnosis and lack of accurate support (incorrect information to persons with dementia and their families potentiates the risk for inappropriate management), crises, poor psychological adjustment to the diagnosis, and reduced coping capacity and ability to forward plan.

Fourth, help families cope with feelings of loss and bereavement as the condition progresses. There is an acknowledgement that family care does not end once 'hands-on' caregiving ceases, and the dementia guidelines support the principle that family carers should be supported during the illness of dementia and into bereavement.

For family carers of people with dementia, the more social support that is received during the years of caregiving, the easier it is to adjust and adapt post-bereavement.

Finally, provide advice on referrals to other appropriate services and liaise with other health care professionals on behalf of the family.

<hr>

SOURCE: ADAPTED FROM *NURSING TIMES*; CITED IN RAHMAN AND DENING (2016).

—— Essential reading ——

Acute care in hospitals

Rahman S. 2015. *Living Better with Dementia*, London: Jessica Kingsley Publishers, pp.152–155.

—— References ——

Aaltonen M, Raitanen J, Forma L, Pulkki J, Rissanen P, Jylhä M. 2014. Burdensome transitions at the end of life among long-term care residents with dementia. J Am Med Dir Assoc, 15(9), 643–648.

ADASS. 2010. Carers as Partners in Hospital Discharge: Improving Carer Recognition, Support and Outcomes within Timely and Supported Discharge Processes (a Review), available at static. carers.org/files/hospital-discharge-final-version-4945.pdf (accessed 3 Oct 2016).

Alzheimer's Society. 2009. *Counting the Cost*, London: Alzheimer's Society, available at www. alzheimers.org.uk/countingthecost (accessed 3 Oct 2016).

Ambulance Service Network/NHS Confederation. 2010. *Factsheet: Seeing Ambulance Services in a Different Light*, London: NHS.

Aminzadeh F, Dalziel WB. 2002. Older adults in the emergency department: a systematic review of patterns of use, adverse outcomes, and effectiveness of interventions. Ann. Emerg. Med, 39(3), 238–247.

Audit Commission. 2009. *More for Less: Are Productivity and Efficiency Improving in the NHS?* London: Audit Commission.

Bamford C, Poole M, Brittain K, Chew-Graham C, et al. 2014. Understanding the challenges to implementing case management for people with dementia in primary care in England: a qualitative study using Normalization Process Theory. BMC Health Serv Res, 14, 549.

Beernaert K, Van den Block L, Van Thienen K, Devroey D, et al. 2015. Family physicians' role in palliative care throughout the care continuum: stakeholder perspectives. Fam Pract, September, cmv072 (e-pub ahead of print).

Bernabei R, Landi F, Gambassi G, Sgadari A, et al. 1998. Randomised trial of impact of model of integrated care and case management for older people living in the community. Br Med J, 316, 148–151.

Bloomer M, Digby R, Tan H, Crawford K, Williams A. 2014. The experience of family carers of people with dementia who are hospitalised. Dementia (London), November, 1471301214558308 (e-pub ahead of print)

Briggs R, Coughlan T, Collins R, O'Neill D, Kennelly SP. 2013. Nursing home residents attending the emergency department: clinical characteristics and outcomes. QJM, 106(9), 803–808.

Brindle N, Holmes J. 2005. Capacity and coercion: dilemmas in the discharge of older people with dementia from general hospital settings. Age Ageing, 34(1), 16–20.

British Geriatrics Society. 2016. British Geriatrics Society comments on contractual arrangements for provision of GP services in Care Homes, available at www.bgs.org.uk/index.php/press-3/4589-bgs-on-gp-services-care-homes (accessed 29 Nov 2016).

Bryan K. 2010. Policies for reducing delayed discharge from hospital. Br Med Bull, 95, 33–46.

Burns E, Nair S. 2014. New horizons in care home medicine. Age Ageing, 43(1), 2–7.

Buswell M, Lumbard P, Prothero L, Lee C, *et al.* 2016. Unplanned, urgent and emergency care: what are the roles that EMS plays in providing for older people with dementia? An integrative review of policy, professional recommendations and evidence. Emerg Med J, 33(1), 61–70.

Callahan CM, Boustani MA, Unverzagt FW, Austrom MG, et al. 2006. Effectiveness of collaborative care for older adults with Alzheimer disease in primary care: a randomized controlled trial. J Am Med Assoc, 295, 2148–2157.

Callahan CM, Tu W, Unroe KT, LaMantia MA, Stump TE, Clark DO. 2015. Transitions in care in a nationally representative sample of older Americans with dementia. J Am Geriatr Soc, 63(8), 1495–1502.

Chenoweth L, Kable A, Pond D. 2015. Research in hospital discharge procedures addresses gaps in care continuity in the community, but leaves gaping holes for people with dementia: a review of the literature. Australias J Ageing, 34(1), 9–14.

Clark PG. 2015. Emerging themes in using narrative in geriatric care: implications for patient-centred practice and interprofessional teamwork. J Aging Stud, 34, 177–182.

Clissett P, Porock D, Harwood RH, Gladman JR. 2013. The challenges of achieving person-centred care in acute hospitals: a qualitative study of people with dementia and their families. Int J Nurs Stud, 50(11), 1495–1503.

Coker E, Papaioannou A, Kaasalainen S, Dolovich L, Turpie, I, Taniguchi A. 2010. Nurses' perceived barriers to optimal pain management in older adults on acute medical units. Appl. Nurs. Res, 23, 139–146.

Coleman EA. 2003. Falling through the cracks: challenges and opportunities for improving transitional care for persons with continuous complex care needs. J Am Geriatr Soc, 51(4), 549–555.

Connolly S, O'Shea E. 2015. The impact of dementia on length of stay in acute hospitals in Ireland. Dementia (London), 14(5), 650–658.

Crilly J, Chaboyer W, Wallis M. 2012. A structure and process evaluation of an Australian hospital admission avoidance programme for aged care facility residents. J Adv Nurs, 68(2), 322–334.

Crilly J, Chaboyer W, Wallis M, Thalib L, Polit D. 2011. An outcomes evaluation of an Australian hospital in the nursing home admission avoidance programme. J Clin Nurs, 20(7–8), 1178–1187.

de Vries K, Drury-Ruddlesden J, Gaul C. 2016. 'And so I took up residence': the experiences of family members of people with dementia during admission to an acute hospital unit. Dementia (London), June, 1471301216656097 (e-pub ahead of print)

Department of Health. 2009. Living well with dementia: A national dementia strategy, London: TSO, available at https://www.gov.uk/government/uploads/system/uploads/attachment_data/file/168220/dh_094051.pdf (accessed 29 Nov 2016).

Department of Health. 2010. *Quality Outcomes for People with Dementia: Building on the Work of the National Dementia Strategy*, London: Stationery Office.

Dutton RP, Cooper C, Jones A, Leone S, Kramer ME, Scalea TM. 2003. Daily multidisciplinary rounds shorten length of stay for trauma patients. J Trauma, 55(5), 913–919.

Elliot R, Adams J. 2011. The creation of a Dementia Nurse Specialist role in an acute general hospital. J Psychiatr Ment Health Nurs, 18(7), 648–652.

Emmett C, Poole M, Bond J, Hughes JC. 2013. Homeward bound or bound for a home? Assessing the capacity of dementia patients to make decisions about hospital discharge: comparing practice with legal standards. Int J Law Psychiatry, 36(1), 73–82.

Freeman G, Hughes J. 2010. Continuity of Care and the Patient Experience, London: The King's Fund, available at https://www.kingsfund.org.uk/sites/files/kf/field/field_document/continuity-care-patient-experience-gp-inquiry-research-paper-mar11.pdf (accessed 29 Nov 2016).

Fry M, Arendts G, Chenoweth L, MacGregor C. 2014. Cognitive impairment is a risk factor for delayed analgesia in older people with long bone fracture: a multicentre exploratory study. International Psychogeriatrics, August, 1–6.

Fry M, Bennetts S, Huckson S. 2011. An Australian audit of ED pain management patterns. Journal of Emergency Nursing, 37, 269–274.

Fry M, Chenoweth L, Arendts G. 2016. Assessment and management of acute pain in the older person with cognitive impairment: a qualitative study. Int Emerg Nurs, 24, 54–60.

Glasby J. 2003. *Hospital Discharge: Integrating Health and Social Care*, Oxford: Radcliffe Publishing.

Glasby J, Lester H. 2004. Delayed hospital discharge and mental health: the policy implications of recent research. Soc Policy Adm, 38, 744–757.

Griffiths P Bridges J, Sheldon H, Thompson R. 2015. The role of the dementia specialist nurse in acute care: a scoping review. J Clin Nurs, 24(9–10), 1394–1405.

Grober E, Sanders A, Hall CB, Ehrlich AR, Lipton RB. 2011. Very mild dementia and medical comorbidity independently predict health care use in the elderly. Journal of Primary Care and Community Health, 3(1), 23–28.

Ham C, Imison C, Jennings M. 2010. *Avoiding Hospital Admissions: Lessons from Evidence and Experience*. London: The King's Fund.

Harwood RH. 2012. Dementia for hospital physicians. Clin Med (Lond), 12(1), 35–39.

Health Foundation. 2013. *Improving Patient Flow: How Two Trusts Focused on Flow to Improve the Quality of Care and Use Available Capacity Effectively: Learning Report*, London: Health Foundation.

Health Foundation. 2014. *My Discharge: A Proactive Case Management for Discharging Patients with Dementia*, London: Health Foundation.

Healthwatch England. 2015. Safely Home: What Happens when People Leave Hospital and Care Settings? Healthwatch England Special Inquiry findings, July.

Holdcroft A, Power I. 2003. Recent developments: management of pain. Br. Med. J, 326(7390), 635–639.

House of Commons Committee of Public Accounts. 2016. *Discharging Older People from Acute Hospitals: Twelfth Report of Session 2016–17 Report, Together with Formal Minutes Relating to the Report Ordered by the House of Commons.*

HSJ. 2015. HSHSJ Workforce: Time for Some Advanced Thinking? The Benefits of Specialist Nurses. An HSJ supplement, 27 February.

Hutchinson AF, Graco M, Rasekaba TM, Parikh S, Berlowitz DJ, Lim WK. 2015. Relationship between health-related quality of life, comorbidities and acute health care utilisation, in adults with chronic conditions. Health Qual Life Outcomes, 13, 69.

Jurgens FJ, Clissett P, Gladman JR, Harwood RH. 2012. Why are family carers of people with dementia dissatisfied with general hospital care? A qualitative study. BMC Geriatr, 12, 57.

Köpke S, McCleery J. 2015. Systematic reviews of case management: too complex to manage? [editorial]. *Cochrane Database of Systematic Reviews*, 1.

Lenzi J, Mongardi M, Rucci P, Di Ruscio E, et al. 2014. Sociodemographic, clinical and organisational factors associated with delayed hospital discharges: a cross-sectional study. BMC Health Serv Res, 14, 128.

Lisk R, Yeong K, Nasim A, Baxter M, et al. 2012. Geriatrician input into nursing homes reduces emergency hospital admissions. Arch Gerontol Geriatr, 55(2), 331–337.

Lutze M, Fry M, Gallagher R. 2015. Minor injuries in older adults have different characteristics, injury patterns, and outcomes when compared with younger adults: an emergency department correlation study. Int Emerg Nurs, 23(2), 168–173.

Manias E. 2012. Complexities of pain assessment and management in hospitalised older people: a qualitative observation and interview study. Int. J. Nurs. Stud, 49(10), 1243–1254.

Manzano-Santaella A, Belinda Goode B. 2011. Delayed discharges in mental health beds. British Journal of Health Care Management, 17(3), 113–119.

Matesanz-Fernández M, Monte-Secades R, Íñiguez-Vázquez I, Rubal-Bran D, Guerrero-Sande H, Casariego-Vales E. 2015. Characteristics and temporal pattern of the readmissions of patients with multiple hospital admissions in the medical departments of a general hospital. Eur J Intern Med, 26(10), 776–781.

McCloskey R. 2011. The 'mindless' relationship between nursing homes and emergency departments: what do Bourdieu and Freire have to offer? Nurs Inq, 18(2), 154–164.

Mytton OT, Oliver D, Mirza N, Lipet J, et al. 2012. Avoidable acute hospital admissions in older people. British Journal of Healthcare Management, 18(11), 597–603.

Natalwala A, Potluri R, Uppal HK, Heun R. 2008. Reasons for hospital admission in dementia patients in Birmingham, UK, during 2002–2007. Dementia and Geriatric Cognitive Disorders, 26(6), 499–505.

Naylor C, Alderwick H, Honeyman M. 2015. *Acute Hospitals and Integrated Care: From Hospitals to Health Systems*, London: King's Fund, available at www.kingsfund.org.uk/sites/files/kf/field/field_publication_file/acute-hospitals-and-integrated-care-march-2015.pdf (accessed 3 Oct 2016).

Naylor C, Imison C, Aldicott R, Buck D, et al. 2015. *Transforming Our Health Care System,* London: King's Fund, available at www.kingsfund.org.uk/sites/files/kf/field/field_publication_file/10PrioritiesFinal2.pdf (accessed 3 Oct 2016).

NHS Benchmarking Network. 2015. *National Audit of Intermediate Care, Summary Report 2015*, available at www.nhsbenchmarking.nhs.uk/CubeCore/.uploads/NAIC/Reports/NAICReport2015FINALA4printableversion.pdf (accessed 3 Oct 2016).

NHS England. 2013. *Delayed Transfers of Care: Statistics for England 2012/13 Annual Report*, available at www.england.nhs.uk/statistics/wp-content/uploads/sites/2/2013/04/Annex-3-Annual-report-2012-13.pdf (accessed 3 Oct 2016).

NHS Institute for Innovation and Improvement. No date. Indicator Construction: Managing Variation in Emergency Admissions.

O'Brien J. 2008. Antipsychotics for people with dementia. BMJ, 337, 64–65.

Oliver D. 2015. Who is to blame for older people's readmission? BMJ, 351, h4244.

Park M, Delaney C, Maas M, Reed D. 2004. Using a nursing minimum data set with older patients with dementia in an acute care setting. Journal of Advanced Nursing, 47, 329–339.

Phelan EA, Debnam KJ, Anderson LA, Owens SB. 2015. A systematic review of intervention studies to prevent hospitalizations of community-dwelling older adults with dementia. Med Care, 53(2), 207–213.

Quinn T. 2011. Emergency hospital admissions from care-homes: who, why and what happens? A cross-sectional study. Gerontology, 57(2), 115–120.

Rahman S, Dening KH. 2016. The need for specialist nurses in dementia care. Nursing Times, 112(16), 14–17.

Reilly S, Miranda-Castillo C, Malouf R, Hoe J, et al. 2015. Case management approaches to home support for people with dementia. Cochrane Database of Systematic Reviews, 1(CD008345).

Robinson CA, Bottorff JL, Lilly MB, Reid C, et al. 2012. Stakeholder perspectives on transitions of nursing home residents to hospital emergency departments and back in two Canadian provinces. J Aging Stud, 26(4), 419–247.

Robinson L, Bamford C, Beyer F, Clark A, et al. 2010. Patient preferences for future care – how can Advance Care Planning become embedded into dementia care: a study protocol. BMC Geriatr, 10, 2.

Roche L, MacCann C, Croot K. 2016. Predictive Factors for the Uptake of Coping Strategies by Spousal Dementia Caregivers: A Systematic Review. Alzheimer Dis Assoc Disord, 30(1), 80–91.

Ross S, Curry N, Goodwin N. 2011. *Case Management: What It Is and How It Can Be Best Implemented*, London: King's Fund.

Royal College of Physicians. 2012. *Hospitals on the Edge? The Time for Action. A Report by the Royal College of Physicians*, available at www.rcplondon.ac.uk/guidelines-policy/hospitals-edge-time-action (accessed 3 Oct 2016).

Royal College of Physicians' Future Hospitals Commission. 2013. *Future Hospital: Caring for Medical Patients*, available at www.rcplondon.ac.uk/projects/outputs/future-hospital-commission (accessed 3 Oct 2016).

Rudolph JL, Zanin NM, Jones RN, Marcantonio ER, et al. 2010. Hospitalization in community-dwelling persons with Alzheimer's disease: frequency and causes. J Am Geriatr Soc, 58(8), 1542–1548.

Sampson EL, Blanchard MR, Jones L, Tookman A, King M. 2009. Dementia in the acute hospital: prospective cohort study of prevalence and mortality. Br J Psychiatry, 195(1), 61–66.

Sampson EL, White N, Lord K, Leurent B, et al. 2015. Pain, agitation, and behavioural problems in people with dementia admitted to general hospital wards: a longitudinal cohort study. Pain, 156(4), 675–683.

Samsi K, Manthorpe J, Nagendran T, Heath H. 2012. Challenges and expectations of the Mental Capacity Act 2005: an interview-based study of community-based specialist nurses working in dementia care. J Clin Nurs, 21(11–12), 1697–1705.

Shepperd S, Lannin NA, Clemson LM, McCluskey A, Cameron ID, Barras SL. 2013. Discharge planning from hospital to home. Cochrane Database Syst Rev, 1(CD000313).

Sherlaw-Johnson C, Smith P, Bardsley M. 2016. Continuous monitoring of emergency admissions of older care home residents to hospital. Age Ageing, 45(1), 71–77.

Skaalvik MW, Normann HK, Henriksen N. 2010. Student experiences in learning person-centred care of patients with Alzheimer's disease as perceived by nursing students and supervising nurses. Journal of Clinical Nursing, 19(17/18), 2639–2648.

Stevenson J, Spencer L. 2002. *Developing Intermediate Care: A Guide for Health and Social Services Professionals*, London: The King's Fund, available at www.kingsfund.org.uk/sites/files/kf/Developing-Intermediate-Care-guide-health-social-services-professionals-Jan-Stevenson-Linda-Spencer-The-Kings-Fund-July-2009.pdf (accessed 3 Oct 2016).

Teno JM, Gozalo PL, Bynum JP, Leland NE, et al. 2013. Change in end-of-life care for Medicare beneficiaries: site of death, place of care, and health care transitions in 2000, 2005, and 2009. JAMA, 309(5), 470–477.

The King's Fund. No date. *Emergency Hospital Admissions for Ambulatory Care-Sensitive Conditions: Identifying the Potential for Reductions*. London: The King's Fund.

Thompson J. 2015. *Delayed Transfers of Care: Join the Queue* (blog, 9 November).

Toot S, Devine M, Akporobaro A, Orrell M. 2013. Causes of hospital admission for people with dementia: a systematic review and meta-analysis. J Am Med Dir Assoc, 14(7), 463–470.

van den Block L, Pivodic L, Pardon K, Donker G, et al. 2015. Transitions between health care settings in the final three months of life in four EU countries. Eur J Public Health, 25(4), 569–575.

Van Doorn C, Gruber-Baldini AL, Zimmerman S, Hebel RJ, et al. 2003. Dementia as a risk factor for falls and fall injuries among nursing home residents. Journal of American Geriatrics Society, 51(9), 1213–1218.

Varney J, Weiland TJ, Jelinek G. 2014. Efficacy of hospital in the home services providing care for patients admitted from emergency departments: an integrative review. Int J Evid Based Healthc, 12(2), 128–141.

Victor C. 1991. *Health and Health Care in Later Life*, Milton Keynes: Open University Press.

Wasson JH, Thomas TA, Bubiz JL, Teno J. 1998. Can we afford comprehensive supportive care for the very old? J Am Geriatr Soc, 46, 829–832.

Wilson A, Parker H. 2005. Hospital in the home: what next? Medical Journal of Australia, 183, 228–229.

Waugh A, Austin A, Manthorpe J, Fox C, et al. 2013. Designing a complex intervention for dementia case management in primary care. BMC Fam Pract, 14, 101.

Chapter 11

SUPPORTING WELL AND INDEPENDENCE

Independence is high when an older person's experience of receiving assistance matches their desired level of choice, social usefulness and autonomy. (O'Connor and Purves, 2009, p.139)

Learning objectives

By the end of this chapter, you will be able to:

»   explain the importance of a 'personal' approach, as demonstrated through various principles and processes such as integrated personal commissioning, personal genomics and personalised medicine

»   describe the role of dementia advisers

»   explain the importance of assistive technology in maintaining independence, including self-care and meaningful activity

»   describe telecare

»   describe issues with GP access, and explain how capacity might be enhanced by community pharmacy

»   describe self-management in dementia and other long-term conditions

»   understand the potential uses of electronic health and care records, and appreciate wider ethical considerations

»   understand the importance of enablement/reablement, including a professional response to sensory impairments as an example

»   appreciate the critical importance of support groups

Introduction

Chronic diseases cannot be completely cured or eliminated and tend to require lengthy, often expensive treatments involving complex, ongoing care. Examples include diabetes, hypertension, heart failure, many cancers and dementia. The work of Margaret Baltes (e.g. Baltes, 1988) suggests that in many care settings, far from promoting independence, dependency is systematically reinforced. The importance of a timely intervention has been advocated by Moniz-Cook and colleagues (2011), and providing support soon after a diagnosis is a key way to promote this agenda.

I emphasised the importance of this work in Chapter 5.

Post-diagnostic support for people with dementia and their families and friends should include activities that enhance or provide social contact and peer support to reduce isolation. Information and opportunities should also be provided to overcome limitations imposed on those affected by the condition and preserve or bolster self-worth by finding ways for them to make a contribution and feel useful (Clare, 2002). These developments in population health management are important. They take away some of the pressure that providers feel to increase the volume of services they deliver, and they better align the interests of patients and physicians (Main and Slywotzky, 2014).

There have been a number of brilliant new initiatives recently. For example, the Health Service Executive and Genio Dementia Programme is currently developing and testing new service models in Ireland which will improve the range and quality of community-based supports for people with dementia. This very much builds on the work of Kitwood (Genio, 2016, p.4):

> Personhood has been used as a fluid narrative in the context of this service design process – a narrative that respects and encourages autonomy, empowerment and social connectivity for people living with dementia, to ensure that they can live fulfilling lives in their community in the face of changing cognitive abilities.

Wellbeing and independence are worthy goals in dementia care

Casual observation of many dementia care settings suggests that there remains a great deal to be achieved. If we do know how to promote independence and wellbeing, then that knowledge will largely not be implemented (Woods, 1999). Growth in the use of technology has implications for health care providers. For example, there is increasing potential to support the shift of some hands-on treatment in primary care clinics and hospitals to home care via the use of digital communication such as e-visits, e-prescriptions and remote monitoring. There is enormous potential for further improvements across many aspects of health care provision – for example,

GP practices, residential and nursing homes, hospitals and, in particular, mental health care – but only if the existing barriers can be overcome (Deloitte, 2015).

Recognising the need to support people with dementia and their families resulted in the development of dementia cafés. The first dementia café was opened in 1997 in the Netherlands, with the original concept described by Miesen and Blom (2001, p.2) as a 'meeting place for persons with dementia, family, carers and other interested parties'. Since 2000, over 20 dementia or memory cafés have opened in the UK following Miesen's model. A key issue for some people with dementia and their carers has been their increasing difficulties travelling (relevant to the practical logistics of dementia-friendly communities). Access difficulties potentially isolate people with dementia and their carers, for example difficulties accessing public transport due to increasing frailty as a comorbidity, or having to stop driving due to increasing cognitive impairment or financial reasons (Kelly and Innes, 2014).

There are a number of important ways in which remote health monitoring might be of benefit to supporting people with dementia, as itemised by McKinsey (2010):

» disease diagnosis, complication management and intervention ahead of acute phenomena, for example predicting impending heart failure through non-intrusive remote monitoring

» treatment compliance, by reminding patients and prompting carers to intervene in cases of non-compliance

» quality of care, by giving patients and carers tools to manage disabilities associated with chronic diseases, for example locator devices for persons with dementia.

Skills for Care and Skills for Health have indicated some of the different ways of working in their seven Common Core Principles for Self-Care, including the need to support and enable individuals to use technology to support self-care (cited in SCIE, 2013).

GP practices have led the way in the shift from paper to digital record-keeping, but they remain slow in adopting technology in their interfacing with patients. Many GP practices already offer telephone appointments, telephone triage, email consultations and text messaging to notify patients of appointments. However, their adoption of telecare and telehealth has been patchy, and the potential for such technology to support primary care in making home care more effective, personalised and convenient is underdeveloped (Deloitte, 2015). Because they have increased access to high-speed internet and smartphones, it is conceivable that many persons living with dementia will use mobile apps to manage health (Dimitrov, 2016). These devices and mobile apps are now increasingly used and integrated with telemedicine and telehealth via the medical Internet of Things. Wearables and mobile apps can support fitness, health education, symptom tracking, collaborative disease management and care coordination.

A personal approach: integrated personal commissioning, personal —— genomics and personalised medicine ——

A recurrent theme in this book has been that the precise definition of 'integrated care' is complex and contested.

A total of 175 definitions of the concept were identified in one recent literature review. Shared by all definitions, integration involves processes that overcome the fragmentation of care through better linkages and coordination of services and seeks to improve outcomes for those with complex needs (Stokes, Checkland and Kristensen, 2016). The notion has emerged that constructs such as personal recovery, patient engagement and consumer involvement are central in health care delivery.

Integrated personal commissioning (IPC) is one of the pillars of the Five Year Forward View. Since its publication, a number of national programmes have been launched in addition to IPC – these are transforming the health and social care system dramatically. These include the New Care Models Programme, the Better Care Fund (introduced in Chapter 2), Transforming Care, further devolution, co-commissioning of primary medical services and most recently Sustainability and Transformation Plans (STPs) (NHS England, 2016). IPC is intended to advance the personalisation agenda of more 'choice' and 'control' (see Figure 11.1).

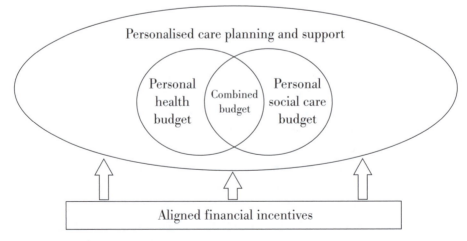

Figure 11.1: Approach to personalised care and support budgets
Source: redrawn from NHS England (2014a, p.8).

However, the legitimacy of the use of information to provide agency and choice can be questioned, as its quality and effectiveness may be limited in terms of dislodging in-built intuitions and preferences, thus ultimately not promoting overall population health (Dawson, 2014). Asymmetric information usually affects the doctor–patient relationship. As a rule, the doctor has relevant information that the patient lacks. Therefore, conventional wisdom tells us, markets fail to operate efficiently (Shmanske, 1996). Buyers and sellers cannot trade efficiently if one side of the transaction can be manipulated or charged excessively because of inferior information; this asymmetry can cause market failure. Besides, the recall of risk information may be particularly problematic in people with dementia and carers.

The use of information pervades all discussions about personal care and medicine. Health care professionals should be aware that each type of genetic risk information may be differentially interpreted and retained by patients and that some patient subgroups may have greater problems with recall than others (Besser et al., 2015). The logic of the market system allowed for new opportunities for purchasers to contract with a range of health and social care providers. However, the dominance of a competitive imperative rather than a collaborative one generally precluded integration. The need for organisations to control costs and protect budgets meant that there was a greater incentive to shift costs to other organisations rather than develop service systems collaboratively.[1]

Integrated personal commissioning is a new voluntary approach to joining up health and social care for adults with complex needs. In future, IPC and personal health budgets will provide essential counterbalances to whole-population commissioning models. Within or alongside overarching place-based models of care, they will enable people who need a more personalised approach to opt out of their local provider for particular services where appropriate, and take increased charge of decision-making for their care (NHS England, 2016).

The goals of this programme are:

» to ensure that people with complex needs and their carers have a better quality of life and can achieve the outcomes that are important to them and their families through greater involvement in their care, with the ability to design support around their needs and circumstances

» the prevention of crises in people's lives that lead to unplanned hospital and institutional care by keeping them well and supporting self-management as measured by tools such as patient activation, thereby ensuring better value for money

» better integration and quality of care, including better user and family experience of care.

---

1   See Goodwin et al. in *International Journal of Integrated Care*, Vol. 1, 1 March 2001, at www.ijic. org (accessed 4 Oct 2016).

IPC is based on two core elements:

» **Care model:** Person-centred care and care planning, combined with an optional personal health and social care budget. The proposed care model will include personalised care and support planning, independent advocacy, peer support and brokerage. People will be able to take as much control as they want, including a clear offer of integrated personal budgets for those who will benefit. Care planning will be based on the strengths and preferences of individuals, instead of a service offer driven by the care system.

» **Financial model:** An integrated, 'year of care' capitated payment model. The IPC financial model attempts to shift incentives towards prevention and coordination of care, by testing an integrated, capitated payment approach.

The potential of genomics is also huge, leading to more precise and faster diagnostic tests, the development of new medical devices that help people lead independent lives, faster clinical trials, new drugs and treatments and, potentially, future new cures. The ethical use of information is intrinsic to personal care and medicine. The future vision of genomics in health care and public health represents a confluence of the development of three important strands: genetic technologies, clinical genetics and genomic health care (Phg Foundation, 2012). A recent paper proposes the following tentative definition of personal utility: 'genomic information has personal utility if and only if it can reasonably be used for decisions, actions or self-understanding which are personal in nature' (Bunnik, Janssens and Schermer, 2015, p.324). The further elaboration on this is crucial (ibid.): 'The proposed definition of personal utility presupposes two things: that a genomic test delivers information (i.e. meaningful information) and that this information can be used or put to use in some reasonable way.'

As a whole, the public should be more informed about the potential benefits but also the limitations of preventive genomics, whereas policy should also address public concerns (Vermeulen et al., 2014). Figure 11.2 illustrates how this approach appears to be much more sophisticated than previous approaches to drug design.

A number of advances have been practice changing (e.g. imatinib mesylate in chronic myeloid leukaemia, herceptin in *erb-B2-positive* breast cancer). Increasingly, we are also seeing the promise of a number of newer approaches, particularly in diseases such as lung cancer and melanoma. However, in this context there is the worrying realisation that many of the early advances cited above that have led to real patient benefit have been supplanted by a culture of marginal, incremental change, whereas transformative benefit is what our patients require (Lawler and Sullivan, 2015). Humans have three major apolipoprotein E (ApoE) alleles (e2, e3 and e4) that produce three ApoE protein isoforms. Because the type of ApoE expressed is related to sporadic Alzheimer's disease risk and familial hyperlipidemia, many clinical studies have utilised ApoE typing in recent years. Serotyping ApoE using mass spectrometry promises highly accurate results while requiring minimal amounts of blood and reagents, resulting in lower costs – this suggests that proteomic-based ApoE serotyping may eventually become a routine clinical laboratory test (Nishimura et al., 2014).

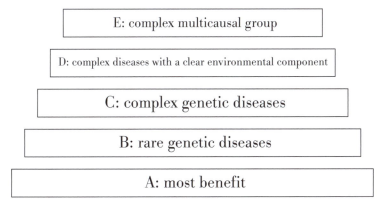

Figure 11.2: Technological advancement towards whole-of-life care

A–E: First, most benefit (**A**). Patients with rare genetic diseases are first then to benefit from genomic sequencing-based testing as affected genes and pathways can be identified (**B**). Utilising electronic health records will improve diagnosis and treatment of complex genetic diseases as informative patient groupings can be achieved more efficiently (**C**). Complex diseases with a clear environmental component, such as diabetes, will benefit from the integration of other omics-based assays (**D**); however, personalised preventive and intervention strategies (**E**) are required to manage the health of this high-burden multicausal group optimally.
Source: based on Bauer et al. (2014, Fig. 1).

Dementia advisers

In 2009, the National Dementia Strategy for England, *Living Well with Dementia* (Department of Health, 2009), was launched. Objective 4 of the strategy sets out the need for 'a Dementia Adviser (DA) to facilitate easy access to appropriate care, support and advice for those diagnosed with dementia and their carers' (Department of Health, 2009, p.11).

The following definition is helpful.

Dementia adviser service is defined as the provision of a service for those diagnosed with dementia and their families who they can approach for help and advice at any stage of the illness. The role of the dementia adviser will vary, but includes supporting those with dementia from the point of diagnosis by providing a single identifiable point of contact that has knowledge of, and direct access to, the whole range of available local services. They help with advice, signposting and enabling contact with other services if needed. (Ipsos MORI, 2016)

The Department of Health, working with Age UK and Ipsos MORI, undertook a project to investigate the provision of services available for older people in England, with a particular interest in understanding dementia adviser services. Ipsos MORI conducted an online survey with those responsible for commissioning dementia services in CCGs and local authorities between October and November 2015.

The following findings were noted in that study:

Dementia advisers communicate with a variety of people and organisations on behalf of the people they support. In almost all cases (95%), participants say that dementia advisers communicate with memory clinic staff/nurses. Dementia advisers also communicate with community social care services (91% of commissioners say this), support groups (89%) and community health services (85%). (Ipsos MORI, 2016)

The evidence pertaining to roles such as dementia advisers arguably suggests that their effectiveness is likely to depend on manageable caseloads, adequate dedicated time and a minimum level of existing service integration (after Knapp et al., 2014). La Fontaine and colleagues (2011) noted that barriers to the effectiveness of the DA role included: the length of time it took to receive referrals; the emotional experience of providing a service to people with complex and emotionally demanding needs; and a lack of services to enable people to live well with dementia. However, these authors also noted that the identification and development of relationships with key players, who in turn were able to support the development of the role through referrals and promotion of the DA to others, were particularly important in enabling the DA to begin to embed the service within the localities.

—— Technology and maintenance of independence –

Persons living better with Alzheimer's disease experience a progressive decline of their condition, with a gradual loss of their independence in daily functioning (Lancioni et al., 2014).

Cognitive difficulties, for which assistance could be appropriate, are often faced by people trying to live with dementia, such as:

» managing medication and finances

» performing daily activities such as preparing food

» using typical communication means to interact with family and friends

» managing orientation and travel within circumscribed and familiar places, such as the home or the day centre

» engaging in recreation activities such as listening to music.

(Lancioni et al., 2014)

More than a decade ago, the White Paper 'Our Health, Our Care, Our Say: A New Direction for Community Services' (Department of Health, 2006) drew attention to the ageing population. It kick-started the debate about investment in preventive and community-based services that aim to keep people ageing well and maintain independence.

People are aspiring to secure more autonomy in their disease management (Draper et al., 2002).

Telecare and telehealth have developed within the context of tackling health and illness issues and as efforts to ensure older people who may be at risk of losing their independence are helped to avoid long-term hospital placements or residential care for as long as possible. Telecare helps people who need health services or social care to continue living at home. It uses technology that can monitor activities and safety, provide virtual home visiting, activate reminder systems, increase home security and convey information.

The NICE (2015) guideline 'Home Care: Delivering Personal Care and Practical Support to Older People Living in Their Own Homes' (NG21)[2] covers the planning and delivery of person-centred care for older people living in their own homes (known as home care or domiciliary care). This guidance aims to promote older people's independence and to ensure safe and consistently high-quality home care services. Its stated audience comprises health and social care practitioners, home care provider organisations, home care managers and workers, older people using or planning to use home care services (and their carers), and commissioners of home care services.

Maintaining independence is the critical factor that the technology aims to address, for example by detecting falls, aids for sensory impairment, medication management, memory prompts and the monitoring of vital signs (Fisk, 2003). Methodological insight is needed for designers to focus on patients' needs and incorporate user requirements into technological design (De Rouck, Jacobs and Leys, 2008). In terms of the home setting, computer-based technology might in future become part of the living environment and household routine (Kerssens et al., 2015). A recent study has indicated that attitudes and the perceived usefulness of computer technology have shifted over time (Simpson and Kenrick, 1997).

---

2   Available at https://www.nice.org.uk/guidance/48 (accessed 28 Oct 2016).

Inexpensive health information technology (e.g. reporting systems for patients' falls) can be successfully implemented in low technology settings (Mei et al., 2013).

Assistive technology (AT) can be defined as 'any device or system that allows an individual to perform a task that they would otherwise be unable to do, or increases the ease and safety with which the task can be performed' (Cowan and Turner-Smith, 1999, p.325).

A variety of assistive technologies have been adopted to help seniors in their daily lives, such as robotics, sensors, computers and the internet (Khosravi and Ghapanchia, 2015). Research illustrating the effectiveness of assistive technologies is scant, however (Fuhrer, 2001; Jutai et al., 2005). Assistive technologies need to be evaluated not only for feasibility and acceptance, but also effectiveness. There are methodological concerns in trialling assistive technologies. One key aspect of designing or assessing technology in this field is the difficulty of recreating 'natural' conditions where types of prompting support can be assessed. Controlled laboratory settings, although convenient for consistent test conditions, can also miss some of the relevant, real-world factors that can impact upon a person's ability to carry out a task (Boyd et al., 2015). The evidence also suggests that consumer health information technologies have the potential to release patients from high hospital care costs, improve health care convenience, promote communication between clinicians and patients, and enhance the accessibility of health care resources for patients (Or and Karsh, 2009).

Everyday technologies play an important role in supporting patients with dementia and their families to continue caring, but further research is needed to determine the most effective and person-centred models for future AT provision. It has been argued that the **mixed economy** landscape, with private AT provision supplementing state provision, is a key feature for the mainstreaming of AT services. Gibson and colleagues (2015) argue that this mixed economy has arisen from more participants using off-the-shelf, privately purchased goods and services, rather than via state services. Furthermore, assistive technologies may need to be reframed. Technological advances are important, but they must be underpinned by industry and service providers following a user-centred approach to design and delivery. For the ARCHIE principles to be realised, the sector requires a shift in focus from product (assistive technologies) to performance (supporting technologies-in-use) (Greenhalgh et al., 2015).

—— Telecare ——

Telecare is a subtype of AT which usually involves the remote monitoring of people living in their own homes, communicating with them at a distance via telephony and the internet (Gibson et al., 2015). Telecare devices include personal alarms, fall detectors, epilepsy sensors, enuresis sensors (detecting bed moisture), large button telephones, and carbon monoxide, gas and flood detectors. These may all be linked to a central alert system, key safes (securely holding house keys but with a code to allow access for carers and emergency services) and Buddi systems (personal tracking system using GPS technology).

New models of care are offering opportunities for innovation to improve the wellbeing of people living with dementia (see Chapter 1), and new models of enhanced self-care for people with dementia and their supporters are now being introduced and promulgated (Moniz-Cook, De Lepeleire and Vernooij-Dassen, 2004). A great example, which I introduced in Chapter 1, is Airedale. Furthermore, the proposed new model from the Nottingham City Clinical Commissioning Group will provide a structured and proactive approach to care. This will be complemented by a number of local innovations, including: mobile working for primary care; access to SystmOne for care homes; remote video consultation between care home residents and GPs; remote access to resident health data through telehealth; and the increased use of telecare. Care home residents, commissioners and providers will work together to aim to ensure that residents have enhanced involvement in decisions about care, the place of care and place of dying, and improve the quality of care for residents through well-coordinated, timely care and the appropriate use of technology.[3]

—— GP access and community pharmacy ——

General practice plays a central role in ensuring the delivery of universal, high-quality care to NHS patients. For most patients, general practice is among their first and most regular points of contact with the NHS. As well as providing advice, diagnosis and treatment directly to patients, GPs act as gatekeepers to services provided by other parts of the NHS and have a role in coordinating these for patients. There are issues about effective GP access (see Box 11.1), but it appears that the fundamental problem seems to be one of adequate resources in the right place.

GP services and primary care are generally expected to change significantly as the NHS makes the Five Year Forward View a reality. More patient care will be delivered locally, and investment in primary and community care will increase. At the same time, the boundaries between primary and other forms of care will blur as integrated models of care, such as Multispeciality Community Providers and combined Primary and Acute Care Systems, develop (Monitor, 2015).

3   See www.nottinghamcity.nhs.uk/news-projects/integrated-care/care-homes-vanguard.html (accessed 4 Oct 2016).

The Health Select Committee has identified a number of problems in access to general practice in England:[4]

» recruitment and retention problems mean that there are not enough GPs to meet demand; for the last decade, demand in general practice has risen faster than capacity

» having good access to general practice is too dependent on where patients live because of variations in staffing levels

» there is unacceptable variation in patients' experiences of getting and making appointments

» it is not always easy for people to find the information they need to access the right medical care

» the Department of Health and NHS England do not have enough information about demand, activity or capacity to support their decisions on general practice.

As far as hospital inpatients admitted as an emergency are concerned, a recent study revealed that patients registered to more accessible general practices were more likely to have been admitted via a GP (as opposed to an A&E department). This suggests that access to general practice is related to the use of emergency hospital services in England (Cowling et al., 2016). Access is difficult to define and there is no consensus as to what constitutes 'appropriate' access or what indicates a high degree of access. In general terms, good access exists when patients can get 'the right service at the right time in the right place' (Chapman et al., 2004, p.374). Gaining access to general practice quickly and conveniently is a high priority for patients and influences their perceptions of the quality of care. However, access should not be confused with speed. Some UK research suggests that it is a higher priority for people to be seen on their day of choice rather than being seen quickly and that more same-day appointments can actually reduce the perceived quality of care (Health Foundation, 2014).

In a large national survey of patients recently, self-reported difficulty in accessing a GP within standard opening hours was associated with the increased use of out-of-hours primary care services, independent of age, sex, ethnicity, deprivation, chronic disease and employment status (Zhou et al., 2015). The relationship between the convenience of opening hours, our strongest predictor, and the use of out-of-hours primary care, was strongest among patients not in employment or education,

---

4   See www.publications.parliament.uk/pa/cm201516/cmselect/cmpubacc/673/67305.htm (accessed 4 Oct 2016).

indicating that reducing the demand for out-of-hours primary care may be done by improving in-hours access (rather than extending opening hours).

Access to primary care and its impact on demand for emergency hospital care is topical in many developed countries (OECD, 2014). Telemedicine, a branch of e-health that uses communication networks to deliver health care services and medical education from one geographical location to another, can help solve the problem of access to geriatric assessments for nursing home residents (Brignell, Wootton and Gray, 2007). The organisation of primary care and patients' perceived communication with their GP were found to be highly correlated with patients' decisions to seek health care for minor or severe complaints, suggesting that the characteristics of health care systems directly influence patients' care-seeking behaviour, potentially leading to the overuse or underuse of health services.

Box 11.1: Good access

Good access is about:

* patients being able to book an appointment quickly, within a reasonable timeframe, and pre-book one if they wish

* patients being able to see a preferred clinician if they wish to wait longer for an appointment

* patient access to reliable information about the practice, so that they can make their own decisions about the access they require

* patients not only being able to book an appointment on the telephone but by other means, such as through the internet, email, TV or by text message; allowing patients to create, amend and cancel their appointments online is becoming a popular alternative

* patients contributing to good access through patient participation groups and other forums; patient participation groups can play an important role in identifying key local support groups

* patients being able to telephone the practice throughout the day.

Source: based on NHS Practice Management Network (2009).

Telemedicine includes real-time teleconsultations linking a physician and patient at different sites without the need to transport the patient to a geriatric centre (Sood et al., 2007). Clay and Stern (2015) reveal that one of the strongest themes emerging from their research is the unnecessary extra workload created by the lack of clear systems and processes for practices and their local hospitals to communicate with each other and their shared patients. In the study from Georgeton and colleagues (2015), the rate of GP adherence to recommendations from geriatric assessments made during teleconsultations for the elderly living in nursing homes is about 84%, which is slightly higher than for the reported rates of 49–79% for the elderly living in a community. One explanation for this was the good relationship between the GP and geriatrician. Good relationships between GPs and geriatricians are necessary for the management of care in nursing homes, because the implementation of recommendations and their outcomes increases the health status of the elderly.

Growing dissatisfaction with access to GP services appears to be growing in tandem with reports of pressures on the GP workforce (NHS England, 2013). As of 31 March 2013, there were 11,495 community pharmacies in England, all offering services without an appointment and many having extended opening hours on weekdays and weekends. Community pharmacy has the potential and the capacity (if the skills-mix issues are addressed) to be the first port of call for more patients, releasing capacity in general practice.

Community pharmacists have an important function in post-diagnostic care and support, working in partnership with local government. Such examples include:

»   public health – pharmacists and their teams already have a track record in delivering public health services, such as promoting and supporting good sexual health and reducing substance misuse within communities

»   support for independent living – by helping people to understand the correct use and management of medicines as well as by providing healthy lifestyle advice and support for self-care, pharmacists and their teams can help contribute to better health, reduce admissions to hospital and help people remain independent for longer.

On 17 December 2015, the Director General of Innovation, Growth and Technology at the Department of Health and the Chief Pharmaceutical Officer sent a letter to Sue Sharpe, the chief executive of the Pharmaceutical Services Negotiating Committee. The letter evidences a strategic need to make enhanced use of pharmacists.

> There is real potential for far greater use of community pharmacy and pharmacists: in prevention of ill health; support for healthy living; support for self-care for minor ailments and long-term conditions; medication reviews in care homes; and as part of more integrated local care models. To this end we need a clinically focussed community pharmacy service that is better integrated with primary care. That will help relieve the pressure on GPs and Accident and Emergency Departments, ensure optimal use

of medicines, better value and better patient outcomes, and contribute to delivering seven day health and care services.[5]

For example, the critical role that medication management plays in treating chronic diseases suggests that the integration of pharmacists into chronic care delivery teams has the potential to improve health outcomes (Schrommer, Doucette and Planas, 2015).

—— Self-management ——————————————

Although self-management has been used in many different chronic health conditions, there is no universally agreed definition (Quinn et al., 2015).

Barlow and colleagues (2002) have defined self-management as the 'individual's ability to manage the symptoms, treatment, physical and psychosocial consequences and lifestyle changes inherent in living with a chronic condition' (p.178).

The goal of disease self-management is to improve health status and health behaviour, reduce utilisation of the health care system and improve patient quality of life in work and home settings (Lorig et al., 2006). Growing evidence suggests that health care is more efficient and effective when patients are actively engaged in their treatment (Singh et al., 2016). It may be challenging for patients diagnosed with chronic conditions to self-manage their illnesses by modifying their lifestyles with little or no additional ongoing support, so it is critical to find ways to provide and promote cost-effective technologies, such as the internet or smartphones (e.g. Archer et al., 2014). Benefits of such an approach can include improved knowledge, self-efficacy, health status and better performance of self-management behaviours (Quinn et al., 2014). One source of self-management support that has received unanimous endorsement from people with dementia and their carers is providing support groups, which could offer companionship as well as information (Toms et al., 2015).

Self-management interventions share the objectives of educating people about the condition, optimising wellbeing, enhancing control over the situation, and enabling people to take more responsibility for managing the condition (Quinn et al., 2014). Historically, there has been relatively little research on the use of self-management in dementia, but now it is overwhelmingly clear that self-management can improve outcomes in integrated care (see Box 11.2), provided they are not used as a 'cover' for chronic underfunding.

A review by De Silva (2011) concluded that self-management techniques can lead to improvements in quality of life, clinical outcomes and health service use in people with long-term conditions. Self-management does not specifically aim to

---

5   See www.gov.uk/government/uploads/system/uploads/attachment_data/file/486941/letter-psnc.pdf (accessed 4 Oct 2016).

improve cognitive functioning, unlike interventions such as cognitive rehabilitation (e.g. Giebel and Challis, 2015). Instead, in self-management the focus is on helping the person to develop the necessary skills and knowledge to manage their condition. On the other hand, offering suitable evidence-based interventions to people with early-stage dementia could delay admission to residential care and add to the cost-effectiveness of services. Participation in self-management programmes also leads to a universal reduction in service costs that remains evident over time (Lorig, Mazonson and Holman, 1993).

The core self-management skills identified by Lorig and Holman (2004) are:

» undertaking problem solving and decision-making

» locating and using resources

» the creation of a partnership between the person and health professional

» making an action plan and taking action.

Weingarten and colleagues (2002) also identified a number of elements that might be included within a self-management programme. These included education, feedback and reminders for patients and health care providers.

Box 11.2: Some properties of self-management programmes

* Self-management has the potential to improve health outcomes in some cases, with patients reporting increases in physical functioning. Most of the time, people manage their own health and wellbeing, rather than health professionals or services taking on this role.

* Self-management can potentially offer personalised coordinated care, support or treatment.

* Self-management can improve patient experience, affording people dignity, compassion and respect, with reports of benefits in terms of greater confidence and reduced anxiety.

* Self-management programmes have been shown to reduce unplanned hospital admissions for chronic obstructive pulmonary disease and asthma, and to improve adherence to treatment and medication, but evidence that this translates into cost savings is more equivocal.

* Self-management programmes can support people to recognise and develop their own strengths and abilities to enable them to live an independent and fulfilling life.

SOURCE: BASED ON NAYLOR ET AL. (2015) AND HEALTH FOUNDATION (2015).

—— Electronic records ——

An electronic health record (EHR) is a computerised health information system where providers record detailed encounter information such as patient demographics, encounter summaries, medical history, allergies, intolerances and lab test histories (Ludwick and Doucette, 2009).

The arrival of the electronic patient record, more than 20 years ago, has delivered enormous benefits, both to clinical practice and research. Despite an increasing quantity of data about patients, few clinicians outside general practice have access to that data in real time and little progress has been made in developing an accessible decision-support system to supplement professional skills. In addition, we need patient records to be mobile, editable and accessible to all those in the care process, including patients themselves and carers.

As is also noted: 'Digital records must support the delivery of care in the community as much as in the hospital – their mobility, extensibility and interoperability is fundamental' (NHS Information Board, 2014, p.27).

It is well documented that paper records often cannot effectively support modern care services. Access may be inefficient or difficult, and data may be inaccurate, illegible, incomplete or out-of-date. In addition, the task of recording arguably takes nursing staff away from their core duty of providing direct care to patients (Yu et al., 2013). Digital care records provide the ability to capture and synthesise insights about a patient's health status produced, for example, by observation, vital signs monitoring and diagnostic testing. This remarkable innovation is indeed a bold vision – as outlined in the National Information Board's 'Personalised Health and Care 2020: Using Data and Technology to Transform Outcomes for Patients and Citizens. A Framework for Action' (2014).

The experience from a number of jurisdictions is that to meet the needs of person-centred care, improve record management, comply with health regulations and support efficient information exchange between health care providers for multidisciplinary collaboration throughout the continuum of care, EHRs are essential in various health care settings to replace paper-based records (Otieno et al., 2008).

Table 11.1 summarises the benefits of EHRs.

Table 11.1: Primary and secondary uses of an electronic health record

Primary uses	Secondary uses
Patient care delivery	Education
Patient care management	Regulation
Patient care support processes	Research
Financial and other administrative processes	Public health and security
Patient self-management	Policy support

Source: adapted from Institute of Medicine (1997).

Those living with complex mental health problems expect high-quality, personalised care coordinated around their individual circumstances. NHS electronic programmes tend not to progress as predicted because they are complex and unpredictable. However, policymakers often persist in thinking that things will soon improve (Greenhalgh et al., 2011).

There is the exciting possibility that records could be harmonised through the integrated health and care records. This would help enormously as 'everyone' could then see whether the blood tests of a resident were 'going off' or 'improving', if the resident found themselves in or out of an acute hospital.

Note that caution should be exercised.

> However, the creation and adoption of integrated digital care records is not an end in itself. It is the backbone upon which increased transparency and participation in our health and care system depend. Having access to the right information at the right time enables excellence. It helps professionals document handovers accurately and makes it easier to share information quickly across multidisciplinary teams and with other providers. (NHS England, 2014b, p.6)

Collaborative care models are team-based, multicomponent interventions to enact system-level medical care delivery, with the goal of improving patient-centred care and providing a pragmatic strategy to deliver integrated health and medical care to patients and families (Galvin, Valois and Zweig, 2014). Trained transdisciplinary care teams deliver care to patients and carers and interface with primary care providers, using comprehensive assessment tools to measure and monitor patient and carer biopsychosocial needs and response to interventions (Towne et al., 2015). However, according to a recent King's Fund reporting *A Digital NHS? An Introduction to the Digital Agenda and Plans for Implementation*, the starting point is that digital technology has the potential to transform the way patients engage with services, improve the efficiency and coordination of care, and support people to manage their health and wellbeing. However, there is a risk that expectations in the high-level vision and goals for digitising the NHS have been set too high (Honeyman, Dunn and McKenna, 2016).

The successful implementation of EHRs would potentially provide a systematic approach to gather and maintain health information and improve the quality and continuity of communication between providers (i.e. physicians, nurses, pharmacies and staff) within and between levels of care (Kuperman, 2011). Such interoperability (e.g. the ability to exchange and interpret shared data) is especially critical for vulnerable or at-risk populations using long-term care who are often involved in complex, interdisciplinary cases and experience frequent transitions (Coleman, 2003). Exchanging electronic health information could improve the quality and efficiency of long-term care by reducing errors and the duplication of health care services. It could also improve the coordination of care between RACFs and other primary care facilities (Brailer, 2005). The evolution and adoption of a comprehensive set of technology and data standards would support interoperability, lower the barriers to innovation and contribute to burden reduction across the care system. With an ageing population's growing demands for health care, RACFs in the US are increasingly expected to provide innovative health care and professional services to improve service quality and gain a competitive advantage on the market (Bhuyan et al., 2014). Introducing EHR systems in RACFs could also cause the adverse effects of: EHR avoidance, access difficulties, increased complexity in information management, an increased documentation burden, a reduction in communication and a lack of follow-up of care (Yu et al., 2013).

Although surveys have consistently shown that health care providers are generally positive about EHRs, there are concerns, such as privacy and security, workflow changes, distractions from direct patient care and other unintended consequences. EHR systems can also result in lower stakeholder 'buy-in', leading to potential rejection of the system (Kirkendall et al., 2013). Despite extensive ethical and technical analyses, concerns still exist, because making health information accessible to and usable by a wide range of health professionals, researchers and planners often conflicts with notions of patient confidentiality and autonomy (Papoutsi et al., 2015). Finally, with patients' prior consent, EHRs can be useful for health research purposes and for policy decisions (if managed appropriately and if the security of data is assured) (European Commission, 2013).

A good example of sharing health and care information in care planning can be found within the model dubbed 'Connecting Care – Wakefield District'. This is a new model of care designed to address social isolation and a shift from fragmented to connected care. The designers will develop a comprehensive approach to proactive assessment and care planning based on the wider determinants of health and life experience.[6] An interesting feature consists of shared records between health and social care organisations.

—— Enablement/reablement ——————

The UK uses the terms **enablement** and **reablement** to describe short-term services with a restorative focus, developed by local authorities with responsibility for adult social care services, as part of their range of home care service provision (Lewin, Alfonso and Alan, 2013). These services are designed to promote personhood, steering integrated dementia policy away from a dependence on the biomedical (neuropsychopharmacological) model.

---

6   See www.connectingcarewakefield.org (accessed 4 Oct 2016).

These services delivered by trained professionals have also been found to be cost-effective (Glendinning et al., 2010). Many people with ill-health, frailty or disability need assistance with personal hygiene, toileting, dressing or feeding to maintain their health and safety at home. In the UK, the provision of adult social care/personal care services is the responsibility of local government (authority) adult care services. Enablement/reablement represents a shift from reactive home care services, to preventive and proactive models of home care service provision based on early intervention and active engagement in reablement (Legg et al., 2015).

As an example, Steeman and colleagues (2006) found that consistent care and follow-up reablement services are essential to live well with dementia. They suggested that care should be proactive and involve people close to the person with dementia so that they have someone to go through the adjustment process with.

—— Sensory considerations in enablement ——

In the real world, you can't enjoy aromatherapy if you have problems with your sense of smell, and you can't enjoy music if you have a hearing impairment, aside from any cognitive problem you may have. A right to **sensory health** is therefore imperative for living better in the community. As cognitive function deteriorates, the world is experienced at a sensory level, with a reduced ability to integrate the sensory experiences to understand the context. There is a paucity of literature on care practice for people with dementia and concurrent visual impairment. What is known, however, is that people with dementia are more likely to require assistance performing activities of daily living and to be in contact with social services (Darba, Kaskens and Lacey, 2015). Similarly, it is known that people with visual impairment often have greater dependency on others due to difficulties with mobility and activities of daily living (Burmedi et al., 2002; Desrosiers et al., 2009).

Impairments in hearing and vision are well-known risk factors for social withdrawal and depression (Haanes et al., 2014). Thus, people with dementia are very sensitive to sensory experiences, and their environment needs to be managed carefully to make it understandable, comfortable and (if possible) therapeutic (Behrman, Chouliaras and Ebmeier, 2014). Hearing aids may reduce the risk of sensory deprivation and have been shown to be acceptable to patients with dementia and their carers (Cohen-Mansfield and Infeld, 2006).

In particular, people with posterior cortical atrophy often have healthy eyes but have sight loss because the area of the brain that interprets visual images has been affected (Crutch et al., 2011). There is thus a need to ascertain the social care and support needs of people with both dementia and visual impairment (Nyman, Innes and Heward, 2016). Health services should take a joined-up approach to the assessment, diagnosis and management of dementia for people with hearing loss and deaf people who use British Sign Language (BSL). The Action on Hearing Loss/ ESRC Deafness, Cognition and Language Resource Centre (2013) estimated that at least £28 million per year could be saved in England by properly managing hearing loss in people with dementia, and thus delaying their admission to residential care. This is calculated by offsetting the cost of community-based provisions for people with severe dementia against the cost of residential care, which would be avoided. Likewise the Quality Standard for people with sight loss and dementia in an ophthalmology department (Royal College of Ophthalmologists, 2015) provides useful statements about what good-quality care should look like (see Box 11.3).

Box 11.3: Quality Standards statements

* **Quality Statement 1.** People with sight loss and dementia receive care from health care professionals appropriately trained in sight loss and dementia.

* **Quality Statement 2.** People with sight loss and dementia, and their carers, are provided with accessible information and the support they require to participate in decisions about their care.

* **Quality Statement 3.** People with sight loss and dementia, and their carers, can safely and effectively attend ophthalmology appointments.

* **Quality Statement 4.** People with sight loss and dementia have a shorter wait in clinic and a longer appointment.

* **Quality Statement 5.** People with sight loss and dementia, and their carers, receive accessible information about vision and eye health.

* **Quality Statement 6.** When people with sight loss and dementia cannot perform a standard vision test, a functional vision assessment is used.

* **Quality Statement 7.** People with sight loss and dementia are referred to local support services via agreed pathways.

SOURCE: ROYAL COLLEGE OF OPHTHALMOLOGISTS (2015). REPRODUCED BY KIND PERMISSION OF THE ROYAL COLLEGE OF OPHTHALMOLOGISTS, WITHOUT ADAPTATION.

A research team carried out a series of case studies (Thomas Pocklington Trust, 2008). This team's remarkable conclusion was that sight loss professionals felt they were not equipped to work with people who had mental health needs, while dementia professionals felt the needs created by sight loss risked being overlooked in mental health services. Increased coordination between mental health and sensory impairment teams would help identify individuals' abilities and needs for support.

—— Support groups ——

A scarcity of public resources means that value for money for interventions for people with dementia requires closer scrutiny (Knapp, Iemmi and Romeo, 2013). People with dementia and their carers say that peer support groups are important as they provide opportunities to speak to other people in a similar situation and provide social interaction.

Peer support groups are organised so that small groups of people who have been similarly affected by dementia can meet and support each other by sharing their experiences and thoughts. Peer support groups can be for people who have recently been diagnosed with dementia (British Psychological Society, 2014).

As the number of people with dementia increases, so too will the number of experienced carers willing to volunteer to support others (Charlesworth et al., 2016). Studies suggest that peer support may lead to direct health care savings by equipping people with coping mechanisms and providing emotional support. This can lessen the risk of crises and potentially avoidable and expensive interventions by the statutory sector. Traditionally, cost-effectiveness and cost–benefit analyses have been used to assess the value for money of health and social care interventions (Willis, Semple and de Waal, 2016).

Meta-analysis studies of specific types of support groups are limited but desperately needed for arguments based on the social return of investment and social value. Some time ago, Chien and colleagues (2011) conducted a review and assessment of the effectiveness of support groups for carers of persons with dementia and examined the impact of support group characteristics. The authors concluded as follows:

> Support groups benefit caregivers and findings of this meta-analysis serve as immediate guidance for group facilitators. Future research should include additional outcome variables with our defined factors on effectiveness collected as demographic characteristic data for comparison. A more comprehensive understanding of the effectiveness of support groups is indicated to enhance outcomes for caregivers and patients. (p.1089)

Tommy Whitelaw from Glasgow was a full-time carer for his mother who had vascular dementia; she died in 2012. Tommy has become a successful campaigner raising awareness of the issues surrounding dementia. He continues to speak to carers' groups, as well as key decision-makers who have influence over the lives of people affected by dementia.[7] Dementia Carer Voices, managed by the Health and Social Care Alliance Scotland (the ALLIANCE), is a Scottish Government-funded project to engage with health and social care professionals and students to promote

---

7   See www.nhsggc.org.uk/about-us/professional-support-sites/dementia-shared-practice/experiences-of-dementia/tommy-whitelaw (accessed 4 Oct 2016).

a fuller understanding of the carer journey, provide a platform where carers can express their views and experiences of caring for a loved one with dementia, and harness the awareness-raising undertaken by Tommy.

Essential reading

Sanderson H, Bailey G. 2013. *Personalisation and Dementia: A Guide for Person-Centred Practice*, London: Jessica Kingsley Publishers.

Sanderson H, Bailey G (with Martin L). 2014. *Making Individual Service Funds Work for People with Dementia Living in Care Homes: How It Works In Practice*, London: Jessica Kingsley Publishers.

Ambient assisted living

Rahman S. 2014. *Living Well with Dementia*, London: CRC Press. Chapter 15, Ambient Assisted Living and the Innovation Culture, pp.253–268.

Assistive technology

Rahman S. 2014. *Living Well with Dementia*, London: CRC Press. Chapter 14, Assistive Technology and Living Well with Dementia, pp.233–252.

References

Action on Hearing Loss/ESRC Deafness, Cognition and Language Resource Centre. 2013. *Why People with Hearing Loss or Deafness Would Benefit from an Integrated Response to Long-Term Conditions*, available at www.ucl.ac.uk/dcal/documents/Joining_Up_long_term_conditions_report.pdf (accessed 2 Oct 2016).

Archer N, Keshavjee K, Demers C, Lee R. 2014. Online self-management interventions for chronically ill patients: cognitive impairment and technology issues. Int J Med Inform, 83(4), 264–272.

Baltes MM. 1988. The etiology and maintenance of dependence in the elderly: three phases of operant research. Behav. Ther, 19, 301–319.

Barlow J, Wright C, Sheasby J, Turner A, Hainsworth J. 2002. Self-management approaches for people with chronic conditions: a review. Patient Education & Counselling, 48, 177–187.

Bauer DC, Gaff C, Dinger ME, Caramins M, et al. 2014. Genomics and personalised whole-of-life health care. Trends Mol Med, 20(9), 479–486.

Behrman S, Chouliaras L, Ebmeier KP. 2014. Considering the senses in the diagnosis and management of dementia. Maturitas, 77(4), 305–310.

Besser AG, Sanderson SC, Roberts JS, Chen CA, et al. 2015. Factors affecting recall of different types of personal genetic information about Alzheimer's disease risk: the REVEAL study. Public Health Genomics, 18(2), 78–86.

Bhuyan SS, Zhu H, Chandak A, Kim J, Stimpson JP. 2014. Do service innovations influence the adoption of electronic health records in long-term care organizations? Results from the U.S. National Survey of Residential Care Facilities. Int J Med Inform, 83(12), 975–982.

Boyd HC, Evans NM, Orpwood RD, Harris ND. 2015. Using simple technology to prompt multistep tasks in the home for people with dementia: an exploratory study comparing prompting formats. Dementia (London), September, 1471301215602417 (e-pub ahead of print).

Brailer DJ. 2005. Interoperability: the key to the future health care system. Health Aff (Millwood), Suppl Web Exclusives: W5–19/W5–21.

Brignell M, Wootton R, Gray L. 2007. The application of telemedicine to geriatric medicine. Age Ageing, 36, 369–374.

British Psychological Society (Division of Clinical Psychology). 2014. *A Guide to Psychosocial Interventions in Early Stages of Dementia*, London: BSP.

Bunnik EM, Janssens AC, Schermer MH. 2015. Personal utility in genomic testing: is there such a thing? J Med Ethics, 41(4), 322–326.

Burmedi D, Becker S, Heyl V, Wahl HW, Himmelsbach I. 2002. Behavioral consequences of age-related low vision. Visual Impairment Research, 4, 15–45.

Chapman JL, Zechel A, Carter YH, Abbott S. 2004. Systematic review of recent innovations in service provision to improve access to primary care. Br J Gen Pract, 54(502), 374–381.

Charlesworth G, Sinclair JB, Brooks A, Sullivan T, Ahmad S, Poland F. 2016. The impact of volunteering on the volunteer: findings from a peer support programme for family carers of people with dementia. Health Soc Care Community, doi: 10.1111/hsc.12341.

Chien LY, Chu H, Guo JL, Liao YM, et al. 2011. Caregiver support groups in patients with dementia: a meta-analysis. Int J Geriatr Psychiatry, 26(10), 1089–1098.

Clare L. 2002. Developing awareness about awareness in early stage dementia: the role of psychosocial factors. Dementia, 1(3), 295–312.

Clay H, Stern R. 2015. *Making time in general practice: Freeing GP capacity by reducing bureaucracy and avoidable consultations, managing the interface with hospitals and exploring new ways of working*, London: Primary Care Foundation and NHS Alliance, available at http://www.nhsalliance.org/wp-content/uploads/2015/10/Making-Time-in-General-Practice-FULL-REPORT-01-10-15.pdf (accessed 29 Nov 2016).

Cohen-Mansfield J, Infeld DL. 2006. Hearing aids for nursing home residents: current policy and future needs. Health Policy, 79, 49–56.

Coleman EA. 2003. Falling through the cracks: challenges and opportunities for improving transitional care for persons with continuous complex care needs. J Am Geriatr Soc, 51(4), 549–555.

Cowan D, Turner-Smith A. 1999. The Role of Assistive Technology in Alternative Models of Care for Older People. In A. Tinker et al. (eds), *Royal Commission on Long-Term Care (Research Volume 2)*, London: The Stationery Office.

Cowling TE, Harris M, Watt H, Soljak M, et al. 2016. Access to primary care and the route of emergency admission to hospital: retrospective analysis of national hospital administrative data. BMJ Qual Saf, August, bmjqs-2015-004338, doi:10.1136/bmjqs-2015-004338 (e-pub ahead of print).

Crutch SJ, Lehmann M, Gorgoraptis N, Kaski D, et al. 2011. Abnormal visual phenomena in posterior cortical atrophy. Neurocase, 17(2), 160–177.

Darba J, Kaskens L, Lacey L. 2015. Relationship between global severity of patients with Alzheimer's disease and costs of care in Spain: results from the co-dependence study in Spain. European Journal of Health Economics, 16(8), 895–905.

Dawson A. 2014. Information, choice and the ends of health promotion. Monash Bioeth Rev, 32(1–2), 106–120.

De Rouck S, Jacobs A, Leys M. 2008. A methodology for shifting the focus of e-health support design onto user needs: a case in the homecare field. Int J Med Inform, 77(9):589–601.

De Silva D. 2011. *Helping People Help Themselves: A Review of the Evidence Considering Whether It Is Worthwhile to Support Self-Management*, London: The Health Foundation.

Deloitte. 2015. *Connected Health: How Digital Technology Is Transforming Health and Social Care*, London: Deloitte.

Department of Health. 2006. Our Health, Our Care, Our Say: A New Direction for Community Services, available at www.gov.uk/government/uploads/system/uploads/attachment_data/file/272238/6737.pdf (accessed 3 Oct 2016).

Department of Health. 2009. *Living Well with Dementia: A National Dementia Strategy*, London: Department of Health, available at www.gov.uk/government/uploads/system/uploads/attachment_data/file/168220/dh_094051.pdf (accessed 3 Oct 2016).

Desrosiers J, Wanet-Defalque MC, Témisjian K, Gresset J, et al. 2009. Participation in daily activities and social roles of older adults with visual impairment. Disabil Rehabil, 31(15), 1227–1234.

Dimitrov DV. 2016. Medical internet of things and big data in healthcare. Healthc Inform Res, 22(3), 156–163.

Draper DA, Hurley RE, Lesser CS, Strunk BC. 2002. The changing face of managed care. Health Affairs, 21, 11–23.

European Commission. 2013. Patient access to Electronic Health Records. Report of the eHealth Stakeholder Group, June 2013, available at https://ec.europa.eu/digital-single-market/en/news/commission-publishes-four-reports-ehealth-stakeholder-group (accessed 29 Nov 2016).

Fisk MJ. 2003. *Social Alarms to Telecare: Older People's Services in Transition*, London: The Policy Press.

Fuhrer MJ. 2001. Assistive technology outcomes research: challenges met and yet unmet. Am. J. Phys. Med. Rehabil, 80, 528–535.

Galvin JE, Valois L, Zweig Y. 2014. Collaborative transdisciplinary team approach for dementia care. Neurodegener Dis Manag, 4(6), 455–469.

Georgeton E, Aubert L, Pierrard N, Gaborieau G, Berrut G, de Decker L. 2015. General practitioners adherence to recommendations from geriatric assessments made during teleconsultations for the elderly living in nursing homes. Maturitas, 82(2), 184–189.

Genio. 2016. Community Supports Model for People with Dementia, available at www.genio.ie/system/files/publications/GENIO_DEMENTIA_PROGRAMME_2015.pdf (accessed 25 Sept 2016).

Gibson G, Dickinson C, Brittain K, Robinson L. 2015. The everyday use of assistive technology by people with dementia and their family carers: a qualitative study. BMC Geriatr, 15, 89.

Giebel C, Challis D. 2015. Translating cognitive and everyday activity deficits into cognitive interventions in mild dementia and mild cognitive impairment. International Journal of Geriatric Psychiatry, 30(1), 21–31.

Glendinning C, Jones K, Baxter K, Rabiee P, et al. 2010. *Home Care Re-Ablement Services: Investigating the Longer-Term Impacts (Prospective Longitudinal Study)*, York: Social Policy Research Unit, available at www.york.ac.uk/inst/spru/research/pdf/Reablement.pdf (accessed 23 Sept 2016).

Greenhalgh T, Procter R, Wherton J, Sugarhood P, Hinder S, Rouncefield M. 2015. What is quality in assisted living technology? The ARCHIE framework for effective telehealth and telecare services. BMC Med, 13, 91.

Greenhalgh T, Russell J, Ashcroft RE, Parsons W. 2011. Why national eHealth programmes need dead philosophers: Wittgensteinian reflections on policymakers' reluctance to learn from history. Milbank, 89(4), 533–563.

Haanes GG, Kirkevold M, Horgen G, Hofoss D, Eilertsen G. 2014. Sensory impairments in community health care: a descriptive study of hearing and vision among elderly Norwegians living at home. J Multidiscip Healthc, 7, 217–225.

Health Foundation. 2014. *Improving Quality in General Practice (No. 23), London:* Health Foundation.

Health Foundation. 2015. *Quick Guide: A Practical Guide to Self-Management Support: Key Components for Successful Implementation.* London: Health Foundation.

Honeyman M, Dunn P, McKenna H. 2016. *A Digital NHS? An Introduction to the Digital Agenda and Plans for Implementation*, London: King's Fund.

Institute of Medicine. 1997. *The Computer-Based Patient Record: An Essential Technology for Health Care* (revised edition), eds. RS Dick, EB Steen and DE Detmer, Washington, DC: National Academy Press.

Ipsos MORI/Social Research Institute. 2016. *Dementia Advisers' Survey,* available at www.gov.uk/government/uploads/system/uploads/attachment_data/file/513191/Dementia_Advisers_Full_Report.pdf (accessed 3 Oct 2016).

Jutai JW, Fuhrer MJ, Demers L, Scherer MJ, DeRuyter F. 2005. Towards a taxonomy of assistive technology device outcomes. Am J Phys Med Rehabil, 84(4), 294–302.

Kelly F, Innes A. 2014. Facilitating independence: the benefits of a post-diagnostic support project for people with dementia. Dementia (London), 17.

Kerssens C, Kumar R, Adams AE, Knott CC, et al. 2015. Personalized technology to support older adults with and without cognitive impairment living at home. Am J Alzheimers Dis Other Demen, 30(1), 85–97.

Khosravi P, Ghapanchi AH. 2016. Investigating the effectiveness of technologies applied to assist seniors: a systematic literature review. Int J Med Inform, 85(1), 17–26.

Kirkendall ES, Goldenhar LM, Simon JL, Wheeler DS, Andrew Spooner S. 2013. Transitioning from a computerized provider order entry and paper documentation system to an electronic health record: expectations and experiences of hospital staff. Int J Med Inform, 82(11), 1037–1045.

Knapp M, Black N, Dixon J, Damant J, Rehill A, Tan S. 2014. *Independent Assessment of Improvements in Dementia Care and Support since 2009*, London: PIRU.

Knapp M, Iemmi V, Romeo R. 2013. Dementia care costs and outcomes: a systematic review. Int J Geriatr Psychiatry, 28(6), 551–561.

Kuperman GJ. 2011. Health-information exchange: why are we doing it, and what are we doing? J Am Med Inform Assoc, 18(5), 678–682.

La Fontaine J, Brooker D, Bray K, Milosevic SK. 2011. *A Local Evaluation of Dementia Advisers, Worcester:* University of Worcester, available at www.worcester.ac.uk/documents/Dementia_Adviser_Service_Final_Report.pdf (accessed 3 Oct 2016).

Lancioni GE, Singh NN, O'Reilly MF, Sigafoos J, et al. 2014. Persons with moderate Alzheimer's disease use simple technology aids to manage daily activities and leisure occupation. Res Dev Disabil, 35(9), 2117–2128.

Lawler M, Sullivan R. 2015. Personalised and precision medicine in cancer clinical trials: panacea for progress or Pandora's Box? Public Health Genomics, 18(6), 329–337.

Legg L, Gladman J, Drummond A, Davidson A. 2015. A systematic review of the evidence on home care reablement services. Clin Rehabil, September, 0269215515603220 (e-pub ahead of print).

Lewin GF, Alfonso HS, Alan JJ. 2013. Evidence for the long-term cost-effectiveness of home care reablement programmes. Clin Interv Aging, 8, 1273–1281.

Lorig KR, Holman H. 2003. Self-management education: history, definition, outcomes, and mechanisms. Ann Behav Med, 26(1), 1–7.

Lorig KR, Mazonson PD, Holman HR. 1993. Evidence suggesting that health education for self-management in patients with chronic arthritis has sustained health benefits while reducing health care costs. Arthritis Rheum, 36, 439–446.

Lorig KR, Ritter PL, Laurent DD, Plant K. 2006. Internet-based chronic disease self-management: a randomized trial. Med Care, 44(11), 964–971.

Ludwick DA, Doucette J. 2009. Adopting electronic medical records in primary care: lessons learned from health information systems implementation experience in seven countries. Int J Med Inform, 78(1), 22–31.

Main T, Slywotzky A. 2014. *Oliver Wyman Report: The Patient-to-Consumer Revolution: How High Tech, Transparent Marketplaces and Consumer Power are Transforming U.S. Health Care*, available at www.oliverwyman.com/content/dam/oliver-wyman/global/en/images/insights/health-life-sciences/2014/October/The-Patient-To-Consumer-Revolution.pdf (accessed 3 Oct 2016).

McKinsey. 2010. *mHealth: A New Vision for Healthcare*, available at www.gsma.com/connectedliving/wp-content/uploads/2012/03/gsmamckinseymhealthreport.pdf (accessed 3 Oct 2016).

Mei YY, Marquard J, Jacelon C, DeFeo AL. 2013. Designing and evaluating an electronic patient falls reporting system: perspectives for the implementation of health information technology in long-term residential care facilities. Int J Med Inform, 82(11), e294–306.

Miesen, BML, Blom, M. 2001. The Alzheimer Café: A guideline manual for setting one up. Translated and adapted from the Dutch Alzheimer's Society document by GMM Jones, available at www.alzheimercafe.co.uk/media/ACIntroductory%20PackACUKJan2014.pdf (accessed 29 Nov 2016).

Monitor. 2015. Improving GP Services: Commissioners and Patient Choice, available at www.gov.uk/government/uploads/system/uploads/attachment_data/file/431317/GP_services.pdf (accessed 3 Oct 2016).

Moniz-Cook E, De Lepeleire J, Vernooij-Dassen M. 2004. Chronic disease management – what can be learned from dementia management? British Medical Journal, 328(7453) 1396-d.

Moniz-Cook E, Vernooij-Dassen M, Woods B, Orrell M, et al. 2011. Psychosocial interventions in dementia care research: the INTERDEM manifesto. Aging & Mental Health, 15(3), 283–290.

Naylor C, Imison C, Aldicott R, Buck D, et al. 2015. *Transforming Our Health Care System – Ten Priorities for Commissioners* (revised edition), London: King's Fund.

NHS England. 2013. *Improving Health and Patient Care through Community Pharmacy – Evidence Resource Pack*, London: NHS.

NHS England. 2014a. Integrated Care Commissioning Prospectus: Making a Reality of Health and Social Care Integration for Individuals, available at https://www.england.nhs.uk/wp-content/uploads/2014/09/item4a-board-0914.pdf (accessed 3 Oct 2016).

NHS England. 2014b. The Integrated Care Fund: Achieving Integrated Health and Care Records, available at www.england.nhs.uk/wp-content/uploads/2014/05/idcr.pdf (accessed 3 Oct 2016).

NHS England. 2016. Integrated Personal Commissioning: Emerging Framework, available at www.england.nhs.uk/healthbudgets/wp-content/uploads/sites/26/2016/05/ipc-emerging-framework.pdf (accessed 3 Oct 2016).

NHS Information Board. 2014. Personalised Health and Care 2020: Using Data and Technology to Transform Outcomes for Patients and Citizens. A Framework for Action, available at www.gov.uk/government/uploads/system/uploads/attachment_data/file/384650/NIB_Report.pdf (accessed 3 Oct 2016).

NHS Practice Management Network. 2009. Improving Access, Responding to Patients: A 'How-To' Guide for GP Practices.

Nishimura M, Satoh M, Matsushita K, Nomura F. 2014. How proteomic ApoE serotyping could impact Alzheimer's disease risk assessment: genetic testing by proteomics. Expert Rev Proteomics, 11(4), 405–407.

Nyman SR, Innes A, Heward M. 2016. Social care and support needs of community-dwelling people with dementia and concurrent visual impairment. Aging Ment Health, May, 1–7 (e-pub ahead of print).

O'Connor D, Purves B (eds). 2009. *Decision-Making: Personhood and Dementia – Exploring the Interface*, London: Jessica Kingsley Publishers.

Or CKL, Karsh B. 2009. A systematic review of patient acceptance of consumer health information technology, J.Am. Med. Inform. Assoc, 16(4), 550–560.

Organisation for Economic Co-operation and Development. 2014. Reviews of Health Care Quality, available at www.oecd-ilibrary.org/social-issues-migration-health/oecd-reviews-of-health-care-quality_22270485T (accessed 29 Nov 2016).

Otieno GO, Hinako T, Motohiro A, Daisuke K, Neiko N. 2008. Measuring effectiveness of electronic medical records systems: towards building a composite index for benchmarking hospitals, Int. J. Med. Inform, 77(10), 657–669.

Papoutsi C, Reed JE, Marston C, Lewis R, Majeed A, Bell D. 2015. Patient and public views about the security and privacy of Electronic Health Records (EHRs) in the UK: results from a mixed methods study. BMC Med Inform Decis Mak, 15, 86.

Phg Foundation. 2012. *Genomics in Medicine*, available at www.phgfoundation.org/file/12095 (accessed 3 Oct 2016).

Quinn C, Anderson D, Toms G, Whitaker R, et al. 2014. Self-management in early-stage dementia: a pilot randomised controlled trial of the efficacy and cost-effectiveness of a self-management group intervention (the SMART study). Trials, 15, 74.

Quinn C, Toms G, Anderson D, Clare L. 2015. A Review of Self-Management Interventions for People With Dementia and Mild Cognitive Impairment. J Appl Gerontol, pii: 0733464814566852.

Royal College of Ophthalmologists. 2015. Quality Standard for People with Sight Loss and Dementia in an Ophthalmology Department, available at www.rcophth.ac.uk/wp-content/uploads/2016/01/Quality-standard-for-people-with-sight-loss-and-dementia-in-an-ophthalmology-department.pdf (accessed 3 Oct 2016).

Schommer JC, Doucette WR, Planas LG. 2015. Establishing pathways for access to pharmacist-provided patient care. J Am Pharm Assoc, 55(6), 664–668.

SCIE. 2013. *Personalisation: A Rough Guide*, available at www.scie.org.uk/publications/guides/guide47/files/guide47.pdf (accessed 3 Oct 2016).

Shmanske S. 1996. Information asymmetries in health services – the market can cope. The Independent Review, I, 2.

Simpson G, Kenrick M. 1997. Nurses' attitudes towards computerization in clinical practice in a British general hospital, Comput. Nurs, 15(1), 37–42.

Singh K, Drouin K, Newmark LP, Rozenblum R, et al. 2016. Developing a Framework for Evaluating the Patient Engagement, Quality, and Safety of Mobile Health Applications Commonwealth Fund, available at www.commonwealthfund.org/publications/issue-briefs/2016/feb/evaluating-mobile-health-apps (accessed 3 Oct 2016).

Sood S, Mbarika V, Jugoo S, Dookhy R, et al. 2007. What is telemedicine? A collection of 104 peer-reviewed perspectives and theoretical underpinnings. Telemed J E Health, 13(5), 573–590.

Steeman E, de Casterlé BD, Godderis J, Grypdonck M. 2006. Living with early-stage dementia: a review of qualitative studies. J Adv Nurs, 54(6), 722–738.

Stokes J, Checkland K, Kristensen SR. 2016. Integrated care: theory to practice. J Health Serv Res Policy, July, 1355819616660581 (e-pub ahead of print).

Thomas Pocklington Trust. 2008. *The Experiences and Needs of People with Dementia and Serious Visual Impairment: A Qualitative Study*. London: Thomas Pocklington Trust.

Toms G, Quinn C, Anderson DE, Clare LX. 2015. Help yourself: perspectives on self-management from people with dementia and their caregivers. Qual Health Res, 25(1), 87–98.

Towne SD Jr, Lee S, Li Y, Smith ML. 2015. Assessment of eHealth capabilities and utilization in residential care settings. Health Informatics J, October, 1460458215610895 (e-pub ahead of print).

Vermeulen E, Henneman L, van El CG, Cornel MC. 2014. Public attitudes towards preventive genomics and personal interest in genetic testing to prevent disease: a survey study. Eur J Public Health, 24(5), 768–775.

Weingarten SR, Henning JM, Badamgarav E, Knight K, et al. 2002. Interventions used in disease management programmes for patients with chronic illness-which ones work? Meta-analysis of published reports. BMJ, 325(7370), 925.

Willis E, Semple AC, de Waal H. 2016. Quantifying the benefits of peer support for people with dementia: A Social Return on Investment (SROI) study. Dementia (London), pii: 1471301216640184.

Woods B. 1999. Promoting well-being and independence for people with dementia. Int J Geriatr Psychiatry, 14(2), 97–105.

Yu P, Qian S, Yu H, Lei J. 2013. Measuring the performance of electronic health records: a case study in residential aged care in Australia. Stud Health Technol Inform, 192, 1035.

Zhou Y, Abel G, Warren F, Roland M, Campbell J, Lyratzopoulos G. 2015. Do difficulties in accessing in-hours primary care predict higher use of out-of-hours GP services? Evidence from an English National Patient Survey. Emerg Med J, 32(5), 373–378.

Chapter 12

DYING WELL

Learning objectives

By the end of this chapter, you will be able to:

» explain the palliative approach, and describe the Gold Standards Framework

» describe the importance of end-of-life care in dementia, including burdensome symptoms, for residential settings and primary care, and barriers to good end-of-life care

» describe anticipatory grief, carer grief or pre-grief

» discuss the case for viewing dementia 'as a terminal illness'

» explain hospices as a great innovation in care

» explain contemporary issues surrounding advance care planning

» discuss principles of pain control in palliative care for people with dementia

» contribute to the design and discussion of palliative and end-of-life care services for people living with dementia

Introduction

A good death is important.

The median length of stay of care home residents before they die has been found to be just under two years (Forder and Fernandez, 2011), but prognostication difficulties in dementia mean that it is difficult to recognise when someone is actually dying (Goodman et al., 2010; van der Steen et al., 2011); increasing longevity means that in advanced industrial societies twice as many people now die with multiple morbidities, frailty and/or dementia at the end of a long life than die of the cancers on which the expertise of palliative care is historically based (Lynn and Adamson, 2003). Although an older person may die *with* dementia, he or she may die *from* another medical condition, for example cancer or heart disease, or as a result of the interplay between another illness and dementia (Cox and Cook, 2002). Variation in the place of death can partly be explained by the way different diseases progress. For cancer, the disease trajectory can be relatively predictable, with patients tending to experience a period of relatively rapid decline at the end of life, whereas dementia has a more gradual deterioration (Lynn and Adamson, 2003). In particular, there is much evidence that people with advanced dementia receive inadequate treatment in some ways (e.g. insufficient pain relief), while also being subject to rather burdensome investigations and treatments in other ways (e.g. hospitalisation which serves no useful purpose) (Hughes et al., 2007).

In a recent nationwide after-death survey, surviving families expressed more dissatisfaction with the NHS than with other sites of care. Poor-quality communication was found to be a barrier to making difficult choices about care for their loved ones with advanced dementia, including resuscitation, hospital transfer, feeding options and treatment of infection (for a review see Einterz et al., 2014).

The Parliamentary ombudsman recently reported on features which constituted a poor death (see Box 12.1).

Box 12.1: Key themes of 'Dying without Dignity'

Key themes are:

1. Not recognising that people are dying, and not responding to their needs.

    If the needs of those who are close to death are not recognised, their care cannot be planned or coordinated, which means more crises and distress for the person and their family and carers.

2. Poor symptom control

    People have watched their loved ones dying in pain or in an agitated state because their symptoms have been ineffectively or poorly managed.

3. Poor communication

    Poor communication is an important element in our complaints about end-of-life care. It is clear that health care professionals do not always have the open and honest conversations with family members and carers that are necessary for them to understand the severity of the situation, and the subsequent choices they will have to make.

4. Inadequate out-of-hours services

    People who are dying and their carers suffer because of the difficulties in getting palliative care outside normal working hours.

5. Poor care planning

    A failure to plan adequately often leads to the lack of coordinated care; for example, GPs and hospitals can fail to liaise.

6. Delays in diagnosis and referrals for treatment

    This can mean that people are denied the chance to plan for end of life and for their final wishes to be met.

SOURCE: FROM PARLIAMENTARY AND HEALTH SERVICE OMBUDSMAN (2015, PP.2–3).

Experts from different countries, care settings and positions have shared concerns about the difficulties of communication within palliative care, the variable integration of services, the problems of securing sustained funding in different reimbursement systems, the complexities of care itself and the time constraints on providing good-quality care (Davies et al., 2014). The National Bereavement Survey (VOICES) was commissioned by the Department of Health and administered by the Office for National Statistics (ONS). It describes the quality of care delivered in the last three months of life for adults who died in England, including variations between different parts of the country and different groups of patients.

Some take-home points from the National Bereavement Survey are shown in Box 12.2.

Box 12.2: National Bereavement Survey

Some key points:

*   3 out of 4 bereaved people (75%) rate the overall quality of end-of-life care for their relative as outstanding, excellent or good; 1 out of 10 (10%) rated care as poor

*   7 out of 10 bereaved people (69%) whose relative or friend died in a hospital rated care as outstanding, excellent or good; this is significantly lower than outstanding, excellent or good ratings of care for those who died in a hospice (83%), care home (82%) or at home (79%)

*   ratings of fair or poor quality of care are significantly higher for those living in the most deprived areas (30%) compared to the least deprived areas (21%)

*   1 out of 3 respondents (33%) reported that the hospital services did not work well together with GP and other services outside the hospital

*   3 out of 4 bereaved people (75%) agreed that the patient's nutritional needs were met in the last two days of life; 1 out of 8 (13%) responded that the patient did not have enough support to eat or receive nutrition

* more than 5 out of 6 bereaved people (86%) understood the information provided by health care professionals, but 1 out of 6 (16%) disagreed they had time to ask questions with health care professionals

* 7 out of 10 respondents (73%) felt hospital was the right place for the patient to die, despite only 3% of all respondents stating patients wanted to die in hospital.

SOURCE: OFFICE FOR NATIONAL STATISTICS (2015). LICENSED
UNDER THE OPEN GOVERNMENT LICENCE V.3.0.

Why are palliative care and —— end-of-life in dementia important? ——

Jennings (2003) has referred to patients with dementia as the 'hot potato that no one in the health care system really wants to touch' (p.S24), emphasising the lack of attention that such patients receive from multiple health care providers as they approach death. Relatively little is known about the ethical issues surrounding palliative care in the context of late-stage dementia (Rabins, Lyketsos and Steele, 1999). Palliative care for people with dementia poses particular challenges to those providing services, who report a lack of confidence in their skills, a sense of helplessness and a need for training (Dening et al., 2012). Although health care systems and funding structures differ greatly between countries, the philosophy behind and the intention to provide good-quality end-of-life care for people remains relatively consistent (van der Steen et al., 2014).

Consensus has emerged that the quality of palliative care for cancer patients is much better and better organised than for people with dementia (Davies et al., 2014). Differences in the attitudes of countries in identifying the time point of the palliative phase are to be expected, because of different cultures and national regulations for such care. However, even within countries and between services, there are different opinions of the definitions of the palliative phase (van Riet Paap et al., 2015). The challenges of providing palliative and end-of-life care to people with dementia may stem in part from the different time course of the illness compared to cancer, but this may partly be because the needs of those who cannot express their own needs much earlier in the illness are fundamentally less easily met (Treloar, Crugel and Adamis, 2009). The **palliative care approach** should be integral to the management of all non-curative diseases. A good death for people with dementia is of considerable importance still, especially in light of the accumulating evidence that the quality of care for people with advanced dementia is so poor (Hughes, Robinson and Volicer, 2005).

Six ambitions have been suggested for palliative and end-of-life care (see Box 12.3).

Box 12.3: Six ambitions for palliative and end-of-life care

* Ambition One: Each person is seen as an individual

* Ambition Two: Each person gets fair access to care

* Ambition Three: Maximising comfort and wellbeing

* Ambition Four: Care is coordinated

* Ambition Five: All staff are prepared to care

* Ambition Six: Each community is prepared to help

SOURCE: NATIONAL PALLIATIVE AND END-OF-LIFE CARE PARTNERSHIP (2015).

One of the ways to monitor the growth of palliative care worldwide has been the development of a system mapping the development of palliative care on a country-by-country basis (Wright et al., 2008). This report measured palliative care development in all countries of the world and classified them using a four-part typology depicting levels of hospice-palliative care development:

» no known hospice-palliative care activity (group 1 countries)

» capacity-building activity (group 2 countries)

» localised hospice-palliative care provision (group 3 countries)

» countries where hospice-palliative care services were reaching a measure of integration with the mainstream health care system (group 4 countries).

The clinical implication of this is that we need to improve dementia care overall. It is an argument against a semantic overemphasis on timely diagnosis. The care of people with dementia needs to cover the full course of the condition (*palliare* means to cover). Palliative care focuses on improving patients' quality of life by alleviating the symptom burden of life-limiting illnesses (Zahradnik and Grossman, 2014).

Van der Steen and colleagues (2014) have attempted to create clearer boundaries for what we mean by palliative care in dementia. They used a Delphi process to generate a set of core domains and then tested these on a wider international panel of experts. Harris highlighted the relevance of palliative care to dementia – since it is a progressive, life-limiting condition with complex needs – but also recognised that these palliative care needs are poorly addressed for people with dementia (Harris et al., 2013). And post-diagnosis, there may be points of critical symbolic significance, for example as a person passes from 'living well with dementia' to the next stage, which might be regarded as that of inexorable decline (Dening and Dening, 2016). The timing of these needs exploring. The expectation now is good-quality, person-centred dementia care that will include adequate liaison with end-of-life specialists when the time is right (Mahin-Babaeia, Hilal and Hughes, 2016).

The rising prevalence of dementia will also have an impact on acute hospitals. Extra resources will be required for intermediate and palliative care and mental health liaison services (Sampson et al., 2009). Health and social care professionals should ascertain carers' perspectives on the situation of a person with dementia and the carer's wishes (Raymond et al., 2014). Goals of integrated care are person-centred, culturally sensitive approaches to providing care that meet a patient's changing needs and respect their preferences regarding end-of-life care (Arcand, 2015). Goals of care help ensure open and ongoing communication between the patient, the proxy decision-maker, the family and care team so that all parties have a clear, shared understanding of what constitutes optimal care for the individual patient. Towards the end of life, it is usually necessary to give priority to palliative care over potentially burdensome life-prolonging treatment.

Comfort care is doing for people what they would do for themselves if they could. A focus on comfort includes attention to knowing the person and executing care practices that support physical, psychological, social and spiritual needs (Long et al., 2012). These comfort principles incorporate strategies to ensure that pain is assessed and addressed and that meaningful connections are maintained for all activities. The recommended approach in patients with advanced dementia and dysphagia is careful hand-feeding for comfort, emphasising the importance of focusing on the patient's comfort in all interactions around nutrition (Palecek et al., 2010). Families of patients tend to be more satisfied with end-of-life care when a comfort care goal was established shortly after admission than when another goal or no goal was established (van Soest-Poortvliet et al., 2015). Nonetheless, not all families have a clear indication of their relative's wishes, and the medical team may hold views that differ from those of the family (Caron, Arcand and Griffith, 2005).

Professionals in care homes may often have limited experience of palliative care services. Hospital staff have often commented that people with dementia were less likely to receive a palliative care referral, although the value of palliative care input has been readily recognised (Lawrence et al., 2011). Specifically, nursing home residents with advanced dementia often undergo aggressive medical care with limited or no benefits. In a comprehensive review of the literature, Volicer noted many negative outcomes associated with this type of care for nursing home residents with advanced dementia. For example, intercurrent infections are a common and almost inevitable consequence of advanced dementia, but antibiotic therapy does not prolong survival and is unnecessary for symptom control (Volicer, 2005). There is a concern, however, that in long-term care settings care is primarily delivered by staff with limited training in dementia-specific care. In addition, staff may be exposed to highly stressful conditions due to the challenging nature of the caring experience, long work hours and low pay (Long et al., 2012). The length of time given in education and the practical experience of caring for dying individuals are independently associated with positive attitudes towards care for the dying among student nurses (Grubb and Arthur, 2016). International experts have now selected a set of 23 quality indicators for the organisation of palliative care that can be implemented in daily practice in order to demonstrate that organisations are providing high-quality and effective palliative care or to identify areas for improvement (van Riet Paap et al., 2014).

The UK Gold Standards Framework (GSF) is a multidimensional programme that supports and trains staff to identify patients requiring palliative or supportive care towards the end of life. It uses a structured approach to recognise when the last year of life may have begun, assess patients' needs, symptoms and preferences and plan care around these, especially supporting people to live and die where they choose (Sampson, 2010). Although not developed specifically for patients with dementia, the GSF developed for care homes attempts to enhance communication between GPs and other specialists, particularly in out-of-hours care. Tailored individual advance care plans are developed for residents, and these have been shown to reduce acute hospital admission and hospital deaths by at least 50% (Gold Services Framework/NHS End of Life Programme, 2008). Advance care planning (ACP) is a key part of the GSF programme. It should be included consistently and systematically so that every appropriate person is offered the chance to have an advance care planning discussion with the most suitable person caring for them (e.g. one of the recommendations in GSF training in care homes, primary care and hospitals).[1]

The general aims of the GSF are that:

» people's symptoms will be as well controlled as possible

» people will be enabled to live well and die well where they choose

» people will experience less fear and anxiety; there will be better information, fewer crises and fewer admissions to hospital

» family carers will feel supported, informed and involved.

(Thomas et al., 2005)

Barriers to palliative care in dementia were perceived to include a deficit in dementia knowledge in health care staff and the public, a resource shortfall within the GP practice and community, poor team coordination alongside inappropriate

---

1   See www.goldstandardsframework.org.uk/advance-care-planning (accessed 4 Oct 2016).

dementia care provision, and disagreements by and within families. In 'General Practitioners' Perceptions of the Barriers and Solutions to Good-Quality Palliative Care in Dementia', a postal survey of GPs across Northern Ireland was conducted with open-ended items soliciting for barriers in their practices and possible solutions (Carter et al., 2015). Regulatory frameworks aim to ensure minimum standards in care homes, and some of the improvements in this care sector might be attributed to a desire to improve end-of-life care. However, the increasing size and competitiveness of this market for providers may also act to improve standards, alongside responding to the wishes of older people and their families (Badger, Thomas and Clifford, 2007).

Dementia as a terminal illness

There is considerable reluctance to view dementia as a terminal illness. The reasons for this, and the consequences, are interesting.

As a carers' organisation, Alzheimer Europe stresses the need to provide support to carers too, particularly as the person with dementia is likely to need a considerable amount of care and the permanent presence of a carer in the last stages. A good relationship between carers and health care professionals is also necessary (Gove et al., 2010). Because there is no curative treatment for these diseases, most affected individuals survive to an advanced stage of dementia, which is under-recognised as a terminal illness (Nourhashémi et al., 2012). Data suggest that acute physical illness, requiring emergency hospital admission, may be an indicator (Morrison and Siu, 2000). Gillick uses the term **terminal phase of life** for elderly people whose functional status is permanently and severely impaired and whose life expectancy is probably a maximum of two years, independent of any concomitant diseases (Christakis and Iwashyna, 1998). This definition of a terminal phase of life deviates from the convention in traditional palliative medicine, where life expectancy is a maximum of six months (Frohnhofen et al., 2011).

There are reports of inadequate quality of care in nursing homes for people in the terminal phase of dementia (Koppitz et al., 2015). However, in Switzerland there is a lack of data about the types and courses of symptoms in clinical practice for people with dementia in their terminal phase. The concern is that this lack of knowledge about these symptoms prevents targeted interventions. Two distinct patterns of symptoms were identified over the last 90 days of life: (a) symptoms occurring with increasing frequency (crescent pattern): anxiety, apathy, breathing abnormalities, feeding problems and pain; and (b) symptoms occurring with decreasing frequency (decrescent pattern): unusual behaviours, mobility difficulties, sleep disturbances, agitation and depressive episodes (Koppitz et al., 2015).

The fact that dementia itself is very rarely mentioned as a cause of death perhaps implies that, unlike cancer for instance, it is not considered an illness that causes death (Sachs, Shega and Cox-Hayley, 2004). However, people who have died with dementia may have had symptoms and health care needs that were similar to those of patients with cancer (McCarthy, Addington-Hall and Altmann, 1997). Having reasonable estimates of life expectancy within the context of the risks and benefits of specific treatments facilitates a discussion with patients and their families with respect to making clinical decisions. Palliative care could greatly improve the care of patients with advanced dementia (Gove et al., 2010). If considered at all, the dementia is probably seen as predisposing or contributing to the terminal pneumonia, rather than being the cause of death in itself (Sachs et al., 2004).

One of the major themes within the international literature is the agreement that dementia is a terminal condition, but there is a distinct lack of a coordinated palliative care philosophy (Gott, Ibrahim and Binstock, 2011) and the difficulties associated with the diagnosis of the terminal stage (Lloyd-Williams and Payne, 2002). The terminal illness status of some residents in advancing stages of dementia is often denied, despite tacit understandings about the progressive nature of the disease and its inevitable clinical outcome (Powers and Watson, 2008). It is argued that failure to recognise dementia as a terminal condition, and the costs attached to accommodating non-cancer patients, may preclude access to palliative care (Field and Addington-Hall, 1999; Sampson et al., 2006). Current research identifies advanced dementia to be the terminal phase of this progressive and incurable condition. However, there has been relatively little investigation into how the family members of people with advanced dementia understand their relative's condition. Andrews and colleagues (2015) recently explored family members' understandings of dementia, whether they were aware that it was a terminal condition, and the ways they developed their understandings. The majority of family members could not recognise the terminal nature of dementia. Relying predominantly on **lay understandings**, they had little access to formal information and most failed to conceptualise a connection between dementia and death.

—— End-of-life care ——

A wide range of care professionals have proposed that functional dependency defined the end of life of people with dementia (Lawrence et al., 2011). Accordingly, and despite the weaknesses in physical care provision, some felt that meeting physical needs and symptoms defined end-of-life care in this population. Kupeli and colleagues (2016) noted that the complex nature of dementia also required highly skilled and experienced staff who were able to identify and manage the complex symptoms of residents who may not have the capacity to communicate their needs. Many researchers have argued that the needs of people with dementia at end of life are not in reality met (McCarthy et al., 1997), and that carers require much more support at this time as they may feel exhausted and alone (Shanley et al., 2011). Both patients and carers have to cope with psychological symptoms such as depressive mood, grief and anxiety about death (Woo et al., 2011). Some outcomes may be intrinsically difficult to measure. Spiritual caring may contribute to wellbeing at the end of life, as shown in palliative populations of mostly cancer patients; spiritual caring in dementia may be a neglected area, with little research available (van der Steen et al., 2014).

Various trajectories have been described by Barclay and colleagues (2014). Four distinct but potentially overlapping trajectories to death were identified:

» the largest group of dying residents experienced **anticipated dying**, with planned provision of end-of-life care in the care home

» others experienced **unexpected dying**, where death occurred in the care home after sudden and unexpected events

» others experienced **uncertain dying**, where decisions were made to admit them to hospital in the context of clinical and diagnostic uncertainty or failure of initial treatment

» a final group experienced **unpredictable dying** in hospital after unexpected events such as a heart attack or hip fracture.

Recognising when a person stops living with dementia and starts dying from it, and the prediction of survival time, can influence decisions to involve specialist palliative care services and the release of resources (Goodman et al., 2010). End-of-life care services, whatever the care setting, aim to support people approaching the end of their life to live as well as possible until they die. End-of-life care is often delivered by a large number and wide variety of generalist staff such as doctors, nurses, allied health professionals and social workers (National Audit Office, 2008).

A recent survey, carried out by Alzheimer Europe in the framework of its three-year EC-funded EuroCoDe Project (European Collaboration on Dementia), revealed a lack of palliative care services for people with dementia in Europe as well as a lack of support for carers who care for people with dementia at home in the final stage of life (Gove et al., 2010).[2] It is important that people with dementia nearing their end of life are identified early to enable better planned and coordinated care in line with their needs and wishes. Compassionate community networks could be argued to be a natural evolution for palliative care, at least in Britain. If dying people are to be perceived holistically, that must mean 'relationally'. If people want

---

2   See www.alzheimer-europe.org/Research/European-Collaboration-on-Dementia (accessed 4 Oct 2016).

to die at home, they must ideally mobilise their networks (Abel et al., 2011). It is a generally accepted belief that people wish to die peacefully. Nevertheless, literature on dying peacefully is rather limited. The concept of dying peacefully is broad, often referred to as tranquillity, which may be connected to various aspects of emotional and spiritual wellbeing, such as feeling close to loved ones and feeling deep inner harmony (De Roo et al., 2014). The recommendations of Alzheimer Europe draw attention to the reduced communicative capacity of people with severe dementia and the necessity to find alternative ways of communicating if their needs are to be recognised and respected (Gove et al., 2010).

End-of-life care in England has been framed by various discourses. The UK Department of Health's 'End-of-Life Care Strategy: Promoting High Quality Care for Adults at the End of Their Life' is an example (Department of Health, 2008). It is a general strategy irrespective of disease, since many principles of care are common for all who are approaching death. Meanwhile, the Netherlands has achieved such a combination via a unique approach, the creation of a new medical speciality, the nursing home physician, who provides dedicated care for people with dementia, towards and at the end of life, specifically in care homes (Lee et al., 2015). However, compared with cancer or other chronic diseases, people with dementia may have different end-of-life needs, including communication and cognitive difficulties (van der Steen, 2010).

It is not surprising for an end-of-life care intervention to achieve an improvement in the process and outcomes of care, when compared with 'usual' care for people with dementia in care homes that are known to have limited access to health care services. The need now is to understand how different interventions address all or some of the uncertainties observed, and whether some are more suited for care home populations than others (Goodman et al., 2015). On the whole, research on end-of-life care for people with dementia has yet to develop interventions that address the particular challenges that dying with dementia pose. There is a need for the investigation of interventions and outcome measures for providing end-of-life care in the settings where the majority of this population live and die (Goodman et al., 2010). Jones and colleagues (2015) describe how, in an iterative process, they used empirical data from a three-year programme of research on end-of-life care in dementia and expert opinion to develop the COMPASSION intervention. The COMPASSION intervention was found to facilitate integrated care at the end of life in advanced dementia. It includes training and support to enable this to occur.

Residential settings

Nursing home patients with the longest duration of stay, or a diagnosis of cancer, were more likely to receive palliative end-of-life drugs on the day of death than those without these characteristics (Jansen, Schaufel and Ruths, 2014). Nursing homes are an increasingly common site of death. Predicted socio-demographic trends show rapid increases in the numbers of people aged over 85 and of single households, with concomitant decreases in the availability of informal carers. These trends mean that nursing homes are likely to remain as important sites of end-of-life care for the foreseeable future (Froggatt, 2001).

People with advanced dementia may reside in nursing homes and at the same time be under the care of acute hospitals, community mental health teams and clinical staff from a range of specialities spanning primary and secondary care. This complicated care system makes adequate communication between care providers, patients and carers very challenging (Sampson et al., 2008). Nursing home staff should initiate conversations about preferences for end-of-life care, assisting patients and relatives in talking about these issues, while being sensitive to diverse opinions and the timing for such conversations. A recent study had a qualitative and explorative design, based on a combination of individual interviews with 35 patients living in six nursing homes and seven focus group interviews with 33 relatives. The data was analysed applying a **bricolage approach** (Gjerberg et al., 2015). Few patients and relatives had participated in conversations about end-of-life care. Most relatives wanted such conversations, while patients' opinions varied. With some exceptions, patients and relatives wanted to be informed about the patient's health condition.

Primary care

Critical factors in improving end-of-life care in nursing homes include developing clinical leadership, developing relationships with GPs, the support of key external advocates and the leverage of additional resources by adopting care pathway tools (Seymour, Kumar and Froggatt, 2011). A large UK study has shown that variability in GP support for care homes, in particular out-of-hours support, can be a challenge to the provision of good-quality end-of-life care (Watson, Hockley and Murray, 2010). While good support from palliative care nurse specialists and GPs can help ensure that key processes remain in place, stable management and **key champions** are vital to ensure that a palliative care approach becomes embedded within the culture of the care home (Finucane et al., 2013).

Burdensome symptoms

Burdensome symptoms present frequently in the last phase of life, as Mitchell and colleagues (2009) have reported. Pain and shortness of breath are the most prevalent symptoms at some point in the process of dementia, with a peak when death approaches. The rates of these symptoms vary widely, from 12% to 76% for pain, and from 8% to 80% for shortness of breath. Care professionals all talk of a holistic approach encompassing the individual's physical, psychological, social, emotional and cultural needs; however, only a minority demonstrate how this was implemented in their everyday work with people with dementia (Lawrence et al., 2011). In terms of physical problems, people with advanced dementia suffer a range of symptoms, similar to those found in the terminal stages of cancer, for example pain and dyspnoea (Sampson, Burns and Richards, 2011). Many of these symptoms remain poorly detected and often go untreated (Shega et al., 2006). Pressure sores, agitation and eating problems (i.e. difficulty swallowing or anorexia) are very common.

Barriers to good end-of-life care

Various factors might act as barriers to good end-of-life care. From semi-structured interviews and focus groups with recently bereaved family carers of a person with dementia and a wide range of health and social care staff, thematic content analysis was used to analyse data and identify barriers (Dening et al., 2012).

Five areas were identified as barriers to providing good end-of-life care:

» the impact of hospitalisation

» care pathways

» advance care planning

» the impact on carers

» staff skills and training.

A wide range of health and social care professionals provided end-of-life care to people with dementia but with little coordination or knowledge of each other's activities or remit. Care was often fragmented and ad hoc, leading to crises and inappropriate hospital admissions. Staff lacked confidence and requested more training. Many of the difficulties have been identified at a national level too. For example, the lack of clear integrated dementia pathways has been highlighted in the English National Dementia Strategy; the UK Alzheimer's Society has also reported on the poor quality of care received by people with dementia in acute hospitals, and advance care planning for people with dementia has not yet become part of routine practice in the UK (Sampson et al., 2012).

Interventions to improve the organisation of palliative care encounter challenges beyond the usual problems of implementing change in health care. Patients in need of palliative care often move between services, have changing (and often increasing) needs for treatment and support, have multiple problems and symptoms, and receive care from a variety of professionals (van Riet Paap et al., 2014). The critical need for integrated working between health practitioners and care home staff is highlighted when considering care for residents with dementia approaching the end of life. Evaluative studies of interventions to improve end-of-life care in care homes have identified certain prerequisites for the successful implementation of end-of-life tools and frameworks in these settings, including the cooperation of GPs with care homes and the confidence of GPs in care home staff to make informed decisions (Amador et al., 2016).

Care home residents, including persons with dementia with a high degree of clinical complexity, require access to well-trained staff able to identify 'avoidable admissions' to hospitals (Gordon, 2015). A palliative and end-of-life care approach is therefore highly relevant here.

Goodman and colleagues (2015) recently used data from three studies on end-of-life care in care homes, including 29 care homes and 205 care home staff, to inform the development of a framework for understanding the essential dimensions of end-of-life care delivery in long-term care settings for people with dementia in care homes. The authors found that 'treatment uncertainty' was evident in three situations: (i) when a resident had been stable with no signs of decline, (ii) when a resident had previously recovered from a similar episode of ill-health, for example a urinary tract infection, and (iii) when the period of deterioration was protracted with weeks and sometimes months of good health between episodes of ill-health.

Care home staff, appropriately 'trained, supported, and empowered (by regulators, managers, and primary care teams' (p.1), therefore potentially have a critical role to play in achieving reductions in ambulance conveyance or hospital admission (Oliver, 2016). Preliminary evidence for this, for example, has come from work undertaken jointly by Walsall CCG and Walsall Healthcare NHS Trust (Roberts, 2015).

Policy

Professional and policy guidance on care for people with dementia nearing the end of life emphasises the importance of advance care planning and coordinated work between health and social care. Quality statements relevant to end-of-life care are useful to advance practice but they have a limited evidence base. High-quality empirical work is needed to establish that the recommendations in these statements are best practice (Candy et al., 2015). As highlighted in the *RCGP Commissioning Guidance in End-of-Life Care* (Thomas and Paynton, 2013), for some with life-limiting conditions such as dementia, this might require planning earlier than the final year.

'NICE Quality Standard 13: End of Life Care for Adults'[3] provides health and social care workers, managers, service users and commissioners with a description of what high-quality end-of-life care looks like, regardless of the underlying condition

---

3   Available at www.nice.org.uk/guidance/qs13 (accessed 4 Oct 2016).

or setting. Delivered collectively, these quality statements should contribute to improving the effectiveness, safety and experience of people approaching the end of life and their families.

—— Anticipatory grief, carer grief or pre-grief ——

The grief and feelings of loss experienced by family members caring for a family member with dementia has received growing attention from researchers (Sanders and Sharp, 2004). Clute and Kobayashi (2012) named this group of mourners 'the invisible people', stating that grief must be honoured for all individuals, including those with intellectual disabilities. Preparedness for death has been identified as an important contributor to family carer bereavement outcomes (Boerner et al., 2015). Carers and the family members of people with dementia often suffer significant levels of distress, burden and in particular **anticipatory or pre-death grief**. Anticipatory grief refers to the process of experiencing the phases of normal bereavement in advance of the loss of a significant person (Theut et al., 1991). It encompasses the mourning, coping, planning and psychosocial reorganisation that are stimulated and begun, in part in response to the awareness of an impending loss (usually death) and in recognition of associated losses in the past, present and future (Rando, 1986).

Rando (2000) points out that the term 'anticipatory grief' is actually a misnomer because although this type of grief encompasses losses that are being anticipated in the future, it also incorporates losses that have already occurred and those that are presently occurring. Anticipatory grief comprises past, present and future losses. Carers cite anticipatory grief as their biggest barrier while caring (Frank, 2008). Pre-death grief is the emotional response as family dementia carers mourn for the psychologically absent patient and anticipate impending losses (Blandin and Pepin, 2015). The unpredictable nature of the disease progression as well as personality changes and the behavioural and psychological symptoms of dementia add to this. Meuser, Marwitt and Sanders (2004) suggest that carer grief, which they define as 'the caregiver's emotional, cognitive, and behavioral reactions to the recognition of personally significant loss' (p.175), is an ever-present stressor in caring for a person with dementia. They argue that it is 'true grief' that is 'relatively indistinguishable from post-death grief in personal impact and meaning' (p.174).

Carers of persons with Alzheimer's disease or related dementias may experience and grieve for a multitude of losses. These can include the loss of the relationship with the care receiver, the loss of closure, the loss of recreational activities, the loss of a future with the care receiver and, in some circumstances, the losses associated with using a nursing home (Williams and Moretta, 1997). Related to the cognitive stress perspective of grief is the unpredictable and intermittent nature of the carer's sense of loss, especially as the care recipient progressively deteriorates as a result of dementia. This phenomenon is captured by Boss (1999) and Blieszner and colleagues (2007), who used the term **ambiguous loss** to describe the kind of loss that a carer may experience as the care recipient fades in and out of realistic consciousness depending, more or less, on the severity and the course of the dementia. Carers and families are described as experiencing anticipatory or pre-death grief; the cognitive deterioration of dementia leads to the loss of personhood, often long before actual bodily death (Meuser and Marwit, 2001).

Because people with advanced or end-stage dementia are likely to lack the capacity to make decisions, carers are frequently expected to act as proxies. If preparing family carers for the death of a loved one is considered integral to good end-of-life care, this notion should be expanded to encompass formal carers who replace or complement family carers (Hebert et al., 2006). Spouses of persons living with dementia both anticipate future loss and grieve for multiple losses occurring during caring – this ultimately influences their bereavement experience.

Table 12.1 summarises grief intervention strategies.

Table 12.1: Overview of grief intervention strategies

Name of the category	Definition
I: Recognition and Acceptance of Loss and Change	The therapist supports the carer in accepting losses associated with the disease and in accepting the new reality. The focus is also on the verbalisation and disclosure of painful emotions associated with these losses.
II: Normalisation of Grief	Some carers assume that it is not right to grieve and therefore avoid it. Many also fear that grieving could lead to depression. The therapist communicates that it is normal and healthy to grieve and explains the difference between normal grief and depression.
III: Redefinition of the Relationship	As the disease progresses, the cognitive abilities and personality of the care recipient change. This has strong implications for the relationship between the carer and care recipient. The intervention is aimed at the recognition of these changes and the redefinition of the spousal or child identity.
IV: Addressing Future Losses	Dementia is a terminal disease. As the disease progresses, the carer anticipates further losses and is confronted with decisions that could increase grief.

SOURCE: ADAPTED FROM MEICHSNER, SCHINKÖTHE AND WILZ (2016, TABLE 1).

—— Pain in palliative care and end-of-life care ——

In a recent study, teams consisting of 84 professionals working in 13 long-term care settings from six countries (France, Germany, Italy, Norway, Poland and the Netherlands) received a case-vignette concerning a person with dementia recently admitted to a nursing home (van Riet Paap et al., 2015). Teams were asked to discuss when they considered people with dementia eligible for palliative care. Most professionals described that palliative care should be provided when a person with dementia shows symptoms indicating that the advanced stage of dementia is approaching the end-of-life phase, such as swallowing disorders, pain or when the body no longer responds to food or liquids. Despite the fact that pain is the most common complaint at the end of life, pain management may be suboptimal for some primary diagnoses (Romem et al., 2015). According to recent NICE guidelines, there is often uncertainty about how long a person has left to live and the signs that suggest that someone is dying can be 'complex and subtle' (NICE, 2015, p.18).

The prevalence of comorbidities in people with dementia often necessitates pain management throughout disease progression and into the final months of life (Klapwijk et al., 2014; Hendriks et al., 2014/2015). Pain and shortness of breath are the most prevalent symptoms at some point in the process of dementia, with a peak when death approaches. Pain, agitation and dyspnoea have been found in varying proportions of patients with dementia, in the last weeks and days before death (Hendriks et al., 2015). The cornerstone of high-quality care at end of life is ensuring that persons are free of pain and other potentially burdensome symptoms (Mitchell, 2015). Patients with advanced dementia often have a decreased ability to communicate their symptoms verbally. Due to this limitation, it is often difficult to understand the cause of distressed responses, but an aetiology and assessment of pain and behavioural symptoms should be considered in the differential diagnosis. Refractory behavioural challenges make the diagnostic process even more challenging (Brecher and West, 2016). Evaluating pain using assessment tools and the role that opioids play in this population will require further research and education. General disagreement in the literature as to whether dementia is a terminal disease also contributes to this treatment discrepancy (Mitchell et al., 2009, 2012).

Nurses often experience difficulties, such as feelings of powerlessness because of difficulties in obtaining adequate prescriptions for analgesics. They also face ethical dilemmas, feelings of inadequacy because analgesia did not have the desired effect and a feeling of not being able to connect with the patient (Brorson et al., 2014). Various factors, including knowledge about the patient, professional experience, the utilisation of pain assessment tools, interpersonal relationships and interprofessional cooperation, served as resources and enabled end-of-life pain relief. A review by Scherder and Ploolij (2012) described the use of a number of pharmaceutical agents routinely used in the management of pain in dementia, but they also proposed that a number of other agents might be more suitable for pain of a more 'central' nature. The authors also concluded: 'Next to pharmacotherapy, non-pharmacological treatment strategies such as transcutaneous electrical nerve stimulation may be effective as long as afferent pathways transmitting the electrical stimulus are still intact' (p.701).

—— Advance care planning ——

People living with a long-term condition, especially those with dementia, may wish to be able to plan ahead, so that if in future they cannot make decisions, their wishes about their care will be known; this process is termed advance care planning (ACP).

ACP is the process whereby patients, in consultation with health care professionals, family members and other loved ones, make individual decisions about their future health care, to prepare for future decisions about medical treatment (Singer, Robertson and Roy, 1996). ACP is the process of discussing and then recording future wishes and preferences for care and treatment. This record comes into effect if one's mental capacity is lost to make important decisions about current or future care. It can include statements as to how one wishes to be treated at end of life. Advance care planning decisions are becoming increasingly important and advocated as the UK experiences a rapidly ageing population.

ACP is often cited as a cornerstone of the strategy to improve end-of-life care for people with dementia. It is a complex issue influenced by many conflicting factors, such as the lack of legal capacity characteristic of advanced dementia, difficulties in working across health and social care boundaries, the perception among relatives and professionals that dementia is not a terminal illness, and the constraints and limitations of different legal systems in different countries (Sampson and Robinson, 2009). The goals of ACP are to avoid crisis-driven decision-making and unwanted and inappropriate treatments. However, Sudore and Fried (2010) suggest that there is a need to shift the focus from what they describe as premature decisions based on incomplete information to preparing individuals and their families (and in this instance, care home staff) for the types of decisions and conflicts they may encounter when they do have to make 'in the moment' decisions.

Demographic trends are changing the modern experience of death and dying. In western Europe, the majority of people with advanced dementia spend the last period of their life in a nursing home (Houttekier et al., 2010). ACP has been defined as a process of formal decision-making that aims to help patients establish decisions about future care that take effect when they lose capacity. It recently gained increased importance in the UK. It is widely acknowledged that the application of ACP is an important component of personalised end-of-life care, and that the recognition and accommodation of preferences expressed in ACP documents allow individuals to have control over the level of health care they receive at end of life (Silvester et al., 2013). Patients with advancing dementia often experience significant comorbidities, such as malnutrition and dehydration. They may have no ACP in place, and this can pose difficult management questions for their families and physicians concerning palliation and end-of-life care (Jethwa and Onalaja, 2015).

A health care professional who knows most about the person living with the condition is in a good position to facilitate the ACP, but may need to involve others where there are multiple comorbidities or specific circumstances. The advance planning of care can be of particular importance for nursing home residents with dementia, considering the loss of decision-making capacity inherent to the disease (Vandervoort et al., 2014a, b). Stewart and colleagues (2011) explored views on ACP in care homes for older people. Staff and family felt that advance care planning provided choice for residents and encouraged better planning, but they also perceived some residents as reluctant to discuss advance care planning.

Although there is growing recognition across the globe that people with dementia are entitled to appropriate palliative care, the weighty question is why so many of them are still exposed to disproportionate hospital interventions when facing death. The reasons for this seeming paradox are multiple, such as the lack of funding, understaffing and sociocultural (i.e. legal) factors influencing medical decision-making (Hertogh, 2006). ACP differs from general care planning in that it is usually used in the context of progressive illness and anticipated deterioration. This has implications for its acceptability to patients. It is a voluntary process and may result in a written record of a patient's wishes, which can be referred to by carers and health professionals in the future. If a patient loses capacity, health and social care professionals should make use of information gleaned from the ACP process to guide them in decision-making (Mullick, Martin and Sallnow, 2013).

Given the high prevalence of persons with dementia that reside in long-term care homes in the United Kingdom and North America, discussing their wishes and treatment preferences is appropriate. Several programmes that promote ACP in long-term care homes have been described and evaluated in the literature. However, little work has been done to assess whether these programmes include the consideration of values important to persons with dementia and their family members (Wickson-Griffiths et al., 2014). There is some evidence as to the effectiveness of ACP in nursing home residents, including but not limited to those with dementia, in terms of improvement in process measures. This refers to the better documentation of preferences, changes in health care utilisation (decreased hospitalisation and increased hospice use) and reduced costs (van der Steen et al., 2014).

During a nursing home stay, there are several crucial moments for talking about ACP (Ampe et al., 2015) (see Figure 12.1). Three moments are of particular importance. First, the time of admission, including the first weeks or months, is considered to be a crucial moment for starting ACP or for updating advance care plans (Volicer et al., 2002, Vandervoort et al., 2014a, b).

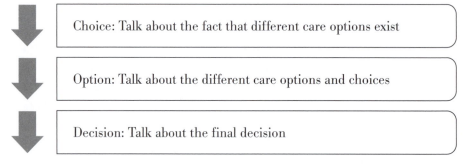

Figure 12.1: Three-step model for shared decision-making

'Choice' means explain that all options are of equal value, check whether resident/ family carer understands that options exist, and check that the resident/family carer knows what options are available. 'Option' means sum up all options, including the option to do nothing, discuss advantages, disadvantages and possible risks of each option, and explore resident's/family carer's preferences. 'Decision' means determine if and to what extent resident/family carer want to be involved in advance care planning, and guide the resident/family carer to a final decision; indicate that it is possible to reconsider the decision. Source: adapted for use from Ampe et al. (2015, Fig. 2, p.1159).

There is considerable ambiguity about initiating ACP in dementia at diagnosis among physicians practising in two different European health care systems and caring for different patient populations. ACP strategies should accommodate not only variations in one's readiness to engage in ACP early on among patients and families, but also among physicians (van der Steen et al., 2010). Better education and executive function predict a willingness to engage in ACP, and these factors are instrumental in a person's ability to acquire knowledge and process information. Initiating ACP discussions early on, increasing efforts at education and providing tailored information are important interventions that facilitate completion of ACP (Tay et al., 2015). The 'right' timing for physicians to take the initiative in planning care for patients with dementia in the last stage of life is unclear. The study by Tay and colleagues (2015) suggests that GPs transfer little to no information about patient wishes and advance treatment decisions when a patient is admitted to a nursing home. GPs also may have difficulties defining the right moment to initiate ACP for patients with dementia. Access to specific health care services or admission to a health care facility for long-term care, such as a nursing home, may trigger the initiating or reviewing of ACP discussions.

The timing of ACP is influenced by barriers such as prognostic uncertainty, the fear of damaging positive coping strategies, the potential workload of having earlier ACP with patients or simply because of an unawareness of the needs of patients (Glaudemans, Moll van Charante and Willems, 2015). Barriers and facilitators for GPs to engage in ACP have been investigated in a systematic review by De Vlaminck and colleagues (2013). Stronger evidence was found for the following barriers: a lack of skills to deal with patients' vague requests, difficulties with defining the right moment, the attitude that it is the patient who should initiate ACP, and the fear of depriving patients of hope. Stronger evidence was found for the following facilitators: accumulated skills, the ability to foresee health problems in the future, skills to respond to a patient's initiation of ACP, personal convictions about who to involve in ACP, a longstanding patient–GP relationship, and the home setting. Finally, ACP appears to be associated with health care savings for some people in some circumstances, such as people living with dementia in the community, people in nursing homes or those in areas with high end-of-life care spending. There is no evidence that ACP is likely to be more expensive (Dixon, Matosevic and Knapp, 2015).

—— Hospices ——

One of the great social innovations of the 20th century, hospice care has transformed both the way society thinks about and the way it cares for people approaching the end of their lives.

The inspiration behind the modern hospice movement was Dame Cicely Saunders (1918–2005) (Ahmed and Siddiqi, 2015). Dementia has emerged as a key issue for hospices as they consider their strategic direction for the future. While few people challenge the belief that dementia is a life-limiting illness, it has struggled to be accorded the same degree of service provision from within the palliative care domain as other life-limiting illnesses (Hospice UK, 2015). The good death constitutes one – and because of its practical implications, perhaps the most important – of the conceptual guidelines for the modern hospice movement. It was the desire to offer marginalised and abandoned patients a peaceful, serene death, with compassionate reception, based on the idea of the **good death**, that initially triggered the movement. The efforts involved in fulfilling this doctrine represent a genuine leitmotif for the professionals involved in its daily practice (Floriani and Schramm, 2012).

The actual lived experience of 'living with dying' is incredibly interesting, and preliminary evidence has revealed a marked heterogeneity in the reactions of people living in anticipation of imminent death in terminal illness. These reactions range from despair to near euphoria, or from loss of meaning to great meaning (Willig, 2015). The hospice movement has had considerable impact on end-of-life and bereavement care in the UK since the 1960s (Hockley, 1997). It stresses the significance of a shared, holistic approach to end-of-life care, where the physical, social and emotional experiences of the patient and their family are central. This approach can be viewed in parallel with the philosophy of integrated care whereby emphasis is placed on providing coordination and continuity in care by adopting a multidisciplinary approach that is viewed through a **patient lens** (Paul, Cree and Murray, 2016). There are several differences between residents of assisted living receiving hospice care and individuals living at home receiving it. A better understanding of these differences could allow hospices to develop guidelines for better coordination of end-of-life care for the assisted living population (Dougherty et al., 2015).

Providing palliative care to people with dementia is perceived as effective and is an increasing feature of care at end of life. A lack of awareness about the role played by palliative care providers including hospices in end-of-life dementia care is a major barrier to its usage (Ryan and Ingleton, 2011). Providing support to families is viewed as the most important aspect of palliative care work in end-of-life dementia care. Meeting the palliative care needs of this growing population is a huge task, since the aim is to optimise the quality of life of people who have complex, incurable and life-threatening health problems by addressing their physical, emotional, psychosocial and spiritual needs (Iliffe et al., 2016).

I will return to this question in Chapter 14.

Hospices as a place of death

Studying the place of death of people with dementia can provide essential information for the planning of end-of-life care services and facilities, because such people are more likely to enter institutional care (Houttekier et al., 2010). The absolute and relative numbers of inpatient hospice deaths in England have increased over time, though numbers remain small. However, it is now recognised that non-cancer conditions such as dementia and chronic respiratory disease have a similar symptom burden to cancer conditions and that hospice care should be provided according to need rather than diagnosis (Sleeman et al., 2016). Most people in Germany, for example, die in institutions; the most common place of death is still the hospital, where more than half of all deaths take place. Only one death in four occurs at home. There is a marked secular trend away from dying at home or in the hospital, in favour of dying in a care or nursing home; death in palliative care units and hospices is also becoming more common (Dasch et al., 2015).

There appears to be a failure to identify dementia as a terminal illness in some quarters, for example by health and social care professionals themselves. This has implications for the type of care which is provided for people with dementia; indeed most people with dementia have, historically, not had access to specialist palliative care (Hughes et al., 2007). Physicians and clinicians have difficulty knowing when the individual with dementia has entered the end stage. The end stage can be quite protracted. This inability to determine terminality results in a high percentage of individuals missing out on the additional benefits of palliation and hospice enrolment (McCarty and Volicer, 2009). Although functional status generally declines in individuals in hospices, this decline is heterogeneous. Some individuals retain some physical and cognitive function until the last day of life (Harris et al., 2013).

It is important to note that, for some people with dementia, the move to a hospice (or any other care setting) can cause unnecessary confusion and distress at a stage in the condition when the person may be less able to cope with change. This may also partially explain why people in the latter stages of dementia rarely use hospice services (Robinson et al., 2005). Another barrier to hospice utilisation for individuals with dementia in nursing homes is a lack of coordination between nursing home and hospice staff. This includes communication gaps between the family, the hospice and nursing home staff as well as a lack of agreement on and implementation of the end-of-life care plan (McCarty and Volicer, 2009). The use of aggressive treatment for people with dementia is common and can include tube feeding and antibiotic treatment for infections (Perl, Khan and Marin, 2002). Another barrier is a lack of continuity of care. Continuity of care is extremely important as changes in health or social care staff can create unnecessary distress (Sampson et al., 2006). While most people grieve after a person has actually died from a terminal illness, the families of those with dementia may experience different stages of loss as the condition progresses, for example when the person with dementia no longer recognises them.

Analyses suggest that patients who receive hospice care while living in a nursing home differ in important ways from hospice patients in other settings. Most notably, these patients are older and have higher rates of dementia (Unroe et al., 2013). A significant part of the work of an Admiral nurse (clinical specialist nurse) is in the community, reaching out to those affected by advanced dementia. Helping the wider health and social care community see dementia through a palliative lens can give a different perspective on it, and enable discussions about emergency health care planning and symptom control (Tolman, 2015).

Britain's hospices have steadily transformed our society's relationship with end-of-life care, demonstrating innovative and responsive developments to new approaches in care. This continues to be the case as hospices plan for the needs of emerging social groups that have, until now, not constituted a core segment of patients, but who represent a steadily growing sector of older people in their final years (Ahmed and Siddiqi, 2015). Recent results identify the reasons for employees to be intrinsically motivated to share their best practices and mistakes (Mura et al., 2013). The results, in fact, support the notion that knowledge sharing can (also) be a self-interested behaviour; that is, a behaviour that leads professionals to help themselves while – and before – helping their organisation. A higher propensity and capacity to promote and implement new ideas, in fact, were facilitated by an active involvement in knowledge-sharing behaviours. Hospices are major employers of professionals who have significant specialist skills and have helped professionals working in other settings to develop similar skills. As such they are ideally placed to be at the forefront of the future provision of end-of-life care, and the development of new models of care and the skills needed to effectively deliver this care (Help the Hospices Commission, 2013).

—— Essential reading ——

Downs M, Middleton-Green L, Chatterjee J, Russell S. 2016. *End of Life Care for People with Dementia: A Person-Centred Approach*, London: Jessica Kingsley Publishers.
Rahman S. 2014. *Living Well with Dementia*, London: CRC Press. Chapter 8, Maintaining Wellbeing in End-of-Life Care for Living Well with Dementia, pp.133–146.

—— References ——

Abel J, Bowra J, Walter T, Howarth G. 2011. Compassionate community networks: supporting home dying. BMJ Support Palliat Care, 1(2), 129–133.
Ahmed S, Siddiqi N. 2015. *Bridging the Gap: Strengthening Relations between Hospices and Muslims of Britain*, Cambridge: Woolf Institute.
Amador S, Goodman C, Mathie E, Nicholson C. 2016. Evaluation of an organisational intervention to promote integrated working between health services and care homes in the delivery of end-of-life care for people with dementia: understanding the change process using a social identity approach. Int J Integr Care, 16(2), 14.
Ampe S, Sevenants A, Coppens E, Spruytte N, et al. 2015. Study protocol for 'we DECide': implementation of advance care planning for nursing home residents with dementia. J Adv Nurs, 71(5), 1156–1168.
Andrews S, McInerney F, Toye C, Parkinson CA, Robinson A. 2015. Knowledge of dementia: do family members understand dementia as a terminal condition? Dementia (London), September, 1471301215605630 (e-pub ahead of print).
Arcand M. 2015. End-of-life issues in advanced dementia. Part 1: goals of care, decision-making process, and family education. Can Fam Physician, 61(4), 330–334.
Badger F, Thomas K, Clifford C. 2007. Raising standards for elderly people dying in care homes. European Journal of Palliative Care, 14(6), 238–241.
Barclay S, Froggatt K, Crang C, Mathie E, et al. 2014. Living in uncertain times: trajectories to death in residential care homes. Br J Gen Pract, 64(626), e576–583.
Blandin K, Pepin R. 2015. Dementia grief: a theoretical model of a unique grief experience. Dementia (London), April, 1471301215581081 (e-pub ahead of print).
Blieszner R, Roberto KA, Wilcox KL, Barham EJ, Winston BL. 2007. Dimensions of ambiguous loss in couples coping with mild cognitive impairment. Fam Relat, 56(2), 196–209.
Boerner K, Burack OR, Jopp DS, Mock SE. 2015. Grief after patient death: direct care staff in nursing homes and homecare. J Pain Symptom Manage, 49(2), 214–222.
Boss P. 1999. *Ambiguous Loss*, Cambridge, MA: Harvard University Press.

Brecher DB, West TL. 2016. Under recognition and undertreatment of pain and behavioral symptoms in end-stage dementia. Am J Hosp Palliat Care, 33(3), 276–280.

Brorson H, Plymoth H, Örmon K, Bolmsjö I. 2014. Pain relief at the end of life: nurses' experiences regarding end-of-life pain relief in patients with dementia. Pain Manag Nurs, 15(1), 315–323.

Candy B, Elliott M, Moore K, Vickerstaff V, Sampson EL, Jones L. 2015. UK quality statements on end-of-life care in dementia: a systematic review of research evidence. BMC Palliat Care, 14, 51.

Caron C, Arcand M, Griffith J. 2005. Creating a partnership with families in decision-making for end-of-life care in Alzheimer disease: the perspective of family caregivers. Dementia, 4, 113–136.

Carter G, van der Steen JT, Galway K, Brazil K. 2015. General practitioners' perceptions of the barriers and solutions to good-quality palliative care in dementia. Dementia (London), April, 1471301215581227 (e-pub ahead of print).

Christakis NA, Iwashyna TJ. 1998. Attitude and self-reported practice regarding prognostication in a national sample of internists. Arch Intern Med, 158, 2389–2395.

Clute MA, Kobayashi R. 2012. Looking within and reaching out: bereavement counsellor perceptions of grieving adults with ID. Am J Hosp Palliat Care (online).

Cox S, Cook A. 2002. Caring for People with Dementia at the End of Life. In J Hockley, D Clark (eds), *Palliative Care for Older People in Care Homes*. Buckingham: Open University Press.

Dasch B, Blum K, Gude P, Bausewein C. 2015. Place of death: trends over the course of a decade – a population-based study of death certificates from the years 2001 and 2011. Dtsch Arztebl Int, 112, 496–504.

Davies N, Maio L, van Riet Paap J, Mariani E, et al. 2014. Quality palliative care for cancer and dementia in five European countries: some common challenges. Aging Ment Health, 18(4), 400–410.

De Roo ML, van der Steen JT, Galindo Garre F, Van Den Noortgate N, et al. 2014. When do people with dementia die peacefully? An analysis of data collected prospectively in long-term care settings. Palliat Med, 28(3), 210–219.

De Vleminck A, Houttekier D, Pardon K, Deschepper R, et al. 2013. Barriers and facilitators for general practitioners to engage in advance care planning: a systematic review. Scand J Prim Health Care, 31(4), 215–226.

Dening KH, Greenish W, Jones L, Mandal U, Sampson EL. 2012. Barriers to providing end-of-life care for people with dementia: a whole-system qualitative study. BMJ Support Palliat Care, 2(2), 103–107.

Dening T, Dening KH. 2016. Palliative care in dementia: Does it work? Maturitas, doi: 10.1016/j.maturitas.2015.10.006.

Department of Health. 2008. End-of-Life Care Strategy: Promoting High Quality Care for Adults at the End of Their Life, available at www.cpa.org.uk/cpa/End_of_Life_Care_Strategy.pdf (accessed 6 Oct 2016).

Dixon J, Matosevic T, Knapp M. 2015. The economic evidence for advance care planning: systematic review of evidence. Palliat Med, 29(10), 869–884.

Dougherty M, Harris PS, Teno J, Corcoran AM, et al. 2015. Hospice care in assisted living facilities versus at home: results of a multisite cohort study. J Am Geriatr Soc, 63(6), 1153–1157.

Einterz SF, Gilliam R, Lin FC, McBride JM, Hanson LC. 2014. Development and testing of a decision aid on goals of care for advanced dementia. J Am Med Dir Assoc, 15(4), 251–255.

Field D, Addington-Hall J. 1999. Extending specialist palliative care to all? Soc Sci Med, 48, 1271–1280.

Finucane AM, Stevenson B, Moyes R, Oxenham D, Murray SA. 2013. Improving end-of-life care in nursing homes: implementation and evaluation of an intervention to sustain quality of care. Palliat Med, 27(8), 772–778.

Floriani CA, Schramm FR. 2012. Routinization and medicalization of palliative care: losses, gains and challenges. Palliat Support Care, 10(4), 295–303.

Forder J, Fernandez JL. 2011. *Length of Stay in Care Homes*, Canterbury: PSSRU.

Frank JB. 2008. Evidence for grief as the major barrier faced by Alzheimer caregivers: a qualitative analysis. Am J Alzheimers Dis Other Demen, 22(6), 516–527.

Froggatt KA. 2001. Palliative care and nursing homes: where next? Palliat Med, 15, 42–48.

Frohnhofen H, Hagen O, Heuer HC, Falkenhahn C, Willschrei P, Nehen HG. 2011. The terminal phase of life as a team-based clinical global judgment: prevalence and associations in an acute geriatric unit. Z Gerontol Geriatr, 44(5), 329–335.

Gjerberg E, Lillemoen L, Førde R, Pedersen R. 2015. End-of-life care communications and shared decision-making in Norwegian nursing homes – experiences and perspectives of patients and relatives. BMC Geriatr, 15, 103.

Glaudemans JJ, Moll van Charante EP, Willems DL. 2015. Advance care planning in primary care, only for severely ill patients? A structured review. Fam Pract, 32(1), 16–26.

Goodman C, Evans C, Wilcock J, Froggatt K, et al. 2010. End-of-life care for community dwelling older people with dementia: an integrated review. Int J Geriatr Psychiatry, 25(4), 329–337.

Goodman C, Froggatt K, Amador S, Mathie E, Mayrhofer A. 2015. End-of-Life care interventions for people with dementia in care homes: addressing uncertainty within a framework for service delivery and evaluation. BMC Palliat Care, 14, 42.

Gordon A. 2015. *Care Home Residents Deserve the Best Care: The Best Care Is Integrated*, available at britishgeriatricssociety.wordpress.com/2015/11/10/care-home-residents-deserve-the-best-carethe-best-care-is-integrated (accessed 3 Oct 2016).

Gott M, Ibrahim AM, Binstock RH. 2011. The Disadvantaged Dying: Ageing, Ageism and Palliative Care Provision for Older People in the UK. In M Gott, C. Ingleton (eds), *Living with Ageing and Dying*, Oxford: Oxford University Press.

Gove D, Sparr S, Dos Santos Bernardo AM, Cosgrave MP, et al. 2010. Recommendations on end-of-life care for people with dementia. J Nutr Health Aging, 14(2), 136–139.

Grubb C, Arthur A. 2016. Student nurses' experience of and attitudes towards care of the dying: a cross-sectional study. Palliat Med, 30(1), 83–88.

Harris P, Wong E, Farrington S, Craig TR, et al. 2013. Patterns of functional decline in hospice: what can individuals and their families expect? J Am Geriatr Soc, 61(3), 413–417.

Hebert RS, Prigerson H, Schulz R, Arnold RM. 2006. Preparing caregivers for the death of a loved one: a theoretical framework and suggestions for future research. J Palliat Med, 9, 1164–1171.

Help the Hospices Commission. 2013. *Future Needs and Preferences for Hospice Care: Challenges and Opportunities for Hospices*, available at www.hospiceuk.org/docs/default-source/default-document-library/future-needs-and-preferences-for-hospice-care-challenges-and-opportunities-for-hospices.pdf (accessed 3 Oct 2016).

Hendriks SA, Smalbrugge M, Galindo-Garre F, Hertogh CM, van der Steen JT. 2015. From admission to death: prevalence and course of pain, agitation, and shortness of breath, and treatment of these symptoms in nursing home residents with dementia. JAMA, 16(6), 475–481.

Hendriks SA, Smalbrugge M, Hertogh CM, van der Steen JT. 2014. Dying with dementia: symptoms, treatment, and quality of life in the last week of life. J Pain Symptom Manage, 47(4), 710–720.

Hertogh CM. 2006. Advance care planning and the relevance of a palliative care approach in dementia. Age and Ageing, 35(6), 553–555.

Hockley J. 1997. 'The evolution of the hospice approach.' In D Clark, J Hockley, S Ahmedzai (eds), *New Themes in Palliative Care*, Buckingham: Open University Press.

Hospice UK. 2015. Hospice enabled dementia care: the first steps, available at https://www.hospiceuk.org/what-we-offer/clinical-and-care-support/hospice-enabled-dementia-care (accessed 29 Nov 2016).

Houttekier D, Cohen J, Bilsen J, Addington-Hall J, Onwuteaka-Philipsen BD, Deliens L. 2010. Place of death of older persons with dementia: a study in five European countries. J Am Geriatr Soc, 58(4), 751–756.

Hughes JC, Jolley D, Jordan A, Sampson EL. 2007. Palliative care in dementia: issues and evidence. Advances in Psychiatric Treatment, 13(4), 251–260.

Hughes JC, Robinson L, Volicer L. 2005. Specialist palliative care in dementia. BMJ, 330(7482), 57–58.

Iliffe S, Davies N, Manthorpe J, Crome P, et al. 2016. Improving palliative care in selected settings in England using quality indicators: a realist evaluation. BMC Palliative Care, 15(1), 1–9.

Jansen K, Schaufel MA, Ruths S. 2014. Drug treatment at the end of life: an epidemiologic study in nursing homes. Scand J Prim Health Care, 32(4), 187–192.

Jennings B. 2003. Hospice and Alzheimer's disease: a study in access and simply justice. Hastings Centre Report Special Supplement, 33, S24–S26.

Jethwa KD, Onalaja O. 2015. Advance care planning and palliative medicine in advanced dementia: a literature review. BJPsych Bull, 39(2), 74–78.

Jones L, Candy B, Davis S, Elliott M, et al. 2015. Development of a model for integrated care at the end of life in advanced dementia: a whole systems UK-wide approach. Palliat Med, September, 0269216315605447 (e-pub ahead of print).

Klapwijk MS, Caljouw MA, van Soest-Poortvliet MC, van der Steen JT, Achterberg WP. 2014. Symptoms and treatment when death is expected in dementia patients in long-term care facilities. BMC Geriatr, 14, 99.

Koppitz A, Bosshard G, Schuster DH, Hediger H, Imhof L. 2015. Type and course of symptoms demonstrated in the terminal and dying phases by people with dementia in nursing homes. Z Gerontol Geriatr, 48(2), 176–183.

Kupeli N, Leavey G, Moore K, Harrington J, et al. 2016. Context, mechanisms and outcomes in end-of-life care for people with advanced dementia. BMC Palliat Care, 15, 31.

Lawrence V, Samsi K, Murray J, Harari D, Banerjee S. 2011. Dying well with dementia: qualitative examination of end-of-life care. Br J Psychiatry, 199(5), 417–422.

Lee RP, Bamford C, Exley C, Robinson L. 2015. Expert views on the factors enabling good end-of-life care for people with dementia: a qualitative study. BMC Palliat Care, 14, 32.

Lloyd-Williams M, Payne S. 2002. Can multidisciplinary guidelines improve the palliation of symptoms in the terminal phase of dementia. International Journal of Palliative Nursing, 8(8), 370–375.

Long CO, Sowell EJ, Hess RK, Alonzo TR. 2012. Development of the questionnaire on palliative care for advanced dementia (qPAD). Am J Alzheimers Dis Other Demen, 27(7), 537–543.

Lynn J, Adamson DM. 2003. *Living Well at the End of Life: Adapting Health Care to Serious Chronic Illness in Old Age*, Santa Monica, CA: Rand.

Mahin-Babaei F, Hilal J, Hughes JC. 2016. The basis, ethics and provision of palliative care for dementia: a review. Maturitas, 83, 3–8.

McCarthy M, Addington-Hall J, Altmann D. 1997. The experience of dying with dementia: a retrospective study. Int J Geriatric Psychiatry, 12, 404–409.

McCarty CE, Volicer L. 2009. Hospice access for individuals with dementia. Am J Alzheimers Dis Other Demen, 24(6), 476–485.

Meichsner F, Schinköthe D, Wilz G. 2016. Managing loss and change: grief interventions for dementia caregivers in a CBT-based trial. Am J Alzheimers Dis Other Demen, 31(3), 231–240.

Meuser TM, Marwit SJ. 2001. A comprehensive, stage-sensitive model of grief in dementia caregiving. Gerontologist, 41, 658–670.

Meuser T, Marwit S, Sanders S. 2004. Assessing grief in family caregivers. In KJ Doka KJ (ed.) Living with Grief: Alzheimer's Disease, Washington, DC: Hospice Foundation of America.

Mitchell SL. 2015. Clinical practice: advanced dementia. N Engl J Med, 372(26), 2533–2540.

Mitchell SL, Black BS, Ersek M, Hanson LC, et al. 2012. Advanced dementia: state of the art and priorities for the next decade. Ann Intern Med, 156(1), 45–51.

Mitchell SL, Teno JM, Kiely DK, Shaffer ML, et al. 2009. The clinical course of advanced dementia. N Engl J Med, 361(16), 1529–1538.

Morrison RS, Siu AL. 2000. Survival in end-stage dementia following acute illness. J Am Med Assoc, 284, 47–52.

Mullick A, Martin J, Sallnow L. 2013. An introduction to advance care planning in practice. BMJ, 347.

Mura M, Lettieri E, Radaell, G, Spiller N. 2013. Promoting professionals' innovative behaviour through knowledge sharing: the moderating role of social capital. Journal of Knowledge Management, 17(4), 527–544.

National Audit Office. 2008. *End of Life Care*, London: The Stationery Office, available at www.nao. org.uk/wp-content/uploads/2008/11/07081043.pdf (accessed 3 Oct 2016).

National Palliative and End-of-Life Care Partnership. 2015. Ambitions for Palliative and End-of-Life Care: A National Framework for Local Action 2015–2020.

NICE. 2015. Care of dying adults in the last days of life, NICE guideline 31, available at https://www.nice.org.uk/guidance/ng31/resources/care-of-dying-adults-in-the-last-days-of-life-1837387324357 (accessed 29 Nov 2016).

Nourhashémi F, Gillette S, Cantet C, Stilmunkes A, et al. 2012. End-of-life care for persons with advanced Alzheimer disease: design and baseline data from the ALFINE study. J Nutr Health Aging, 16(5), 457–461.

Office for National Statistics. 2015. National Survey of Bereaved People (VOICES), available at www. ons.gov.uk/peoplepopulationandcommunity/healthandsocialcare/health caresystem/bulletins/ nationalsurveyofbereavedpeoplevoices/2015-07-09 (accessed 3 Oct 2016).

Oliver D. 2016. Keeping care home residents out of hospital. BMJ, doi: 10.1136/bmj.i458.

Palecek EJ, Teno JM, Casarett DJ, Hanson LC, Rhodes RL, Mitchell SL. 2010. Comfort feeding only: a proposal to bring clarity to decision-making regarding difficulty with eating for persons with advanced dementia. J Am Geriatr Soc, 58(3), 580–584.

Parliamentary and Health Service Ombudsman. 2015. Investigations by the

Parliamentary and Health Service Ombudsman into Complaints about End-of-Life Care.

Paul S, Cree VE, Murray SA. 2016. Integrating palliative care into the community: the role of hospices and schools. BMJ Support Palliat Care, August, bmjspcare-2015-001092. doi:10.1136/ bmjspcare-2015-001092 (e-pub ahead of print).

Perl D, Khan K, Marin DB. 2002. Palliative and aggressive end-of-life care for patients with dementia. Psychiatric Services, 53(5), 609–613.

Powers BA, Watson NM. 2008. Meaning and practice of palliative care for nursing home residents with dementia at end of life. Am J Alzheimers Dis Other Demen, 23(4), 319–325.

Rabins PV, Lyketsos CG, Steele CD. 1999. Practical dementia care, New York: Oxford University Press.

Rando TA. 1986. A Comprehensive Analysis of Anticipatory Grief: Perspectives, Processes, Promises, and Problems. In TA Rando (ed.), *Loss and Anticipatory Grief*, New York: Lexington Books.

Rando TA. 2000. Anticipatory Mourning: A Review and Critique of the Literature. In TA Rando (ed.), *Clinical Dimensions of Anticipatory Mourning: Theory and Practice in Working with the Dying, Their Loved Ones, and Their Caregivers*, Champaign, IL: Research Press.

Raymond M, Warner A, Davies N, Iliffe S, Manthorpe J, Ahmedzhai S. 2014. Palliative care services for people with dementia: a synthesis of the literature reporting the views and experiences of professionals and family carers. Dementia (London), 13(1), 96–110.

Roberts S. 2015. Reducing hospital admissions: a new integrated model for care homes. British Geriatrics Society blog, available at http://britishgeriatricssociety.wordpress.com/2015/07/29/ reducing-hospital-admissions-a-new-integrated-model-for-care-homes (accessed 15 Dec 2016).

Robinson L, Hughes J, Daley S, Keady J, Ballard C, Volicer L. 2005. End-of-life care and dementia. Reviews in Clinical Gerontology, 15, 135–148.

Romem A, Tom SE, Beauchene M, Babington L, Scharf SM, Romem A. 2015. Pain management at the end of life: a comparative study of cancer, dementia, and chronic obstructive pulmonary disease patients. Palliat Med, 29(5), 464–469.

Ryan T, Ingleton C. 2011. Most hospices and palliative care programmes in the USA serve people with dementia; lack of awareness, need for respite care and reimbursement policies are the main barriers to providing this care. Evid Based Nurs, 14(2), 40–41.

Sachs GA, Shega JW, Cox-Hayley D. 2004. Barriers to excellent end-of-life care for patients with dementia. J Gen Intern Med, 19, 1057–1063.

Sampson E, Mandal U, Holman A, Greenish W, Dening KH, Jones L. 2012. Improving end of life care for people with dementia: a rapid participatory appraisal. BMJ Support Palliat Care, 2(2), 108–114.

Sampson EL. 2010. Palliative care for people with dementia. Br Med Bull, 96, 159–174.

Sampson EL, Robinson L. 2009. End-of-life care in dementia: building bridges for effective multidisciplinary care. Dementia, 8(3), 331–334.

Sampson EL, Blanchard MR, Jones L, Tookman A, King M. 2009. Dementia in the acute hospital: prospective cohort study of prevalence and mortality. Br J Psychiatry, 195(1), 61–66.

Sampson EL, Burns A, Richards M. 2011. Improving end-of-life care for people with dementia. Br J Psychiatry, 199(5), 357–359.

Sampson EL, Gould V, Lee D, Blanchard MR. 2006. Differences in care received by patients with and without dementia who died during acute hospital admission: a retrospective case note study. Age and Ageing, 35(2), 187–189.

Sampson EL, Thuné-Boyle I, Kukkastenvehmas R, Jones L, et al. 2008. Palliative care in advanced dementia: a mixed methods approach for the development of a complex intervention. BMC Palliat Care, 7, 8.

Sanders S, Sharp A. 2004. The utilization of a psychoeducational group approach for addressing issues of grief and loss in caregivers of individuals with Alzheimer's disease: a pilot program. J Social Work Long-Term Care, 3, 71–89.

Scherder EJ, Plooij B. 2012. Assessment and management of pain, with particular emphasis on central neuropathic pain, in moderate to severe dementia. Drugs Aging, 29(9), 701–706.

Seymour JE, Kumar A, Froggatt K. 2011. Do nursing homes for older people have the support they need to provide end-of-life care? A mixed methods enquiry in England. Palliat Med, 25(2), 125–138.

Shanley C, Russell C, Middleton H, Simpson-Young V. 2011. Living through end-stage dementia: the experiences and expressed needs of family carers. Dementia, 10(3), 325–340.

Shega JW, Hougham GW, Stocking CB, Cox-Hayley D, Sachs GA. 2006. Management of noncancer pain in community-dwelling persons with dementia. J Am Geriatr Soc, 54, 1892–1897.

Silvester W, Fullam RS, Parslow RA, Lewis VJ, et al. 2013. Quality of advance care planning policy and practice in residential aged care facilities in Australia. BMJ Support Palliat Care, 3(3), 349–357.

Singer PA, Robertson G, Roy DJ. 1996. Bioethics for clinicians: 6. Advance care planning. CMAJ, 155, 1689–1692.

Sleeman KE, Davies JM, Verne J, Gao W, Higginson IJ. 2016. The changing demographics of inpatient hospice death: Population-based cross-sectional study in England, 1993–2012. Palliat Med, 30(1), 45–53.

Stewart F, Goddard C, Schiff R, Hall S. 2011. Advanced care planning in care homes for older people: a qualitative study of the views of care staff and families. Age Ageing, 40(3), 330–335.

Sudore RL and Fried TR. 2010. Redefining the 'planning' in advance care planning: preparing for end-of-life decision making. Ann Intern Med, 153, 256–261.

Tay SY, Davison J, Jin NC, Yap PL. 2015. Education and executive function mediate engagement in advance care planning in early cognitive impairment. J Am Med Dir Assoc, 16(11), 957–962.

The Gold Standards Framework. 2008. NHS End-of-Life Care Programme, available at www.goldstandardsframework.org.uk (accessed 3 Oct 2016).

Theut SK, Jordan L, Ross LA, et al. 1991. Caregiver's anticipatory grief in dementia: a pilot study. Int J Aging Hum Dev, 33, 113–118.

Thomas K, Paynton D. 2013. RCGP Commissioning Guidance in End-of-life Care, London: RCPG.

Thomas K, Sawkins N, Meehan H, Griffin T, Newell C. 2005. The Gold Standards Framework Starter Pack for the Gold Standards Framework in care homes Phase 2, Birmingham: GSF Team.

Tolman S. 2015. Admiral Nursing in a Hospice, available at www.ehospice.com/uk/Default/tabid/10697/ArticleId/14477 (accessed 3 Oct 2016).

Treloar A, Crugel M, Adamis D. 2009. Palliative and end-of-life care of dementia at home is feasible and rewarding: results from the 'Hope for Home' study. Dementia, 8(3), 335–347.

Unroe KT, Sachs GA, Dennis ME, Hickman SE, et al. 2013. Hospice use among nursing home and non-nursing home patients. J Gen Intern Med, 30(2), 193–198.

van der Steen JT. 2010. Dying with dementia: what we know after more than a decade of research. J Alzheimers Dis, 22, 37–55.

van der Steen JT, Heymans M, Steyerberg E, Kruse R and Mehr D. 2011. The difficulty of predicting mortality in nursing home residents. European Geriatric Medicine, 2(2), 79–81.

van der Steen JT, Radbruch L, Hertogh CM, de Boer ME, et al. 2014. White paper defining optimal palliative care in older people with dementia: a Delphi study and recommendations from the European Association for Palliative Care. Palliat Med, 28(3), 197–209.

Vandervoort A, Houttekier D, Stichele RV, van der Steen JT, Van den Block L. 2014a. Quality of dying in nursing home residents dying with dementia: does advanced care planning matter? A nationwide postmortem study. PLoS ONE, 9(3), e91130.

Vandervoort A, Houttekier D, Van den Block L, van der Steen JT, Vander Stichele R, Deliens L. 2014b. Advance care planning and physician orders in nursing home residents with dementia: a nationwide retrospective study among professional caregivers and relatives. Journal of Pain and Symptom Management, 47(2), 245–256.

van Riet Paap J, Mariani E, Chattat R, Koopmans R, et al. 2015. Identification of the palliative phase in people with dementia: a variety of opinions between health care professionals. BMC Palliat Care, 14, 56.

van Riet Paap J, Vernooij-Dassen M, Dröes RM, Radbruch L, et al. 2014. Consensus on quality indicators to assess the organisation of palliative cancer and dementia care applicable across national health care systems and selected by international experts. BMC Health Serv Res, 14, 396.

van Soest-Poortvliet MC, van der Steen JT, de Vet HC, Hertogh CM, Deliens L, Onwuteaka-Philipsen BD. 2015. Comfort goal of care and end-of-life outcomes in dementia: a prospective study. Palliat Med, 29(6), 538–546.

Volicer L. 2005 End-of-Life Care for People with Dementia in Residential Care Settings, London: Alzheimer's Association, available at www.alz.org/national/documents/endoflifelitreview.pdf (accessed 3 Sept 2016).

Volicer L, Cantor MD, Derse AR, Edwards DM, et al. 2002. Advance care planning by proxy for residents of long-term care facilities who lack decision-making capacity. Journal of the American Geriatrics Society, 50(4), 761–767.

Watson J, Hockley J, Murray S. 2010. Evaluating effectiveness of the GSFCH and LCP in care homes. End Life Care J, 4(3), 42–49.

Wickson-Griffiths A, Kaasalainen S, Ploeg J, McAiney C. 2014. A review of advance care planning programmes in long-term care homes: are they dementia-friendly? Nursing Research and Practice, Article ID 875897.

Williams C, Moretta B. 1997. Systematic understanding of loss and grief related to Alzheimer's disease. In KJ Doka (ed.) Living with grief when illness is prolonged, Washington, DC: Hospice Foundation of America.

Willig C. 2015. 'My bus is here': a phenomenological exploration of 'living-with-dying'. Health Psychol, 34(4), 417–425.

Woo J, Lo R, Cheng JO, Wong F, Mak B. 2011. Quality of end-of-life care for non-cancer patients in a non-acute hospital. J Clin Nurs, 20(13–14), 1834–1841.

Wright M, Clark D, Wood J, Lynch T. 2008. Mapping levels of palliative care development: a global view. J Pain & Symptom Mgmt, 35(5), 469–485.

Zahradnik EK, Grossman H. 2014. Palliative care as a primary therapeutic approach in advanced dementia: a narrative review. Clin Ther, 36(11), 1512–1517.

Chapter 13

LIVING WELL AT HOME

Learning objectives ————————————————

By the end of this chapter, you will be able to:

- » describe how different care environments compare, including the importance of enhancing living at home
- » explain the significance of living alone with dementia at home
- » describe the interdependence of care services, and outline the critical importance of social care
- » describe skills training for carers
- » describe ambient assistive living
- » describe other approaches to improving wellbeing for living at home, including pets and robots
- » describe the notion of successful 'ageing in place'
- » describe home care or domiciliary care
- » explain the relevance of the international approach of community-based rehabilitation, and explain Buurtzorg as an example of social innovation and entrepreneurship
- » identify the need for respite services

—— Introduction ————————————————————

Because of the great need for long-term care, the economic impact of dementia is tremendous. There is international variation in this, for example private vs non-private funding, statutory or non-statutory, sometimes with blurred boundaries. Like in many other countries, health policy in Germany, for example, aims at avoiding or postponing patients' admission to nursing homes by giving priority to care in the community over nursing home care (Social Security Code XI) (König et al., 2014).

In persons living better with dementia, residence at home depends on the size and the strength of the family networks but also on the availability of care services, which varies across countries and regions. Family carers are at the centre of primary care and health and social care strategies, as research and government guidelines have emphasised the need for continued research and resourcing for carers, offering financial, practical and emotional support. Carers of persons with dementia living at home adopt a variety of caring styles that vary in quality; poor quality of care increased the risk of long-term care placement, as expected, but high-quality care was not related to placement (McClendon and Smyth, 2013, 2015).

The quality of life (QoL) of people with dementia, living at home or in an institution, is influenced by several clinical variables, including: cognitive deficits, behavioural and psychological disorders, degree of autonomy and the extent of dementia progression. However, the impact of these variables respectively is not well documented (Misotten et al., 2009). Based on recent data from Germany, community-based dementia care is cost-saving from the taxpayer's perspective due to substantially lower long-term care expenditures (Schwarzkopf et al., 2013). Health care spending is comparable, but community-living and institutionalised individuals present characteristic service utilisation patterns. This apparently reflects the existence of setting-specific care strategies. However, the bare economic figures do not indicate whether these different concepts affect the quality of care provision and disregard patient preferences and carer-related aspects.

An excellent guide which will be of particular interest to friends and family about the course of dementia from pre-diagnosis to end of life is by Pulsford and Thompson (2013). It is entitled *Dementia: Support for Family and Friends*.

Living alone at home

The wider public, and people with dementia more specifically, have expressed a preference to remain living at home (WHO, 2012).

As a consequence of the timely diagnosis and drug treatment of today, the number of persons with dementia who live at home for a longer period of time after diagnosis is increasing (Svanström and Sundler, 2015). The WHO and many government policies have prioritised the need for people with dementia to be enabled to remain living at home for as long as possible (Kirk et al., 2016). With increasing numbers of older people living alone, there is concern for older people living alone with dementia (Moriarty and Webb, 2000). It is worth noting that the presence of dementia did not alter the association of living alone and the risk of hospitalisation in a cohort from the Pacific Northwest (Ennis et al., 2014).

Feeling at home is a fundamental aspect of human existence (Dekkers, 2011) that is often taken for granted (Gillsjö and Schwartz-Barcott, 2011). Maximising care at home aims to improve the quality and appropriateness of care as part of a rebalancing of the focus away from institutional care to reablement. The aim is also to improve flexibility and responsiveness in order to minimise the need to admit people to hospital at times of crisis, and delay or avoid transfer to a care home.

Previous research describes three types of people who live alone with dementia: those who live alone and have the support of people who live nearby; those who live alone and receive support from people who live far away; and those who live alone and have no family to provide assistance (Newhouse et al., 2001). Health care professionals have important roles in the care of community-dwelling older people with dementia and their families, including: (a) education, (b) crisis intervention and management, and (c) support (de Witt and Ploeg, 2014). A contemporary study in the UK reported that outpatient services, GP appointments and home care were the most frequently used services among older people with dementia living alone (Miranda-Castillo, Woods and Orrell, 2010). **Living alone**, **social isolation** and **loneliness** are terms used interchangeably, although they are different, but related, concepts (Victor et al., 2005). Dementia specifically has also been linked with a decreasing number of social engagements in later life (Saczynski et al., 2006). However, living at home may enable people to experience a better QoL by remaining engaged within known social and physical environments (Luppa et al., 2008).

In research, more focus has been on the situation of people with dementia who live with a spouse. As the care needs of those living with a spouse become manifest, they are more likely to get round-the-clock support and the help needed to maintain a structured everyday life (Vikström et al., 2005; Hellström, Nolan and Lundh, 2007). Health care professionals, it has been suggested, have a critical and unique role in facilitating acceptance of home care services by older people living alone with dementia, and this is especially important for older people with dementia who live alone and who have a strong desire to remain in their homes for as long as possible (Gilmour, 2004; Harris, 2006). For example, an international systematic review reported an increased risk of and a shorter time to placement in a care home among older people with dementia living alone (Luppa et al., 2008). An international systematic review found that enabling people to remain at home has economic and cost advantages, with the direct costs of institutionalised dementia care being on average three times higher than the direct costs for when someone lives at home (Schaller et al., 2015). In the UK, people with dementia who have a co-resident carer are 20 times less likely than those who live alone to be admitted to a care home (Banerjee et al., 2003).

Interdependence and the critical
—— importance of social care ——

Roles within social care are changing. For example, in *The Guardian* Ewan King wrote in December 2015: 'The push for integration of health and care means we need more people who can work across both sectors. The expansion of personal budgets is leading to the creation of new kinds of jobs to support service users with their personal care and support.'

And Lyn Romeo, Chief Social Worker, also wrote in *The Guardian* in December 2015:

> The NHS is missing a trick if it fails to recognise the role and contribution social workers can make in an integrated health and care system, improving outcomes for people, keeping them safe and reducing expenditure across health and care as a whole. The new models of care all require input and leadership from skilled social workers and allied health professionals, working alongside doctors and nurses in true multidisciplinary partnerships with patients.

Social care is typically used to describe community-based care from the many sectors that lie outside health services (the NHS). Typically, social care services encompass residential care in care homes (with or without nursing), home care (domiciliary care) and day services. People pay for this care themselves or it is funded by local authorities (Hussein and Manthorpe, 2012). Poor coordination and collaboration have been identified by many governments as a major and growing weakness of contemporary health care systems. Better integrated care for elderly individuals is one field of particular importance (Holmas, Islam and Kjerstad, 2013). The experience of Norway is that most patients would like to leave hospital as soon as possible and return home or move to adequate nursing facilities (Dam et al., 2016).

The influential article by Hussein and Manthorpe (2012) specifically reported on the secondary analysis of a new national workforce dataset from England covering social care employees. Secondary analysis of this dataset was undertaken using 457,031 unique workers' records. There were some important differences between the dementia care workforce and other parts of the social care workforce in respect of the dementia care workforce being more likely to be female, part-time, less qualified agency staff. There is now undeniably an increasing emphasis on the importance of considering the impact of services on outcomes and QoL in health and social care policy, practice and research (Towers et al., 2015).

Social work is undoubtedly crucial to modern mental health services too, and there is widespread acknowledgement that social work is at the heart of person-centred, integrated dementia care. Excellent social work can transform the lives of people with mental health conditions, and remains an essential, highly valued part of multidisciplinary and multiagency systems of support. As Allen (2014, p.5) states: 'Social workers also manage some of the most challenging and complex risks for individuals and society, and take decisions with and on behalf of people within complicated legal frameworks, balancing and protecting the rights of different parties.' This includes, but is not limited to, their vital role as the core of the approved mental health professional workforce.

Finally, the needs of the person with dementia tend to be the focus of everyone involved with a family, from friends and relatives to health and social care professionals. The spotlight is rarely on the carer and how their life has changed (Skills for Care/Dementia UK, 2012). There has historically been a shift in the theoretical debates about the ways in which organisations deliver the state's objectives of providing health and social care services for its citizens, focusing on issues of welfare governance and the encouragement of partnership working between organisations (Rummery and Coleman, 2003).

—— Enhancing care at home ——

Chronicity in care, which involves health promotion, prevention, self-management, disease control, treatment and disease palliation as applied to patients with dementia, requires interdisciplinary teams formed by professionals who provide distinct health and social care services and ensure continuity of care with patient and family commitment (Innes, 2002; Martin et al., 2008). Medical complexity is important to measure when accounting for **carer strain**. Large numbers of untrained, and usually unpaid, carers provide nursing care at home, and the nature of these tasks is an important contributor to their levels of strain; nursing complexity is important to consider when assessing carers' needs and developing policy and programming to assist them (Moorman and Macdonald, 2013). Interventions based on the assumption that family members and other home carers provide only or mostly personal care fail to address major stressors in carers' experience.

To improve home care for individuals with dementia, health professionals should educate and support carers. Before specific interventional recommendations can be made, further research addressing the limitations of current studies is needed (Zabalegui et al., 2014). One solution to avoid a collapse in the coping ability of hospitals is to perform patient care in home environments through home care services (Bastiani et al., 2013). Most persons with dementia live at home and are cared for by family members. As the disease progresses, however, physical features of the home environment may represent a safety hazard or barrier to performing daily activities of living, particularly at the moderate stage of the disease process. Recommending environmental modifications to enhance safe functioning at home has become a routine part of clinical practice in home care and rehabilitation (Gitlin et al., 2010).

Previous studies on the prevalence of the long-term use of antipsychotics among persons with dementia have mainly focused on specific settings of care such as nursing homes, specialised care units and mental health services. The long-term use of antipsychotics is frequent among community-dwelling persons with Alzheimer's disease in Finland (Koponen et al., 2015). Duration of use is not in line with the guidelines recommending the time-limited use of antipsychotics there. In a small qualitative study, the old age psychiatrists interviewed reported that guidelines are difficult to implement in clinical practice (Wood-Mitchell et al., 2008). They felt pressure to prescribe psychotropics for distressed responses because of a lack of viable alternatives and a lack of resources and time to implement non-pharmacological treatment approaches. These factors may also explain why the duration of antipsychotic use is so often not in line with current treatment guidelines. One of the major issues is ensuring continuity of care between primary and secondary settings, and this can lead to political sensitivities in prescribing and deprescribing.

As most persons with Alzheimer's disease reside in the community, an intervention designed for the home setting is especially advantageous. It is possible that a simple exercise intervention can be administered by an exercise physiologist and adverse events assessed at each visit. Individualised home-based rehabilitation programmes might be able to enable improved mobility recovery after hip fracture over standard care. To be efficacious in reducing or reversing disability after hip fracture, rehabilitation needs to be individualised, include many components, be progressive and span a sufficiently long period (Salpakoski et al., 2014). It is crucial that the personnel provide person-centred care and are able to meet the needs of the people living with dementia and their next of kin, to help to give them a new everyday life (Söderhamn et al., 2013).

Carers and skills training

Carers provide unpaid care by looking after an ill, older or disabled family member, friend or partner. It could be a few hours a week or round-the-clock, in your own home or down the motorway. Some 6.5 million people in the UK are carers, and this number continues to rise. Every year over 2.1 million adults become carers, and almost as many people find that their caring responsibilities come to an end (Carers UK, 2014).

There is a huge number of carers in the UK (see Table 13.1).

Table 13.1: Carer statistics

(a) Figures taken from the official census data for 2001 and 2011

Data for England and Wales	2001	2011
Total number of unpaid carers	5,217,805	5,800,246
1–19 hours per week unpaid carers	3,555,822 (6.8%)	3,665,072 (6.5%)
20–49 hours per week unpaid carers	573,647 (1.1%)	775,189 (1.4%)
50 hours or more per week unpaid carers	1,088,336 (2.1%)	1,359,985 (2.4%)

b) 2011 data breakdown by age

Carer	All categories: Provision of unpaid care	Provides no unpaid care	Provides unpaid care: Total	Provides 1–19 hours' unpaid care a week	Provides 20–49 hours' unpaid care a week	Provides 50 or more hours' unpaid care a week
All categories: Age	56,075,912	50,275,666	5,800,246	3,665,072	775,189	1,359,985
Age 0–15	10,579,132	10,460,165	118,967	96,102	11,953	10,912
Age 16–24	6,658,636	6,334,669	323,967	235,228	51,526	37,213
Age 25–34	7,520,524	7,016,723	503,801	318,461	78,642	106,698
Age 35–49	11,931,776	10,418,856	1,512,920	974,190	212,712	326,018
Age 50–64	10,162,771	8,102,070	2,060,701	1,422,761	256,692	381,248
Age 65 and over	9,223,073	7,943,183	1,279,890	618,330	163,664	497,896

SOURCE: OFFICE FOR NATIONAL STATISTICS,
LICENSED UNDER THE OPEN GOVERNMENT LICENCE V.3.0.[1]

What emerged from a systematic review by Bunn and colleagues (2012) is the striking complexity and variety of responses to becoming a person with dementia, and how this makes diagnosing and supporting this group particularly challenging. In addition, there is the effect on carers.

The Care Act 2014 now makes integration, cooperation and partnership a legal requirement for local authorities and all agencies involved in public care, including the NHS, independent or private sector organisations, some housing functions and the CQC. Section 6 of the Act provides for a general duty to cooperate. Section 7 of the Act provides for cooperation in specific cases and includes caveats for specific cases when cooperation is not possible (NHS England, 2016a, b).

Over the past 20 years, many initiatives have been developed to support people with dementia living in the community and their carers (Knight, Lutzky and Macofsky-Urban, 1993). However, one shortcoming of such services is that they

---

1   Data available at https://www.ons.gov.uk/census (accessed 28 Oct 2016).

are often very fragmented. As a consequence, family carers, and even professionals, are not always aware of what is available (Dröes et al., 2004). By investigating older family carers' specific needs and perceptions of QoL, meaningful evidence may be generated for researchers and primary health and social care professionals to quantify the experience of caring in old age. Above all, it has the potential to facilitate and drive the implementation and evaluation of social and health interventions with older family carers, as well as ensuring the necessary allocation of resources and services available for this population (de Oliviera, Vass and Aubeduck, 2015). It has repeatedly been shown that mutuality, defined as the positive quality of the carer–care receiver relationship, and preparedness, defined as carers' perceived readiness for the tasks and stresses of caring, were found to predict carer role strain (Yang, Liu and Shyu, 2014). Interventions focused on the enhancement of caring satisfaction by increasing the understanding of the disease should be especially addressed to carers without a consanguinity relationship and with high levels of subjective burden and to those managing care recipients with mild or moderate stages of dementia (de Labra et al., 2015).

The quality of the caring relationship has been shown to influence motivation for care, with carers who describe a positive prior relationship being more likely to be motivated by an intrinsic desire to maintain QoL for individuals with dementia, rather than an extrinsic motivation based on obligation (Quinn, Clare and Woods, 2009). The demand on informal carers to support people with dementia at home will therefore increase. It is important for informal carers to develop and maintain competence in this challenging task, as their help is crucial for people with dementia to remain at home as long as possible (Andren and Elmstahl, 2008). Many carers who experience caring pressures and mental health problems are known not to utilise support services to meet their needs, but telecoaching according to the principles of Dementelcoach combined with respite care (psychogeriatric day care) have been found to be more effective in reducing carer stress and health complaints in informal carers of community-dwelling people with dementia than telecoaching or day care only (MacNeil Vroomer et al., 2012).

In the UK, one-to-one social support is commonly provided through voluntary sector-based befriending services. Britain has a long tradition of voluntary action, and the emphasis on partnership in recent government policies has given voluntary, community and users' organisations a more central role in the delivery of services (HM Treasury, 2002). In common with many carers' services, befriending schemes are not taken up by all carers, and providing access to a befriending scheme is not effective in improving wellbeing (Charlesworth et al., 2008). Befriending leads to a non-significant trend towards improved carer QoL, and there is a non-significant trend towards higher costs for all sectors. It is unlikely that befriending is a cost-effective intervention from the point of view of society (Wilson et al., 2009). Information and support interventions are delivered via a number of formats. Of these, only group interventions (underpinned by psychoeducational theoretical foundations) appear to positively impact on depression in carers. The extent to which these benefits are clinically (rather than just statistically) significant remains uncertain (Thompson et al., 2007). Family carers of people with dementia may take on this role without understanding how it will evolve or how to obtain support.

There is considerable worldwide concern to develop accessible, sustainable and cost-effective interventions for carers to enable them to function and remain longer in the caring role in a more meaningful and productive and less stressful manner (Au et al., 2015). A recent review by Gallagher-Thompson and colleagues identified a variety of evidence-based, non-pharmacological interventions on a global basis. These programmes include the following: individual and family counselling, psychoeducation programmes, specialised skills training and psychotherapy, as well as interventions using technology such as telephones/smartphones and internet/online support (Gallagher-Thompson et al., 2012).

One concern is that when overall resources are insufficient to provide for a policy such as interventions for carers at an individual level, a form of rationing takes place (see Box 13.1).

Box 13.1: NHS rationing strategies

* Rationing by denial

* Rationing by selection

* Rationing by delay

* Rationing by deterrence

* Rationing by deflection

* Rationing by dilution

SOURCE: ADAPTED FROM KLEIN AND MAYBIN (2012, P.4).

—— Ambient assistive living ——

The use of ambient assistive living (AAL) technologies aims to empower people with dementia and relieve the burden of their carers (Aloulou et al., 2013). The emerging field of AAL has positioned itself to enable older adults, including individuals living with dementia, to age-in-place (i.e. at home and in their communities) through the support of intelligent and pervasive computing (also referred to as smart home) technologies (Hwang et al., 2012).

Among others, AAL technologies have been utilised in: mobile emergency response systems; fall detection systems; video surveillance systems; activities of daily living (ADL) monitoring systems; reminders issuing systems (e.g. for medication intake); chronic disease management and rehabilitation; mobility and automation assistive tools; and systems that ease the connection and communication with peers, family and friends (Dasios et al., 2015). Over the last few years, several projects have been funded and works have been published to demonstrate the effectiveness of assistive technologies that are integrated in end-users' domestic environments to increase the quality of domiciliary care and reduce the workload of carers who assist persons with Alzheimer's disease (Cavallo, Aquilano and Arvati, 2015).

AAL technologies can be used to assist people with dementia and their carers. AAL consists of a set of ubiquitous technologies – for example, sensors, actuators, interaction devices – embedded in the living space of the patient to monitor and react to his or her contextual needs by providing computerised assistive services. Today, these technologies are used in diverse health care applications and are expected to increase the efficacy and efficiency of health care providers (Bardram et al., 2006). Using the latest technology, AAL technologies aim to provide individuals living with dementia with the means to actively live their daily lives, protect their dignity, feel safe, maintain their capacities, sustain their integration with their communities and help their caregivers in monitoring and preventing avoidable complications in consecutive treatment (Novitzky et al., 2015).

Other approaches

Animal-assisted therapy

Incorporating research into evidence-based practice has a long history in the health care professions, but only relatively recently has it become popular. Therapeutic recreation specialists have traditionally made treatment decisions based on their educational background, client assessment and client and family preferences (Richeson, 2003). Animal-assisted therapy (AAT) promotes mental health through contact between the animal and the person, encouraging independence and improving the patient's QoL. This type of therapy began in the US as a treatment or a form of care in the 1970s (Kanamori et al., 2001). AAT most commonly involves interaction between a client and a trained animal, facilitated by a human handler, with a therapeutic goal such as providing relaxation and pleasure, or incorporating activities into physical therapy or rehabilitation (e.g. brushing a dog with a stroke-affected limb) (Filan and Llewellyn-Jones, 2006).

The benefits of AAT are on the whole quite widely well known. Box 13.2 lists some common benefits of certified dog therapy.

Box 13.2: Examples of 'abilities' that can be trained with a certified therapy dog

* Improved cognition (e.g. in memory, language, problem solving, attention, planning)

* Increased wellbeing, social interaction and self-esteem

* Improved movement and balance

SOURCE: BASED ON NORDGREN AND ENGSTRÖM (2014, TABLE 1).

The therapeutic possibilities of companion animals have been described by Baun and McCabe (2003) with reference to the stage of dementia and the positive effect on carers. While medication has a role in the management of more severe behaviour problems, there has been a growing call to focus on psychosocial methods as alternative or supplementary interventions, particularly given the potential for the adverse effects of medication. Despite a substantial literature on psychosocial interventions in dementia, some of which has been reviewed in this book in Chapters 4 and 5, the number of rigorously controlled studies is limited (Bird et al., 2002). When used in dementia care, AAT takes advantage of the human–animal bond to reduce behavioural and/or psychological symptoms and to increase social engagement and communication (Nordgren and Engström, 2012, 2014).

—— Robots ——————————————————————

AAT is not always possible. Animals are often not allowed in nursing homes or day care centres, due to the risk of injury to patients, staff or visitors, the possibility of allergic reactions and the potential nuisance of cleaning up after the animals (Valentí Soler et al., 2015).

Robots have fewer needs (if a robot can be said to have needs at all) for space, time or care. Their sensors can respond to environmental changes, simulating interaction with the patient. They can monitor patients or be used in therapy. Other potential benefits of therapy with robots are that there are no known adverse effects, specially trained personnel are not required and they can repeat the script in the same way as many times as it is required without tiring. In a trial lasting several days, Marx et al. (2008) showed that the duration of engagement of an older person with a real dog was similar to that with a robotic dog (Marx et al., 2008, discussed in Chu et al., 2016).

The evidence base for such technological interventions has previously been classified as follows (Khosravi and Ghapanchi, 2016):

» general ICT

» robotics

» telemedicine

» sensor technology

» medication management applications

» video games.

Robotics is a 'rapidly growing area of technology that provides services such as the operation of appliances and various other tasks that support the elderly's daily living. Robots respond to an individual's needs such as those elderly individuals who need to maintain mobility or social connectedness' (Khosravi and Ghapanchi, 2016, p.20).

A lack of stimulation can be particularly detrimental to people with dementia as it adversely affects their mood, increases their level of agitation and results in a high use of pharmaceutical interventions (Hwang et al., 2012). To counter these issues, researchers have been investigating the use of companion robotic animals as a means to comfort, engage and stimulate social interaction with dementia (Moyle et al., 2016).

Human-interactive robots for psychological enrichment, which provide services by interacting with humans while stimulating their minds, are rapidly spreading. Such robots not only entertain but also render assistance, guide, provide therapy, educate, enable communication and so on (Shibata and Wada, 2011). Robotic pets, also called emotional or therapeutic robots, have recently been introduced as companions for people with cognitive impairment and/or physical problems.

However, please note: 'it should be pointed out that current robots are poor substitutes for human company. Robots may not exhibit the worst sides of human behavior, but neither are they capable of real compassion and empathy or understanding' (Sharkey, 2014, p.65).

—— Successful ageing in place ——

Longer life expectancies will place unprecedented pressure on health and social services, while ageing has already been identified as an emerging threat to the fiscal stability of developed and developing countries alike (McCurry, 2015). Given that most older adults prefer to live at home in the community for as long as possible, health care organisations and policymakers are increasingly supporting the notion of ageing in place, providing the resources necessary to allow older adults to remain in their homes and communities. The shift away from institutionalised care may alleviate the financial pressures of caring for the burgeoning elderly population while optimising health outcomes and prolonging independence (Young et al., 2015). In the ENABLE-AGE Project, researchers used the term **healthy ageing** to address selected aspects of physical, mental and social health that are assumed to be particularly relevant to housing (Iwarsson et al., 2007). Among the core concepts chosen for the project were *independence in daily activities* and *subjective wellbeing* (Iwarsson, Wahl and Nygren, 2004).

Better understanding of the values and contexts that inform elders' definitions of successful ageing can be used to inform clinical care and preventive programmes in more meaningful ways (Ng et al., 2009). Common to all will be inevitable disability in their ability to perform ADL required for independent living (Ciro, 2014). Retention of ADL performance is associated with personal, familial and financial benefits, such as increased QoL, decreased carer burden and reduced care costs, as well as societal benefits such as a reduction in institutional rates largely paid for by national health programmes (Desai, Grossberg and Sheth, 2014). Having people remain in their homes and communities for as long as possible also avoids the costly option of institutional care and is therefore favoured by policymakers, health providers and by many older people themselves (WHO, 2007).

—— Home care and living at home ——

Home care, also known as domiciliary care, is a term for support provided in the home by careworkers to assist someone with their daily life. Enabling people to remain at home helps them maintain personal independence, comfort and contact with their local community. Home care is flexible, with just the right amount of assistance given at any one time. For most older people, autonomy is important for good QoL, as well as being able to live independently in their own homes unless limited by very poor health. Even if institutionalised, participation in their own care is important (Smebye, Kirkevold and Engedal, 2016). Home care provision grew out of the home help service, introduced after the Second World War. Cultural and demographic changes over time saw the average age of service users increase until, by the 1960s, older people accounted for 90% of the clientele of the service (Godfrey et al., 2000).

As it has been reported that two-thirds of all people with dementia live in their own home in the UK, either alone or with family carers, it is vital that domiciliary home care providers are able to demonstrate good practice by ensuring that all new employees receive training and ongoing support (Carers UK, 2014). The training and development received will enable workers to easily identify any difficulties that they may encounter while providing care and support to people with dementia (Skills for Care, 2014). Home care agencies are required to comply fully with health and safety legislation to identify and minimise risks to people receiving care and their careworkers (Carers UK, 2014). A recent study by Janssen and colleagues (2016) showed that ADL impairment, not living together with the carer and the higher age of the care recipient increased the likelihood of receiving formal home care in memory clinic visitors with mild cognitive impairment (MCI) and dementia. ADL impairment and having a dementia diagnosis increased the likelihood of receiving informal care. Therefore, these factors are relevant to take into account in addition to the diagnosis for care planning.

People's homes now dominate the landscape of long-term care, as increasing numbers of the chronically ill and disabled are cared for outside institutional sites. Services which sustain and support people with dementia to live in their own homes do not operate in isolation: people with dementia and their carers are likely to have a range of needs, and so are likely to be simultaneously engaged with and using health services and other community-based care services (Weber, Pirraglia and Kunik, 2011).

The search for the meaning of home is long-standing and ongoing. The idea of **home** is well known from everyday experience, plays a crucial role in all kinds of narratives about human life, but is hardly ever systematically dealt with in the philosophy of medicine and health care (Dekkers, 2011). Feeling at home is particularly important for individuals with dementia who experience an increased need for familiarity, permanency, affiliation and autonomy in the face of disruptions, dependencies, disappointments and alienation often caused by the disease. It is noteworthy, despite cognitive losses, that a sense of home remains salient in the minds of individuals with dementia in even advanced stages (Frank, 2005). While care in institutions is provided in the relatively standardised spaces of clinics and hospitals designed around professional care practices and equipment needs, care at home is provided in spaces designed for other purposes, of varying sizes and conditions, and where there are strong associations with the notions of privacy and family life (Dyck et al., 2005).

An overview of domiciliary care is given in Box 13.3.

Box 13.3: Examples of useful tips for managers of domiciliary care

* Work in harmony with health and social care services.

* Involve and support family carers where you can. Train all your workers to be 'carer aware' – carers may need as much support as the person diagnosed. Work closely with the other partners in the person's care – see, for example, A Triangle of Care.

* Provide continuity of care for the person with dementia – this will enable new workers to build a solid foundation with them. Consistency and continuity are as important for carers as they are for people who need care and support.

* Promote the independence of care recipients.

* Person-centred care is challenging to get into everyday care; attention to detail on support plans and their formulation process is key to working this way. Life history is very important, but this needs to be combined with knowledge about an individual's health conditions, their social psychology and their personality.

* Treat home care staff as professional experts and support their career development. Involve staff in planning their own learning and development. Ensure employees have the expertise, support and tools they need. Research and use the excellent resources and training materials available. Finally, empower staff to be inspirational – to think *outside the box*, be flexible and communicate what works best.

SOURCE: BASED ON SKILLS FOR CARE (2014).

Services should be flexible to meet the needs of each client. These can include personal care, such as assistance with bathing, dressing, eating and medication; and home help, covering all aspects of day-to-day housework, shopping, meal preparation and household duties. Therefore, in many cases, home care provides help with ADL, as these abilities start to deteriorate from the early stages of dementia onwards (Giebel, Sutcliffe and Challis, 2015). But the scope also includes companionship services that can involve everything from escorting clients on visits or appointments to simple conversation and good company. Home support services also include befriending services or transport day care, while respite for carers is also an option to alleviate informal carer stress duties (Sutcliffe et al., 2016). Researchers now know that place matters (Golant, 2003), and 'it is better, more enjoyable, easier, and less adaptionally costly to grow old in some places than in others' (Golant, 1984, p.2).

Home health care has become an attractive alternative to hospital-based care for a number of reasons. It may be more economically viable as the home setting may be more cost-effective (Naylor et al., 1999; National Association for Home Care and Hospice, 2010). The option to receive home health care is also consistent with the concept of ageing in place. UNISON, the largest public service union, conducted a survey of home care workers entitled 'Time to Care' to help address this imbalance and to illustrate the reality of home care work. The online survey, which was open to home care workers who were either UNISON members or non-members, attracted 431 responses between June and July 2012. This survey found that home care workers were often forced to rush their work or leave early, and also found that the majority of respondents did not receive set wages, making it hard to plan and budget (UNISON, 2012). It is generally felt that most home care visits should be at least half an hour long to enable carers to provide the personalised and dignified care that elderly patients need when being supported to stay in their own home, as a guideline on social care services from NICE indicates (Torjesen, 2015). The wellbeing of this part of the workforce has inevitably come under scrutiny given the potential abuse of zero-hour contracts in certain jurisdictions.

Health care professionals who are charged with delivering health care services in the home setting daily encounter substantial obstacles and challenges. Technological support and other interventions have the potential to alleviate health care providers of these burdens, but only if the designers of such technologies and interventions have a comprehensive understanding of the challenges and the needs of health care providers (Beer et al., 2014). Health care is moving from the hospital to the home. Home health care is described as a range of medical and therapeutic services delivered at a care recipient's home for the purpose of promoting, maintaining or restoring health or maximising the level of independence, while minimising the effects of disability and illness, including terminal illness (Jones, Harris-Kojetin and Valverde, 2012). Problem-solving therapy (PST) is a structured, research-based intervention developed by Mynors-Wallis et al. (1997). It is based on cognitive behavioural therapy principles that follow a logical sequence to identify, prioritise, explicitly define and develop solutions for key problems. The primary persons involved in home health care can be subdivided into two groups: the health care provider (formal or informal individuals providing health care) and the health care recipient (individuals receiving care).

For individuals with dementia, the home environment can promote a sense of personhood, continuity and normalcy in the face of major life events, often experienced as a result of multiple losses in the cognitive, functional and social domains of their lives (Sixsmith and Sixsmith, 1991). A large number of patients with Alzheimer's disease, predominantly females, live alone with severe cognitive and functional impairment. The amount of home-help services used did not reflect cognitive severity, suggesting that home help did not meet the needs related to cognitive deterioration. Increased knowledge of how community-based services can better accommodate the care needs of solitary-living individuals with Alzheimer's is essential (Wattmo, Londos and Minthon, 2014).

—— Community-based rehabilitation ——

> Rehabilitation achieves this by focusing on the impact that the health condition, developmental difficulty or disability has on the person's life, rather than focusing just on their diagnosis. It involves working in partnership with the person and those important to them so that they can maximise their potential and independence, and have choice and control over their own lives. It is a philosophy of care that helps to ensure people are included in their communities, employment and education rather than being isolated from the mainstream and pushed through a system with ever-dwindling hopes of leading a fulfilling life. (NHS England, 2016b, p.5)

How we create these spaces and respond to them will determine the most appropriate places to call home. At the same time, there is a need for researchers to examine new environments that are designed to provide a 'more appropriate', or rather, 'preferred', living environment for younger people with complex health needs (Muenchberger et al., 2011). The WHO and other UN-affiliated bodies have promoted community-based rehabilitation (CBR) since at least 1979, particularly as a strategy to make rehabilitation available to persons with disabilities in low- and middle-income countries (Helander et al., 1989). The WHO guide itself is a superb introduction (WHO, 2010).

CBR is currently implemented in over 90 countries. It was first initiated by the WHO following the International Conference on Primary Health Care in 1978 and the resulting Declaration of Alma-Ata (WHO, 2010). One way of promoting health and delivering preventive care to older people is through regular home visiting. Several studies of home visits by teams based at general practices have shown promising results, with home visitors identifying a large number of previously unmet medical and social needs. Health visitors are well placed to promote the health of older people and to provide surveillance and support (Elkan et al., 2000). Community nurses can be employed by NHS trusts, GPs, charities such as Dementia UK or private providers delivering NHS services. However, their numbers are falling. The Royal College of Nurses has warned that community nurses working in the NHS in England have almost halved in a decade – from 12,620 in 2003 to 6656 in 2013 (Salman, 2016).

Within the framework of the WHO's International Classification of Functioning, Disability and Health, an individual's health state is understood as a vector of capacities to function in a set of domains that range from hearing, seeing and moving around to cognition and affect (Chatterji et al., 2015). Health-related rehabilitation is delivered along a continuum of care ranging from hospital care to rehabilitation in primary care and community settings, and includes measures to enable a person to achieve and maintain optimal functioning in interaction with his or her environment (Skempes, Stucki and Bickenbach, 2015). Significantly, CBR has evolved in recognition of the Convention on the Rights of Persons with Disabilities, including a declaration that CBR should be grounded in human rights principles. One of these principles is 'empowerment, including self-advocacy', whereby empowerment implies the involvement of persons with disabilities in all matters of their concern (Cleaver and Nixon, 2014).

The CBR matrix of the WHO is shown in Figure 13.1.

A recurrent theme of this book has been the need to promote reablement – termed 'restorative care' in Australia, New Zealand and the US – as a service intervention that is being adopted across high-income countries as an alternative to more costly institutional care. It aims to promote independence and help older people to remain in their own home for as long as possible (Aspinal et al., 2016). Reablement is a time-limited, person-centred, home-based intervention for older people who are at risk of functional decline, often after an accident or period of illness (Glendinning et al., 2010).

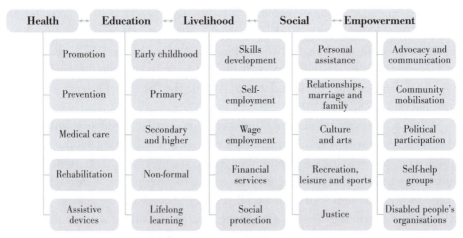

Figure 13.1: The CBR matrix

In light of the evolution of community-based rehabilitation (CBR) into a broader multisectoral development strategy, a matrix was developed in 2004 to provide a common framework for CBR programmes. The matrix consists of five key components – the health, education, livelihood, social and empowerment components.
Source: Reproduced by kind permission of WHO (2010, p.25).

The history of this approach is a long and distinguished one. Portage is a small town in Wisconsin, US, where the first home teaching scheme began in 1969. It was originally developed to support children with special needs and their families living in rural areas. This method of providing help to parents of children with special needs is now in use in many parts of the UK and around the world. In Japan, the government has promoted the development of a broad network of services aimed at assisting family members in providing in-home care and developing systems for community-based, rather than institutional, care of frail elderly (Campbell and Ikegami, 2003).

National governments now, therefore, do have opportunities to take or retake the lead to ensure that community support and the social inclusion of persons with severe mental illness health problems are not just ideological slogans, but solid policy (van Hoof et al., 2015). Especially in times of economic crisis, there is a challenge involved in keeping the social inclusion and community support of persons with severe mental health problems on the national policy agenda (Knapp et al., 2009). Housing satisfaction is an important component of wellbeing, continuity and autonomy in later life (Wahl, 2001). Many people can experience a good life in a care home or equivalent, but most prefer home life for its quality, self-determination and economy (Challis et al., 2002). Thus, investment in models that maintain life at home and avoid relocation directly or indirectly (via a general hospital admission) is required.

Community rehabilitation is unsurprisingly being unlocked in the new models of care. The NHS Newcastle Gateshead CCG and Gateshead Council are working together to enhance health within care homes through the Provider Alliance Network (PAN) to deliver the Gateshead Integrated Community Bed and Home-Based Care Service.[2] It is envisaged that PAN will provide holistic care and seamless support across the traditional health and social care boundaries, and will also oversee and connect health care for a population who are cared for and supported in long- and short-term-stay community beds as well as helping those individuals in their family home undertaking reablement, rehabilitation and recovery services.

Buurtzorg, social innovation, complexity and leadership

To be considered an innovation, a process or outcome must meet two criteria:

» The first is novelty: although innovations need not necessarily be original, they must be new to the user, context or application.

---

2   Available at dementiaroadmap.info/gateshead/resources/gateshead-care-home-project/#.V8sxi2 VX _FI (accessed 4 Oct 2016).

» The second criterion is improvement: to be considered an innovation, a process or outcome must be either more effective or more efficient than pre-existing alternatives.

Furthermore, as I discussed in Rahman (2014), successful innovations are ones which diffuse and get adopted very effectively.

To this list of improvements we add more sustainable or more just ones. By sustainable we mean solutions that are environmentally as well as organisationally sustainable – those that can continue to work over a long period of time (Phllis Jr, Deiglmeier and Miller, 2008). Reframing the narrative from one emphasising individual traits to one emphasising complex adaptive systems arguably makes much better sense of the non-linear, dynamic relationships between multiple stakeholders for collective action in this type of context (Schwandt, Holliday and Pandit, 2009). Social innovation has been described as innovation 'for the greater good' (Tidd and Bessant, 2014, p.353).

Founded in the Netherlands in 2006/07, the Dutch home care provider Buurtzorg Nederland has attracted widespread interest for its innovative use of self-governing nurse teams. Buurtzorg is Dutch for Neighbourhood Care and is a highly successful, award-winning model of quality home care. One particular reason why complexity thinking should be ideally suited to social entrepreneurship research is that 'complexity management is coupled to ethics or values – the need to encourage a diversity and autonomous action implies a respect for other people (and their ideas) and a high level of trust' and a common vision (Pidd, 2004, p.41). Home care in the Netherlands is provided to patients needing temporary services following hospital discharge, patients with chronic conditions requiring medical services, people with dementia, and individuals in need of end-of-life care.

Rather than relying on different types of personnel to provide individual services – the approach taken by most home health providers – Buurtzorg expects its nurses to deliver the full range of medical and support services to clients. The latter point has sparked particular interest in the UK where a key challenge is meeting the needs of an ageing population increasingly susceptible to comorbidity and complex long-term conditions (RCN, 2015). Several organisations are experimenting with self-managed team structures and decentralisation of decision-making at the level of frontline nurses and nurse assistants, but implementing the vision of Buurtzorg requires a more holistic approach. Buurtzorg teams care for patients in need of home, hospice and dementia care, working with the family, primary care providers and community resources to help patients maintain their independence in the least restrictive environment possible (Nandram, 2012).

Buurtzorg was set up by Jos de Blok (himself a former nurse), who envisaged a reformed district nursing system in the Netherlands. Prior to Buurtzorg, home care services in the Netherlands were fragmented, with patients being cared for by multiple practitioners and providers. However, the presumption that the chief driver of success in such programmes lies in the special 'heroic' attributes of their founders stands in opposition to a complex systems framing of the process wherein it is the nonlinear interdependencies inherent in the system that are crucial, and not any single actor (Goldstein, Hazy and Silberstang, 2008). In many high-income countries, integration of services is hampered by the fragmented supply of health and social care services as a result of specialisation, differentiation, segmentation and decentralisation (Stange, 2009). Ongoing financial pressures within the health sector have led to home care providers cutting costs by employing a low-paid and poorly skilled workforce who are unable to properly care for patients with comorbidities, leading to a decline in patient health and satisfaction.

Buurtzorg's answer to this problem was to give its district nurses far greater control over patient care – a factor which it attributes as key for its rapid growth. Some home care services require nursing expertise, but many others, such as help with ADL (e.g. dressing, bathing or toileting), can be provided by less trained, less expensive personnel (Monsen and de Blok, 2013). Nurses lead the assessment, planning and coordination of patient care with one another. The model consists of small self-managing teams of a maximum of 12 professionals (comprising both nurses and other allied health professionals). These teams provide coordinated care for a specific catchment area, typically consisting of between 40 and 60 patients. Their organisational structure aligns with the neurophysiological drivers of successful social functioning, fostered by an environment of mutual trust and collaboration that includes reward systems, communication systems, decision processes, information flow and remuneration systems (Monsen and de Blok, 2013).

It is fascinating to ask what really drives social entrepreneurship and innovation such as Buurtzorg – surely more than just 'capping costs'?

A compelling statement is provided by Tidd and Bessant (2014): 'In many ways the public sector represents a major application field for social innovation […] while there may be concerns about costs and using resources wisely, the fundamental driver is around social change' (p.357).

Respite services

Respite services may be delivered informally by family and friends or may entail the use of a formal service. There are different types of formal respite services, such as in-home services, adult day care centres, residential aged care facilities (RACFs) and hospitals (Neville et al., 2015). The type is determined by the needs of the carer and the person with dementia and the availability of services in the locality.

Caring for someone with dementia can be emotionally and physically demanding, but also exceptionally rewarding. Respite care is any intervention designed to give rest or relief to carers. It is not clear what positive and negative effects such care may have on them, or on people with dementia. Services such as respite, either in the home of an individual with dementia, in a day care centre or in a residential facility, can temporarily ease carers' physical and emotional workload (Stirling et al., 2012). While many people with dementia require institutional care, having a co-resident carer improves the likelihood that people can live at home. Although caring can have positive aspects, carers still report a high need for respite (Phillipson, Jones and Magee, 2014). The provision of respite is consistently identified by carers of people with dementia as one of their critical unmet needs (Brodaty, Thomson and Fine, 2005). For carers, respite services offered them normality and freedom and enabled them to engage freely in a sort of normal life (Ashworth and Baker, 2000).

To support respite use, there is a need for local action to be augmented at a community or population level by strategies to address attitudinal and resource barriers that influence subgroups of the carer population who may be more vulnerable to service non-use (Phillipson et al., 2014). Recent systematic reviews conclude that use of respite programmes may support carers of people with dementia to continue in their caring situation for longer (Eagar et al., 2007; Parker et al., 2008). Defining the content of day care centre services for adults may be a challenge, as the term often describes a building rather than the service or the aims of the interventions offered (Manthorpe and Moriarty, 2014). A day care centre service offers communal care, with paid or voluntary carers present, in a setting outside the users' own home. Individuals come or are brought to use the services, which are available for at least four hours during the day, and return home on the same day (Tester, 2001).

In a Cochrane review, 'Respite Care for People with Dementia and Their Carers', the three studies that compared respite care to no respite care found no evidence of any benefit of respite care for people with dementia or for their carers on any outcome, including rates of institutionalisation and carer burden (Maayan, Soares-Weiser and Lee, 2014). It has been noted that there is variation in the models of day services used by different countries, and some comparative research in this area may be beneficial to gain a global perspective (Iecovitch and Biderman, 2013). Existing day programmes are not always well utilised by those they are intended to serve. As Iecovitch and Biderman (2013) state, regardless of the important goals of adult day services, they need to be utilised to be of benefit.

—— Essential reading ——

Brooker D, Latham I. 2015. *Person-Centred Dementia Care, Second Edition: Making Services Better with the VIPS Framework*, London: Jessica Kingsley Publishers.

Pulsford D, Thompson R. 2013. *Dementia: Support for Family and Friends*, London: Jessica Kingsley Publishers.

References

Allen R. 2014. The Role of the Social Worker in Adult Mental Health Services, London: The College of Social Work, available at http://cdn.basw.co.uk/upload/ http://cdn.basw.co.uk/upload/basw_112306-10.pdf basw_112306-10.pdf (accessed 29 Nov 2016).

Aloulou H, Mokhtari M, Tiberghien T, Biswas J, Phua C, Kenneth Lin JH, Yap P. 2013. Deployment of assistive living technology in a nursing home environment: methods and lessons learned. BMC Med Inform Decis Mak, 8(13), 42.

Andrén S, Elmståhl S. 2008. The relationship between caregiver burden, caregivers' perceived health and their sense of coherence in caring for elders with dementia. J Clin Nurs, 17(6), 790–799.

Ashworth M, Baker AH. 2000. 'Time and space': carers' views about respite care. Health and Social Care in the Community, 8(1), 50–56.

Aspinal F, Glasby J, Rostgaard T, Tuntland H, Westendorp RG. 2016. New horizons: reablement – supporting older people towards independence. Age Ageing, May, afw094 (e-pub ahead of print).

Au A, Gallagher-Thompson D, Wong MK, Leung J, et al. 2015. Behavioral activation for dementia caregivers: scheduling pleasant events and enhancing communications. Clin Interv Aging, 10, 611–619.

Banerjee S, Murray J, Foley B, Atkins L, Schneider J, Mann A. 2003. Predictors of institutionalisation in people with dementia. J Neurol Neurosurg Psychiatry, 74(9), 1315–1316.

Bardram J, Hansen T, Mogensen M, Soegaard M. 2006. Experiences from real-world deployment of context-aware technologies in a hospital environment. UbiComp 2006: Ubiquitous Computing, 369–386.

Bastiani E, Librelotto GR, Freitas LO, Pereira R, Brasil MB. 2013. An approach for pervasive homecare environments focused on care of patients with dementia: CENTERIS 2013 – Conference on ENTERprise Information Systems/PRojMAN 2013 – International Conference on Project MANagement/HCIST 2013 – International Conference on Health and Social Care Information Systems and Technologies. Procedia Technology, 9, 921–929.

Baun MM, McCabe BW. 2003. Companion animals and persons with dementia of the Alzheimer's type: therapeutic possibilities. American Behavioral Scientist, 47, 42–51.

Beer JM, McBride SE, Mitzner TL, Rogers WA. 2014. Understanding challenges in the front lines of home health care: a human-systems approach. Appl Ergon, 45(6), 1687–1699.

Bird M, Llewellyn-Jones RH, Smithers H, Korten A. 2002. Psychosocial Approaches to Challenging Behaviours in Dementia: A Controlled Trial, Canberra: Commonwealth Department of Health and Ageing.

Brodaty H, Thomson C, Fine M. 2005. Why caregivers of people with dementia and memory loss don't use services. International Journal of Geriatric Psychiatry, 20, 537–546.

Bunn F, Goodman C, Sworn K, Rait G et al. 2012. Psychosocial factors that shape patient and carer experiences of dementia diagnosis and treatment: a systematic review of qualitative studies. PLoS Med, 9(10), e1001331.

Campbell JC, Ikegami N. 2003. Japan's radical reform of long-term care. Social Policy & Administration, 37(1), 21–34.

Carers UK. 2014. Facts about Carers, available at www.carersuk.org/for-professionals/policy/policy-library/facts-about-carers-2014 (accessed 3 Oct 2016).

Cavallo F, Aquilano M, Arvati M. 2015. An ambient assisted living approach in designing domiciliary services combined with innovative technologies for patients with Alzheimer's disease: a case study. Am J Alzheimers Dis Other Demen, 30(1), 69–77.

Challis D, von Abendorff R, Brown P, Chesterman J, Hughes J. 2002. Care management, dementia care and specialist mental health services. International Journal of Geriatric Psychiatry, 17, 315–325.

Charlesworth G, Shepstone L, Wilson E, Reynolds S, et al. 2008. Befriending carers of people with dementia: randomised controlled trial. BMJ, 336(7656), 1295–1297.

Chatterji S, Byles J, Cutler D, Seeman T, Verdes E. 2015. Health, functioning, and disability in older adults – present status and future implications. Lancet, 385(9967), 563–575.

Chu MT, Khosla R, Khaksar SM, Nguyen K. 2016. Service innovation through social robot engagement to improve dementia care quality. Assist Technol, April (e-pub ahead of print)

Ciro CA. 2014. Maximizing ADL performance to facilitate aging in place for people with dementia. Nurs Clin North Am, 49(2), 157–169.

Cleaver S, Nixon S. 2014. A scoping review of 10 years of published literature on community-based rehabilitation. Disabil Rehabil, 36(17), 1385–1394.

Dam AE, de Vugt ME, Klinkenberg IP, Verhey FR, van Boxtel MP. 2016. A systematic review of social support interventions for caregivers of people with dementia: are they doing what they promise? Maturitas, 85, 117–130.

Dasios A, Gavalas D, Pantziou G, Konstantopoulos C. 2015. Hands-on experiences in deploying cost-effective ambient-assisted living systems. Sensors (Basel), 15(6), 14487–14512.

de Labra C, Millán-Calenti JC, Buján A, Núñez-Naveira L, et al. 2015. Predictors of caregiving satisfaction in informal caregivers of people with dementia. Arch Gerontol Geriatr, 60(3), 380–388.

de Oliveira DC, Vass CD, Aubeeluck A. 2015. Ageing and quality of life in family carers of people with dementia being cared for at home: a literature review. Quality in Primary Care, 23(1), 18–30.

de Witt L, Ploeg J. 2014. Caring for older people living alone with dementia: health care professionals' experiences. Dementia (London), February (e-pub ahead of print).

Dekkers W. 2011. Dwelling, house and home: towards a home-led perspective on dementia care. Med Health Care Philos, 14(3), 291–300.

Desai AK, Grossberg GT, Sheth DN. 2004. Activities of daily living in patients with dementia: clinical relevance, methods of assessment and effects of treatment. CNS Drugs, 18(13), 853–875.

Dröes RM, Breebaart E, Meiland FJ, Van Tilburg W, Mellenbergh GJ. 2004. Effect of Meeting Centres Support Program on feelings of competence of family carers and delay of institutionalization of people with dementia. Aging Ment Health, 8(3), 201–211.

Dyck I, Kontos P, Angus J, McKeever P. 2005. The home as a site for long-term care: meanings and management of bodies and spaces. Health Place, 11(2), 173–185.

Eagar K, Owen A, Williams K, Westera A, et al. 2007. *Effective Caring: A Synthesis of the International Evidence on Carer Needs and Interventions. Wollongong: Centre for Health Service Development*, University of Wollongong.

Elkan R, Robinson JJ, Blair M, Williams D, Brummell K. 2000. The effectiveness of health services: the case of health visiting. Health Soc Care Community, 8(1), 74–78.

Ennis SK, Larson EB, Grothaus L, Helfrich CD, Balch S, Phelan EA. 2014. Association of living alone and hospitalization among community-dwelling elders with and without dementia. J Gen Intern Med, 29(11), 1451–1459.

Filan SL, Llewellyn-Jones RH. 2006. Animal-assisted therapy for dementia: a review of the literature. Int Psychogeriatr, 18(4), 597–611.

Frank J. 2005. Semiotic Use of the Word 'Home' among People with Alzheimer's Disease: A Plea for Selfhood? In GD Rowles, H Chaudhury (eds), *Home and Identity in Late Life: International Perspectives*, New York: Springer.

Gallagher-Thompson D, Tzuang YM, Au A, Brodaty H, et al. 2012. International perspectives on nonpharmacological best practices for dementia family caregivers: a review. Clin Gerontol, 35(4), 316–355.

Giebel CM, Sutcliffe C, Challis D. 2015. Activities of daily living and quality of life across different stages of dementia: a UK study. Aging & Mental Health, 19(1), 63–67.

Gillsjö C, Schwartz-Barcott D. 2011. A concept analysis of home and its meaning in the lives of three older adults. International Journal of Older People Nursing, 6(1), 4–12

Gilmour H. 2004. Living alone with dementia: Risk and the professional role. Nursing Older People, 16, 20–24.

Gitlin LN, Winter L, Dennis MP, Hodgson N, Hauck WW. 2010. A biobehavioral home-based intervention and the wellbeing of patients with dementia and their caregivers: the COPE randomized trial. JAMA, 304(9), 983–991.

Glendinning C, Jones K, Baxter K, Rabiee P, et al. 2010. *Home Care Reablement Services: Investigating the Longer-Term Impacts (Prospective Longitudinal Study)*, York: Social Policy Research Unit, available at php.york.ac.uk/inst/spru/pubs/1882 (accessed 3 Oct 2016).

Godfrey M, Randall T, Long A, Grant M. 2000. *Review of Effectiveness and Outcomes: Home Care*, Exeter: Centre for Evidence Based Social Services, University of Exeter.

Golant SM. 1984. *A Place to Grow Old: The Meaning of Environment in Old Age*. New York: Columbia University Press.

Golant SM. 2003. Conceptualizing time and behavior in environmental gerontology: a pair of old issues deserving new thought. The Gerontologist, 43, 638–648.

Goldstein JA, Hazy JK, Silberstang J. 2008. Complexity and social entrepreneurship: a fortuitous meeting. Emergence, Complexity and Organization, 10(3), 9–24.

Harris PB. 2006. The experience of living alone with early stage Alzheimer's Disease: What are the person's concerns? Alzheimer's Care Quarterly, 7, 84–94.

Helander E, Mendis P, Nelson G, Goerdt A. 1989. *Training in the Community for People with Disabilities*, Geneva: World Health Organization.

Hellstrom I, Nolan M, Lundh U. 2007. Sustaining 'couple hood': spouses' strategies for living positively with dementia. Dementia: The International Journal of Social Research and Practice, 6(3), 383–409.

HM Treasury. 2002. *The Role of the Voluntary and Community Sector in Service Delivery: A Cross Cutting Review*, London: Stationery Office.

Holmas TH, Islam MK, Kjerstad E. 2013. Interdependency between social care and hospital care: the case of hospital length of stay. Eur J Public Health, 23(6), 927–933.

Hussein S, Manthorpe J. 2012. The dementia social care workforce in England: secondary analysis of a national workforce dataset. Aging Ment Health, 16(1), 110–118.

Hwang SS, Kim Y, da Yun Y, Kim YS, Jung HYJ. 2012. Exploration of the associations between neurocognitive function and neuroleptics side effects. Psychiatr Res, 46, 913–919.

Iecovitch E, Biderman A. 2013. Attendance in adult day care centers of cognitively intact older persons: reasons for use and nonuse. Journal of Applied Gerontology, 32(5), 561–581.

Innes A. 2002. The social and political context of formal dementia care provision. Ageing Soc, 22, 483–499.

Iwarsson S, Wahl HW, Nygren C. 2004. Challenges of cross-national housing research with older people: Lessons from the ENABLE-AGE project. European Journal of Ageing, 1, 79–88

Iwarsson S, Wahl HW, Nygren C, Oswald F, et al. 2007. Importance of the home environment for healthy aging: conceptual and methodological background of the European ENABLE-AGE Project. Gerontologist, 47(1), 78–84.

Janssen N, Handels RL, Koehler S, Ramakers IH, et al. 2016. Combinations of Service Use Types of People with Early Cognitive Disorders. J Am Med Dir Assoc, 17(7), 620–625.

Jones AL, Harris-Kojetin L, Valverde R. 2012. Characteristics and use of home health care by men and women aged 65 and older in the United States. National Health Statistics Reports,52.

Kanamori M, Suzuki M, Yamamoto K, Kanda M, et al. 2001. A day care programme and evaluation of animal-assisted therapy (AAT) for the elderly with senile dementia. Am J Alzheimers Dis Other Demen, 16(4), 234–239.

Khosravi P, Ghapanchi AH. 2016. Investigating the effectiveness of technologies applied to assist seniors: a systematic literature review. Int J Med Inform, 85(1), 17–26.

King E. 2015. *Social Care Jobs Are Changing to Meet the Needs of Our Time, The Guardian*, 7 December, available at www.theguardian.com/social-care-network/2015/dec/07/social-care-jobs-changing-integration (accessed 3 Oct 2016).

Kirk E, Burrows L, Kent B, Abbott R, Warren A. 2016. Facilitators and barriers to remaining at home for people with dementia who live alone: a protocol for a systematic review of qualitative evidence. JBI Database System Rev Implement Rep, 14(4), 20–29.

Klein R, Maybin J. 2012. *Thinking about Rationing*, London: King's Fund.

Knapp M, McDaid D, Medeiros H, the MHEEN Group. 2009. Balance of care (deinstitutionalisation in Europe): results from the Mental Health Economics European Network (MHEEN). Int J Integr Care, 9, e41.

Knight BG, Lutzky SM, Macofsky-Urban F. 1993. A meta-analytic review of interventions for caregiver distress: recommendations for future research. The Gerontologist, 33(2), 240–248.

König HH, Leicht H, Brettschneider C, Bachmann C, et al. 2014. The costs of dementia from the societal perspective: is care provided in the community really cheaper than nursing home care? J Am Med Dir Assoc, 15(2), 117–126.

Koponen M, Taipale H, Tanskanen A, Tolppanen AM, et al. 2015. Long-term use of antipsychotics among community-dwelling persons with Alzheimer's disease: a nationwide register-based study. Eur Neuropsychopharmacol, 25(10), 1706–1713.

Luppa M, Luck T, Brähler E, König HH, Riedel-Heller SG. 2008. Prediction of institutionalisation in dementia. Dementia and Geriatric Cognitive Disorders, 26, 65–78.

Maayan N, Soares-Weiser K, Lee H. 2014. Respite care for people with dementia and their carers. Cochrane Database of Systematic Reviews, 1, CD004396.

MacNeil Vroomen J, Van Mierlo LD, van de Ven PM, Bosmans JE, et al. 2012. Comparing Dutch case management care models for people with dementia and their caregivers: The design of the COMPAS study. BMC Health Serv Res, 12, 132.

Manthorpe J, Moriarty J. 2014. Examining day centre provision for older people in the UK using the Equality Act 2010: findings of a scoping review. Health and Social Care in the Community, 22(4), 352–360.

Martin S, Kelly G, Kernohan WG, McCreight B, Nugent C. 2008. Smart home technologies for health and social care support. Cochrane Database Syst Rev, 4(CD006412).

Marx MS, Cohen-Mansfield J, Regier NG, Dakheel-Ali M, Srihari A, Thein K. 2008. The impact of different dog-related stimuli on engagement of persons with dementia. American Journal of Alzheimer's Disease and Other Dementias, 25(1), 37–45.

McClendon MJ, Smyth KA. 2013. Quality of informal care for persons with dementia: dimensions and correlates. Aging Ment Health, 17(8), 1003–1015.

McClendon MJ, Smyth KA. 2015. Quality of in-home care, long-term care placement, and the survival of persons with dementia. Aging Ment Health, 19(12), 1093–1102.

McCurry J. 2015. Japan will be model for future super-ageing societies. Lancet, 386(10003), 1523.

Miranda-Castillo C, Woods B, Orrell M. 2010. People with dementia living alone: What are their needs and what kind of support are they receiving? International Psychogeriatrics, 22, 607–617.

Missotten P, Thomas P, Squelard G, Di Notte D, et al. 2009. Impact of place of residence on relationship between quality of life and cognitive decline in dementia. Alzheimer Disease and Associated Disorders, 23, 395–400.

Monsen KA, de Blok J. 2013. Buurtzorg: nurse-led community care. Creat Nurs, 19(3), 122–127.

Moorman SM, Macdonald C. 2013. Medically complex home care and caregiver strain. Gerontologist, 53(3), 407–417.

Moriarty J, Webb S. 2000. *Part of Their Lives: Community Care of Older People with Dementia*, Bristol: The Policy Press.

Moyle W, Jones C, Sung B, Bramble M, et al. 2016. What effect does an animal robot called cuddler have on the engagement and emotional response of older people with dementia? A Pilot Feasibility Study. Int J of Soc Robotics, 8, 145.

Muenchberger H, Sunderland N, Kendall E, Quinn H. 2011. A long way to Tipperary? Young people with complex health conditions living in residential aged care: a metaphorical map for understanding the call for change. Disabil Rehabil, 33(13–14), 1190–1202.

Mynors-Wallis L, Davies I, Gray A, Barbour F, Gath D. 1997. A randomised controlled trial and cost analysis of problem-solving treatment for emotional disorders given by community nurses in primary care. Br J Psychiatry, 170, 113–119.

Nandram S. 2012. In search for the spiritual innovation at the Dutch elderly home care organization Buurtzorg Nederland. Amity Case Research Journal, 16.

National Association for Home Care and Hospice. 2010. Basic Statistics about Home Care, available at www.nahc.org/assets/1/7/10hc_stats.pdf (accessed 3 Oct 2016).

Naylor MD, Brooten D, Campbell R, Jacobsen BS, et al. 1999. Comprehensive discharge planning and home follow-up of hospitalized elders: a randomized clinical trial. JAMA, 281(7), 613–620.

Neville C, Beattie E, Fielding E, MacAndrew M. 2015. Literature review: use of respite by carers of people with dementia. Health Soc Care Community, 23(1), 51–53.

Newhouse BJ, Niebuhr L, Stroud T, Newhouse E. 2001. Living alone with dementia: Innovative support programs. Alzheimer's Care Quarterly, 2(2), 53–61.

Ng TP, Broekman BF, Niti M, Gwee X, Kua EH. 2009. Determinants of successful aging using a multidimensional definition among Chinese elderly in Singapore. The American Journal of Geriatric Psychiatry, 17(5), 407–416.

NHS England. 2016a. An integrated approach to identifying and assessing Carer health and wellbeing, available at https://www.england.nhs.uk/wp-content/uploads/2016/05/identifying-assessing-carer-hlth-wellbeing.pdf (accessed 29 Nov 2016).

NHS England. 2016b. Commissioning guidance for rehabilitation, London: TSO, available at https://www.england.nhs.uk/wp-content/uploads/2016/04/rehabilitation-comms-guid-16-17.pdf (accessed 29 Nov 2016).

Nordgren L, Engström G. 2012. Effects of animal-assisted therapy on behavioral and/or psychological symptoms in dementia: a case report. Am J Alzheimers Dis Other Demen, 27(8), 625–632.

Nordgren L, Engström G. 2014. Animal-assisted intervention in dementia: effects on quality of life. Clin Nurs Res, 23(1), 7–19.

Novitzky P, Smeaton AF, Chen C, Irving K, et al. 2015. A review of contemporary work on the ethics of ambient assisted living technologies for people with dementia. Sci Eng Ethics, 21(3), 707–765.

Parker D, Mills S, Abbey J. 2008. Effectiveness of interventions that assist caregivers to support people with dementia living in the community: a systematic review. Int J Evid Based Healthc, 6(2), 137–172.

Phillipson L, Jones SC, Magee C. 2014. A review of the factors associated with the non-use of respite services by carers of people with dementia: implications for policy and practice. Health Soc Care Community, 22(1), 1–12.

Phills Jr JA, Deiglmeier K, Miller T. 2008. Rediscovering social innovation. Stanford Social Innovation Review (Fall).

Pidd M (ed.). 2004. *Systems Modelling: Theory and Practice*, Chichester: John Wiley and Sons Ltd.

Pulsford D, Thompson R. 2013. Dementia: Support for Family and Friends, London: Jessica Kingsley Publishers.

Quinn C, Clare L, Woods B. 2009. The impact of the quality of relationship on the experiences and wellbeing of caregivers of people with dementia: a systematic review. Aging Ment Health, 13(2), 143–154.

Rahman S. 2014. Living Well with Dementia, London: CRC Press.

RCN. 2015. RCN Policy and International Department Policy Briefing 02/15 August 2015: The Buurtzorg Nederland (home care provider) model Observations for the United Kingdom (UK), available at https://www2.rcn.org.uk/__data/assets/pdf_file/0003/618231/02.15-The-Buurtzorg-Nederland-home-care-provider-model.-Observations-for-the-UK.pdf (accessed 29 Nov 2016).

Richeson NE. 2003. Effects of animal-assisted therapy on agitated behaviors and social interactions of older adults with dementia. Am J Alzheimers Dis Other Demen, 18(6), 353–358.

Romeo L. 2015. *Why the NHS Needs Social Workers on Board*, available at www.theguardian.com/society/2015/dec/08/nhs-social-workers-on-board-health-care (accessed 23 Sept 2016).

Rummery K, Coleman A. 2003. Primary health and social care services in the UK: progress towards partnership? Soc Sci Med, 56(8), 1773–1782.

Saczynski JS, Pfeifer LA, Masaki K, Korf ESC., et al. 2006. The Effect of Social Engagement on Incident Dementia: The Honolulu-Asia Aging Study. American Journal of Epidemiology, 163(5), 433–440.

Salman S. 2016. *'Pillars of the Community': Why the NHS Needs More District Nurses*, available at www.theguardian.com/healthcare-network/2016/feb/25/district-nursing-community-nurses-career (accessed 23 Sept 2016).

Salpakoski A, Törmäkangas T, Edgren J, Kallinen M, et al. 2014. Effects of a multicomponent home-based physical rehabilitation program on mobility recovery after hip fracture: a randomized controlled trial. J Am Med Dir Assoc, 15(5), 361–368.

Schaller S, Mauskopf J, Kriza C, Wahlster P, Kolominsky-Rabas PL. 2015. The main cost drivers in dementia: a systematic review. Int J Geriatr Psychiatry, 30(2), 111–129.

Schwandt DR, Holliday H, Pandit G. 2009. The complexity of social entrepreneurship systems: social change by the collective. Complexity Science and Social Entrepreneurship, 191–210.

Schwarzkopf L, Menn P, Leidl R, Graessel E, Holle R. 2013. Are community-living and institutionalized dementia patients cared for differently? Evidence on service utilization and costs of care from German insurance claims data. BMC Health Serv Res, 13, 2.

Sharkey A. 2014. Robots and human dignity: a consideration of the effects of robot care on the dignity of older people, Ethics Inf Technol, 16, 63, doi:10.1007/s10676-014-9338-5

Shibata T, Wada K. 2011. Robot therapy: a new approach for mental health care of the elderly – a mini-review. Gerontology, 57(4), 378–386.

Sixsmith AJ, Sixsmith JA. 1991. Transitions in home experience in later life. The Journal of Architectural and Planning Research, 8(3), 181–191.

Skempes D, Stucki G, Bickenbach J. 2015. Health-related rehabilitation and human rights: analyzing states' obligations under the United Nations Convention on the Rights of Persons with Disabilities. Arch Phys Med Rehabil, 96(1), 163–173.

Skills for Care. 2014. Better Domiciliary Care for People with Dementia.

Skills for Care/Dementia UK. 2012. Dementia: Workers and Carers Together. A Guide for Social Care Workers on Supporting Family and Friends and Carers of People with Dementia.

Smebye KL, Kirkevold M, Engedal K. 2016. Ethical dilemmas concerning autonomy when persons with dementia wish to live at home: a qualitative, hermeneutic study. BMC Health Serv Res, 16, 21.

Söderhamn U, Landmark B, Eriksen S, Söderhamn O. 2013. Participation in physical and social activities among home-dwelling persons with dementia – experiences of next of kin. Psychol Res Behav Manag, 6, 29–36.

Stange KC. 2009. The problem of fragmentation and the need for integrative solutions. Annals of Family Medicine, 7(2), 100–103.

Stirling C, Leggett S, Lloyd B, Scott J, et al. 2012. Decision aids for respite service choices by carers of people with dementia: development and pilot RCT. BMC Med Inform Decis Mak, 12, 21.

Sutcliffe CL, Giebel CM, Jolley D, Challis D. 2016. Experience of burden in carers of people with dementia at the margins of long-term care. International Journal of Geriatric Psychiatry, 31(2), 101–108.

Svanström R, Sundler AJ. 2015. Gradually losing one's foothold – a fragmented existence when living alone with dementia. Dementia (London), 14(2), 145–163.

Tester S. 2001. Day Service for Older People. In C Clark (ed.), *Adult Day Service and Social Inclusion: Better Days*, London: Jessica Kingsley Publishers.

Thompson CA, Spilsbury K, Hall J, Birks Y, Barnes C, Adamson J. 2007. Systematic review of information and support interventions for caregivers of people with dementia. BMC Geriatr, 7, 18.

Tidd J, Bessant J. 2014. Strategic Innovation Management, New Jersey: John Wiley & Sons.

Torjesen I. 2015. Home care visits should be at least 30 minutes long, NICE says. BMJ, 351, h5057.

Towers AM, Holder J, Smith N, Crowther T, et al. 2015. Adapting the adult social care outcomes toolkit (ASCOT) for use in care home quality monitoring: conceptual development and testing. BMC Health Serv Res, 15, 304.

UNISON. 2012. *Time to Care: A UNISON Report into Homecare*, available at www.unison.org.uk/content/uploads/2013/11/On-line-Catalogue220152.pdf (accessed 23 Sept 2016).

Valentí Soler M, Agüera-Ortiz L, Olazarán Rodríguez J, Mendoza Rebolledo C, et al. 2015. Social robots in advanced dementia. Frontiers in Aging Neuroscience, 7, 133.

van Hoof F, Knispel A, Aagaard J, Schneider J, Beeley C, Keet R, van Putten M. 2015. The role of national policies and mental health care systems in the development of community care and community support: an international analysis. J Ment Health, 24(4), 202–207.

Victor CR, Scambler SJ, Bowling A, Bond J. 2005. The prevalence of, and risk factors for, loneliness in later life; a survey of older people in Great Britain. Ageing and Society, 25, 3, 357–376.

Vikström S, Borell L, Stigsdotter Neely A, Josephsson S. 2005. Caregivers' self-initiated support towards their partners with dementia when performing an everyday occupation together. OTJR Occupation Participation Health, 25, 34.

Wahl HW. 2001. Environmental influences on aging and behavior. In JE Birren, KW Schaie (eds) *Handbook of the psychology of aging* (5th ed.), New York: Academic Press.

Wattmo C, Londos E, Minthon L. 2014. Solitary living in Alzheimer's disease over 3 years: association between cognitive and functional impairment and community-based services. Clin Interv Aging, 9, 1951–1962.

Weber SR, Pirraglia PA, Kunik ME. 2011. Use of services by community-dwelling patients with dementia: a systematic review. Am J Alzheimers Dis, 26(3), 195–204.

Wilson E, Thalanany M, Shepstone L, Charlesworth G, et al. 2009. Befriending carers of people with dementia: a cost utility analysis. Int J Geriatr Psychiatry, 24(6), 610–623.

Wood-Mitchell A, James IA, Waterworth A, Swann A, Ballard C. 2008. Factors influencing the prescribing of medications by old age psychiatrists for behavioural and psychological symptoms of dementia: a qualitative study. Age Ageing, 37(5), 547–552.

World Health Organization (WHO). 2007, Global age-friendly cities project, available at www.who.int/ageing/projects/age_friendly_cities_network/en (accessed 3 Oct 2016).

World Health Organization (WHO). 2010. Community-Based Rehabilitation: CBR Guidelines, available at apps.who.int/iris/bitstream/10665/44405/9/9789241548052_introductory_eng.pdf (accessed 3 Oct 2016).

World Health Organization (WHO). 2012. Dementia: A Public Health Priority, available at extranet.who.int/agefriendlyworld/wp-content/uploads/2014/06/WHO-Dementia-English.pdf (accessed 3 Oct 2016).

Yang CT, Liu HY, Shyu YI. 2014. Dyadic relational resources and role strain in family caregivers of persons living with dementia at home: a cross-sectional survey. Int J Nurs Stud, 51(4), 593–602.

Young Y, Kalamaras J, Kelly L, Hornick D, Yucel R. 2015. Is aging in place delaying nursing home admission? J Am Med Dir Assoc, 16(10), 900.e1–6.

Zabalegui A, Hamers JP, Karlsson S, Leino-Kilpi H, et al. 2014. Best practices interventions to improve quality of care of people with dementia living at home. Patient Educ Couns, 95(2), 175–184.

— Chapter 14 ——————————————————————

CONCLUSION

Learning objectives ——————————————————

In this chapter, you are encouraged to reflect on how you might evaluate the relative importance of the biomedical model, personhood and person-centred care and human rights in providing integrated care for people with dementia.

— Introduction ——————————————————————

> Thirty years ago, Roy Griffiths in his landmark inquiry into the management of the NHS declared that 'if Florence Nightingale were carrying her lamp through the corridors of the NHS today she would almost certainly be searching for the people in charge'. It was the right diagnosis for the time. (Timmins, 2015, p.5)

This chapter will look at the following:

»   contemporary challenges in integrated care pathways

»   quality in integrated care

»   dignity and its measurement

»   uncertainty and ambiguity about a complex future

»   moving forward from here.

A useful definition of **integration** is provided by the WHO:

> The management and delivery of health services so that clients receive a continuum of preventive and curative services, according to their needs over time and across different levels of the health system. (WHO, 2008)

This needs to be considered in tandem with what the 'core purpose' of health systems might be, including for people with dementia and their carers:

> The core purpose of a health system should be to maximize the health of the population. When the main challenge is managing long-term conditions, maintaining health rather than delivering health care per se should be the goal. (Mountford and Davie, 2010, p.2407)

As I mentioned in the Preface, each person with dementia and their carers are entitled to the highest standards in person-centred integrated care.

One leap forward would be for all care settings to acknowledge and act on dementia being a terminal illness deserving a palliative approach at some stage.

The trend in current evidence clearly indicates that organisational integration will not deliver benefits if professions and practitioners do not change the way they work (Ham and Curry, 2011). This has clear implications for NHS organisations involved in the Transforming Community Services programme where community services have been integrated with other organisations. People may be living for longer, and this is to be certainly welcomed, but often they are living with several complex conditions that need constant care and attention. However, this is not only about older people, because a 'convenient' media myth is that older people and people with dementia are 'bankrupting' the NHS and social care. Children born with complex conditions are now living to adulthood, while those with learning disabilities and other groups have lifelong needs (National Collaboration for Integrated Care and Support, 2013). Integrated care refers to many different models of care, yet underlying these is a model where the patient's journey through the system of care should be made as simple as possible (Greaves et al., 2013).

It is now necessary to think about the standard definitions of integration used in management circles, and how these can be reconciled with different tranches in dementia, such as respecting personhood, human rights and the biomedical model. I will refer to some topics which I have explored in this book and I hope to demonstrate that this synthesis is incredibly interesting but very difficult.

—— Care pathways – time for a second look? ——

I first introduced the concept of the care pathways in Chapter 1. Put simply, a journey is what a family might take; conversely, a pathway includes all the resources needed to make that journey.

There are substantial problems in getting a gestalt view of the whole, instead of a piecemeal analysis of the components of any integrated health care system. The whole is much more than the sum of its parts. Unfortunately, there are substantial barriers to effective system leadership, and one may have the impression that system leadership is vital wherever integrated care takes place, for example devolved cities or sites of new models of care. Barriers to system leadership typically include money, training, misaligned financial incentives and the current system architecture, and not least regulation. They are also often interconnected in a complex way, which makes it difficult to break into bits (Timmins, 2015).

It may seem reasonable to suggest that the use of information/communications technologies and systems tools could lead to higher productivity, better-quality care and improved patient satisfaction (Reid et al., 2005). The NHS and social care sector are making progress in these issues by using, for example, personal integrated commissioning and electronic health care records. I surveyed the development of electronic records in Chapter 11.

Clinical pathways are essentially document-based tools that provide a link between the best available evidence and clinical practice. They provide recommendations, processes and timeframes for the management of specific medical conditions or interventions. To date, the dominant focus of quality measurement and reporting has been on processes and inputs in care, not on patient outcomes. Process measures can have advantages in that they are often easier to measure than outcomes; they require less risk adjustment and there are examples – arguably – where a favourable patient outcome has resulted despite a defective process (or where an unfavourable outcome has followed a faultless process) (Mountford and Davie, 2010).

Clinical pathways have been implemented worldwide, but the evidence of their impact from single trials is contradictory (Rotter et al., 2010). Specifically, Rotter and colleagues (2010) have observed considerable variation in study design and settings, preventing the statistical pooling of results for length of stay and hospital costs. Generally, poor reporting prevented the identification of characteristics common to successful clinical pathways.

There are various types of integration, shown in Box 14.1.

Integrated care pathways (ICPs) are ones which uniquely record deviations from planned care in the form of 'variances'. An ICP is intended to act as a guide to treatment and an aid to documenting a patient/client's progress. Clinicians are free to exercise their own professional judgements as appropriate, but any alteration to the practice identified within an ICP should be noted as a **variance**. The complexity of the health care industry allows for many opportunities to reduce variability by standardising many processes (Centre for Policy on Ageing, 2014).

Box 14.1: Five types of integration

* **Systemic:** coordinating and aligning policies, rules and regulatory frameworks

* **Normative:** developing shared values, culture and vision across organisations

* **Organisational:** coordinating structures, governance systems and relationships

* **Administrative:** aligning back-office functions, budgets and financial systems

* **Clinical:** coordinating information and services and integrating patient care within a single process; for example, developing extended clinical roles, guidelines and interprofessional education, or facilitating the role of patients in shared decision-making

SOURCE: SHAW, ROSEN AND RUMBLED (2011, TABLE 3, P.7).

It is worth noting that ICPs may involve formidable cultural conflicts; for example:

> The application of such methodologies to clinical care, however, may seem less intuitive because of the dynamic presentation of diseases and patients' response to medical treatment. Clinical care has historically been seen as highly individualized, with clinical judgment and medical decision-making solely owned by each health care provider and tailored specifically to each individual patient. (Buchert and Butler, 2016, p.318)

In the contemporary literature, care pathways based on a single medical condition have also been found to be unsuitable for this patient group. This is because disease-based care pathways are founded in studies that largely exclude patients with comorbid conditions; following clinical guidelines for individual diseases for patients with comorbidity might even lead to potential treatment conflicts (Røsstad et al., 2013). The under-recognised impact of comorbidity has been an important theme in my book.

Sleeman and colleagues (2015) have been able to understand the views of health care professionals through their qualitative research involving surveys of staff members from a single tertiary referral centre intensive care unit, producing some very elegant and striking conclusions.

They have proposed a model with four noteworthy components, outlined below and in Figure 14.1:

> **strong symbolic value:** potentially legitimises death as an outcome

» **benefits:** processes of care are clear, consistent and comprehensive

» **harms:** potential dangers due to tick boxing and poor decision-making

» **weak evidence:** not enough education or evidence.

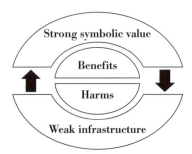

Figure 14.1: Sleeman's model of perception of an integrated care
plan at end of life, with four noteworthy components

Source: Sleeman et al. (2015).

Nonetheless, some overall conclusions about the effectiveness of clinical care pathways are helpful (Centre for Policy on Aging, 2014):

» Care pathways are most effective in contexts where the trajectory of care is predictable.

» Clinical pathways are associated with reduced in-hospital errors/ complications and improved documentation without impacting on the length of stay and hospital costs.

» In general, care pathways report a positive impact on clinical outcomes, cost reduction, patient satisfaction, teamwork and process outcomes, but these positive findings are not universal.

» Care pathways have the potential of enhancing cross-setting collaboration and rebalancing care between hospital and local community provision, but there is very little evidence of the use of care pathways in the community.

These four relatively predictable trajectories of care ICPs can be effective in supporting proactive care management and ensuring that patients receive relevant clinical interventions and/or assessments in a timely manner (Allen et al., 2009). This can lead to improvements in service quality and efficiency without adverse consequences for patients. As emphasised in this book, however, the time course of a post-diagnostic life with dementia can be variable. One important constraint was reported to be a 'cultural aversion' among doctors that arises at least in part from the implication that pathways require multidisciplinary teamwork which will prejudice medical autonomy (Hindle and Yazbeck, 2005). In other words, pathways challenge clinical professional subcultures.

—— Quality in integrated care ——————

In 2001, the US Institute of Medicine's (IOM) *Crossing the Quality Chasm: A New Health System for the 21st Century* defined good-quality care as safe, effective, patient-centred, timely, efficient and equitable (Institute of Medicine, 2001). Value in health care is frequently created by concentrating on doing a few things well for a certain group of people, not trying to do everything for all patient groups. The fact that outcomes tend to be professionally focused and not patient-focused means that outcomes may actually have more *technical* relevance than relevance to patients' lives and functional status. Moreover, the many different clinical indicators used in medical practice do not always discern the aspects of health that patients consider important, or their relative value to patients. One is sometimes sadly reminded of the apocryphal surgeon's observation that the 'operation was a success but the patient died', indicating an existential gap between the views of clinicians and patients on health care (Devlin, 2010).

The precise definition of quality in health care is beyond the scope of this book, and the reader is strongly recommended to look elsewhere for a complete discussion of this topic.

However, quality can be variously measured in care pathways:

» improving the coordination and integration of care

» improving the quality of care, including from a patient perspective

» improving the management of chronic conditions

» understanding how quality in one part of the health care system impacts on other health care services

» lowering costs and improving productivity

» planning and developing health care services.

However, the discussion should revolve around more than the mere 'cost' of dementia. While the G8 Global Dementia Summit saw a financial investment and innovation in dementia research, one is left wondering where the value management of people currently living with dementia lies.

Take, for example, Muir Gray's comment (2011, p.33):

Elinor Ostrom has spent decades studying 'the tragedy of the commons' – how common wealth, forests or grazing land or fishing rights, can be destroyed if all the individuals who use them increase their use by an amount so small that it does not appear to make any difference. Her message of hope is that the tragedy is not inevitable, and that there are many examples where people acting together can preserve and increase the value of the common wealth. This is a message that clinicians and patients need to heed.

I first mentioned Ostrom in my discussion of co-production in Chapter 2.

Achieving high value for patients must become the overarching goal of health care delivery for dementia, with value defined as the health outcomes achieved per pound spent; this goal would benefit all actors in the system and can promote the economic sustainability of the health care system increases. In a comprehensive, publicly funded system like the UK's NHS facing a 'financial gap', there is an overriding imperative to deliver maximum health benefit per pound spent, and to maintain health rather than delivering health care per se should be the goal (see, for example, Mountford and Davie, 2010). Long-term conditions provide a particular opportunity to maximise value over time for individual patients and for the health system, since these patients experience greatest morbidity and incur the highest costs (Mountford and Davie, 2010).

The relationship between costs, outcomes and value for patients is shown in Figure 14.2.

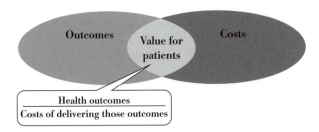

Figure 14.2: Costs, outcomes and value for patient

A recent King's Fund document, *Better Value in the NHS: The Role of Changes in Clinical Practice*, summarised useful advice (Alderwick et al., 2015). For example, it was reviewed that teams should measure their work, involve patients in work to improve care and also take time to understand the experience of patients, including responding to patient feedback. Alderwick and colleagues (2015) specifically refer to 'The Point of Care Foundation's Schwartz Rounds' as an example of how this can be done.[1]

Nick Black has emphasised that patient opinion is paramount in this new age of integrated care:

---

1   See https://www.pointofcarefoundation.org.uk/our-work (accessed 4 Oct 2016).

[…] those who assess hospitals must listen more to those who receive and deliver care. Patients, their relatives and friends, and staff have much to contribute and really want to help. If patients and nurses at Mid Staffordshire and junior doctors at Tameside had been listened to, subsequent events might have been avoided. Some websites show one way that such views can be collected. (Black, 2013, p.1)

Technology now has the potential to improve integrated care massively. At the moment, palliative patients with complex needs are cared for by multiple service providers. In addition, there is no consensus between geographical areas in the provision of key services, with delivery by different professionals or organisations and effectively a 'postcode lottery' for care. The mismatch of the needs of patients with individual services is exacerbated by poor coordination across different settings, resulting in huge frustration for patients, service users and carers.

There is considerable scope for innovation here. The Coordinate My Care record is electronic and displays the patient's diagnosis, prognosis, current problems, anticipated problems, advance care plan, resuscitation status and wishes (Smith et al., 2012). Such work, arguably, would not have been possible without the investment in research in palliative and end-of-life care, such as the literature I reviewed in Chapter 12.

Evidence shows that the systematic use of information from patient-reported outcome measures (PROMs) leads to better communication and decision-making between doctors and patients and improves patient satisfaction with care (Nelson et al., 2015). Nelson and colleagues (2015) argue that the extent to which these systems can improve care will depend on how effectively clinicians respond to the patient voice.

In the US, the National Quality Strategy (NQS), introduced in 2011 by the Agency for Healthcare Research and Quality on behalf of the US Department of Health and Human Services, set six clear improvement priorities to achieve better care, more affordable care and healthier communities (reviewed in Burstin, Leatherman and Goldmann, 2016). This national strategy offered an organising framework upon which to evolve health care measurement.

The priorities are:

» making care safer by reducing harm caused during the delivery of care

» ensuring that all persons, and their families, are engaged as partners in their care (e.g. advance care planning)

» promoting effective communication and coordination of care (e.g. patient experience of care)

» promoting the most effective prevention and treatment practices for the leading causes of mortality (e.g. primary percutaneous coronary intervention within 90 minutes of hospital arrival)

» working with communities to promote widespread use of best practices to enable healthy living (e.g. avoidable hospitalisation for asthma)

» making quality care more affordable for individuals, families, employers and governments by developing and spreading new health care.

One concern across a number of jurisdictions, however, is the *relative inability* of routine measurement systems to capture differences according to race, ethnicity, language, health literacy or insurance status; this has hampered efforts to improve equity (Burstin et al., 2016). Given the huge amount of literature on prevention and risk reduction, this is an important concern.

—— Dignity ——————————————————————

The managerial approach can sit extremely uneasily with clinical outcomes. Each day, clinicians must convince commissioners about the value of their work. Dignity is a key moral and philosophical concept in the care of people with dementia, many of whom are vulnerable (The Nuffield Council on Bioethics, 2009; Gastmans, 2013). It can be seen as a barometer of the 'moral compass' of dementia policy (Moody, 1998).

People with dementia have experienced big changes in their lives, directly related to their dementia, and indirectly related, for example in having to move from their own home to a nursing home (Heggestad and Slettebø, 2015). Dignity crosscuts a number of different areas of dementia care. Previous research has shown that life storytelling may promote the identity and self-esteem of people who suffer from dementia (McKeown, Clarke and Repper, 2006). All care professionals are encouraged to develop their skills and attitudes in environments where dignity is respected; to learn to practise so dignity is not impeded; to involve users and respect their preferences; and to learn how to change the environment so it does not threaten older people's dignity (Askham, 2005; Manthorpe et al., 2010).

Positioning theory proposes that interactions are based on the taking of 'positions', clusters of rights and duties to act in certain ways and impose particular meanings which enable or prohibit access to certain storylines (for a discussion, please see Stevens et al., 2013). It is argued that 'malignant positioning' can contribute to the creation of a climate that allows mistreatment to take place or fails to stop its development.

I considered malignant positioning in some depth in my discussion of abuse in Chapter 9.

Dignity is seen as an important component of quality of life (QoL) (Tranvåg, Petersen and Nåden, 2013), and this is tricky to measure. This book has shown the importance of spirituality as an approach that seeks to give meaning to life, to set values and sometimes seek transcendence, resulting in a spiritual identity. Spirituality and religion may even have some effect on cognitive decline, though this is currently uncertain, and help people use coping strategies to deal with their dementia and have better QoL (Agli, Bailly and Ferrand, 2015). But the precise definition of dignity keeps on recurring. Frequently associated with quality of care, dignity, as it applies in nursing facilities, is defined as a 'feeling experienced by residents', as well as a 'status conferred on residents' (Kane et al., 2003). Dignity as a concept in bioethics has been often criticised as too imprecise, even allowing the concept of human dignity to be applied in somewhat contradictory ways. There is also a 'human rights objection' to genetic research; the important position at stake in opposing some forms of genetic research is that of the human being (Chan, 2015). For those who believe that each of us has a spirit or a soul, a genetic 'reduction' of a human being would be objectionable.

The biomedical model and the doctor–patient relationship are certainly not immune from analysis, and what is 'normative' may be questioned. Medical communication in Western-oriented countries is dominated by concepts of shared decision-making and patient autonomy. In interactions with persons with dementia in the Roma community, for example, behavioural patterns rarely seem to be achieved because culture and ethnicity have often been shown as barriers in establishing an effective and satisfying doctor–patient relationship. The Roma community opposes informing terminal patients about their condition, widely practising a 'conspiracy of silence' (Roman et al., 2013). In Western cultures, despite an increasing emphasis on personhood, it is *not normal* for a physician to ask a patient with dementia about their religious or sexual beliefs; this can even contravene regulatory professional codes. In the biomedical model, reasons for deferring or avoiding disclosure include diagnostic uncertainty, the fear of stigmatisation, cultural preferences and competing expectations between patients and their companion(s), but components of a practical, patient-centred dementia disclosure include diagnostic education, discussing management goals and the provision of realistic hope with a focus on non-abandonment in the pursuit of dignity (Passmore, 2013).

In this book, I set out the case for how non-pharmacological psychosocial interventions in dementia care could improve QoL. These include life story work, reminiscence therapy, music therapy, humour therapy and aromatherapy. The variety of psychosocial interventions that are available may help people with dementia to build coping strategies, reduce distress, provide interpersonal connections and optimise remaining abilities (Johnston and Narayanasamy, 2016). But even doll therapy, akin to therapeutic 'lying' or covert medication, might not be 'dignity reducing'; for example, see Higgins' review (Higgins, 2010), which argues that doll therapy *preserves* dignity since the intervention can allow someone with dementia to take on a familiar role which may have been rewarding for them earlier in life.

I have considered some of the ethical issues to do with therapeutic lying in Chapter 5.

—— Measuring care and measuring dignity ——

There's an old adage that 'if you can't measure it, don't measure it'. Liz Ryan (2014), writing on the Forbes blogpost, comments:

> Who ripped business, a human activity as creative and inspiring as producing a Broadway show (which, of course, is business) or planting a garden or having a baby, and shoved it into a grey metal box labelled Formal, Stiff, Slow, Rulebound and Boring?

Ryan then remarks that the vast majority of things are actually measurable, and that 'measurable is our drug in the business world'. A similar concern is now rapidly emerging for metrics in health care.

Metrics in management can be used for 'corrective action'. Human dignity concerns our status and our equal worth, but also the ways in which various forms of degradation can flow from state power, and the distinctively dehumanising aspects of bad government practices (Riley, 2015). It is no surprise then that dignity can be used as a tool by regulators to see how good care is. Dignity's multiple meanings are rooted in the diverse sources of the idea, and this arguably reflects contemporary confusion about its definition. In the ancient Roman context, *dignitas* referred to the hierarchical concept of a person's status in society, whereas *dignitas hominis* referred to an account of man's elevated standing in the universe because of his ability to reason (Steinmann, 2016). Despite this, there has been some success in operationalising 'dignity'. For example, personal dignity relates to a sense of worthiness, is individualistic, tied to personal goals and social circumstances, and can be taken away or enhanced by circumstances or acts by others; this can be distinguished from 'basic dignity' which is the inherent dignity of each human being and can be regarded as a universal and inalienable moral quality (Albers et al., 2011).

Persons who are cared for in long-term care facilities are vulnerable to losing their personal dignity; arguably, an instrument measuring factors that influence dignity can be used to better target dignified care for an individual patient, but no such instrument is yet available for the long-term care setting. Oosterveld-Vlug and colleagues (2014) have described the creation of the Measurement Instrument for Dignity Amsterdam for Long-Term Care Facilities and assessed its validity and intra-observer agreement. Providing person-centred, dignity-conserving care for hospitalised patients is central to many health care policies and essential to the provision of effective palliative care. Issues that are more tangible to resident dignity, such as being treated with respect and compassion, and having opportunities to engage with others, are possibly not adequately captured in current NHS quality-of-care indicators (Thompson, McArthur and Doupe, 2016). Dignity-conserving care is highlighted as a necessary element of all health care and a responsibility of all health care professionals (Gallagher et al., 2008). Johnston and colleagues (2015) have discussed the design of the Patient Dignity Question, 'What do I need to know about you as a person to take the best care of you that I can?', based on empirical research about patients' perceptions of their dignity at end of life to help health care professionals understand the patient as a person.

Person-centred care has been identified as a key factor for upholding dignity in health and social care, and dementia care mapping (DCM) is a method that has been specifically developed to improve person-centred care (Bradford Dementia Group, 2005). Dementia care mapping developed from the pioneering work of Tom Kitwood on person-centred care. In his final book, *Dementia Reconsidered*, Kitwood (1997) described DCM as 'a serious attempt to take the standpoint of the person with dementia, using a combination of empathy and observational skill' (quoted in Brooker, 2005, p.4). A recent study has provided a sound argument for investigating the effectiveness of the DCM approach, and the extent to which it is associated with improvements in person-centred care and dignity (Woolley et al., 2008). But this precision is in marked contrast to the vague public perception of dignity. Even medical ethicists have the potential to provide precision. Human dignity belongs to human beings in Kant's conception because, on the one hand, they are *homo noumenon* – that is, free persons subject only to reason's universal legislation. As *homo phaenomenon*, on the other hand (sensible beings subject to natural causality), human beings possess no such distinction from (other) animals (Rothhaar, 2010). In the real world, valuing people is one of the four core features of enriched care planning described below:

> Enriched care planning is a means to an end which is delivering person-centred care. Person-centred care is care that values people regardless of age or cognitive ability; is individualised recognising that each individual is unique; includes the perspective of the person as central to all care planning; values the person as being able to live a life that has meaning and provides a supportive social environment to enable people to experience relationships. (May, Edwards and Brooker, 2009, p.15)

This is the heart of person-centred care, which I introduced in Chapter 1.

The development of specific tools to 'measure' dignity may, however, fly in the face of personhood. Many health care providers are reluctant to claim this particular aspect of care, which is variously referred to as spiritual care, whole person care, psychosocial care or dignity-conserving care. This reluctance is often framed in terms of a lack of expertise, for example resources including time, or attention as to how much time this might consume; however, 'when personhood is not affirmed, patients are more likely to feel they are not being treated with dignity and respect' (Chochinov, 2007, p.184). An unintended consequence might be to promote an organisational culture which is entirely counterproductive to respect for personhood. It is argued, for example, that 'abuse and neglectful practice thrives when staff focus on tasks, procedures and processes in preference to the experiences, choices and aspirations of individual service users' (Heath and Phair, 2009, p.143).

Yet it is precisely this focus on human rights-based approaches which is supposed to mitigate against abuse and neglect. Dignity furthermore interfaces with human rights. The first of the 30 articles which comprise the Universal Declaration of Human Rights pronounces: 'All human beings are born free and equal in dignity and rights. They are endowed with reason and conscience and should act towards one another in a spirit of brotherhood'.[2]

The notion of human rights necessarily presupposes persons to whom these rights apply. This influential construction of rights makes that presumption explicit by specifying a particular understanding of personhood: a person with rights has the capacity for reason and conscience (Fryson and Cromby, 2013).

I introduced the critical importance of rights-based approaches in Chapter 2. This interfaces in turn with the agenda of personalisation:

> ...we are all fundamentally, irreconcilably, both relational and interdependent, and this actual interdependence – and not some ideological construction of independence – should be the starting point for any conceptualisation of the human condition. (Fryson and Cromby, 2013, p.1165)

Possibly it is wrong to place too much weight on the logic and detail of any of these preambulatory formulations. They are intended as rhetorical devices, not solid philosophies; they probably represent political compromises (as argued by Waldron, 2013). But arguably these traditionalist conceptions of personhood can be challenged by awkward medical ethical dilemmas; should an embryo or foetus, without any likeness to human beings, share the same dignity and rights as persons (e.g. Tsai, 2001)? And yet dignity is pervasive across many strands of dementia care and support. In the parallel field of disability ethics, this research revealed that what constitutes an adequate home environment was one that enabled and promoted social dignity by providing access to essential conditions:

---

2   See www.un.org/en/universal-declaration-human-rights (accessed 23 Sept 2016).

...the ability to form and sustain meaningful relationships; access to community and civic life; access to control and flexibility of daily activities; access to opportunities for self-expression and identity affirmation; access to respectful relationships with attendants; access to opportunities to participate in school, work or leisure; and access to physical, psychological and ontological security. (Smith and Caddick, 2015, p.4186)

Uncertainty and ambiguity about a complex future

Dementia health, care and wellbeing are incredibly complex taken as a whole, because of the intricate links in a network between actors who are fundamentally interdependent. It may appear that the biomedical approach offers more certainty than personhood; even the issue of personal utility which I discussed in Chapter 11 demonstrates considerable uncertainty.

Interpreting human rights can also be difficult, for example in justifying whether CCTV in a care home is a necessary and proportionate response compared to the right to privacy of a resident. In formulating a strategy for integrated care for dementia, the delivery of health and social care has been further complicated by the rules of the market. There was concern when Sir David Nicholson challenged the accepted dogma that 'competition drives up quality' (as reported by West, 2013). Nicholson had been referring to section 75 of the Health and Social Care Act 2012, which put competition at the core of the latest legislation for the NHS. The issue was raised elegantly by Greaves and colleagues (2015, p.181):

Proponents of the [Health and Social Care] Act claim new alternative providers will be able to innovate, stimulate competition and improve quality. Opponents have suggested that there is a risk that they will hinder integrated care, select the easiest services and patients and focus on maximising profit ahead of performance.

The idea of people competing with one another to promote the health, wellbeing and care of people with dementia and carers seems wholly counterintuitive. So it is very likely that a fundamentally new approach in the legal infrastructure is needed, as well as a shift in societal attitudes.

Ben Hecht, on the Harvard Business Review blog (20 January, 2013), commented in a blogpost entitled 'Collaboration Is the New Competition':

Leaders and organizations are acknowledging that even their best individual efforts can't stack up against today's complex and interconnected problems. They are putting aside self-interests and collaborating to build a new civic infrastructure to advance their shared objectives. It's called collective impact and it's a growing trend across the country.

Collaboration in research, say in pooling the results of harmonised studies, or in interpreting 'big data', might yield faster and more reliable results for both neurochemical and care research. Currently, there is too much danger of reinventing the wheel, especially with both papers and national reports being regurgitated at regular intervals, without adequate replication or follow-up.

And with so many professional disciplines involved (e.g. geriatric psychiatry, social work, neurology, liaison psychiatry, the community geriatrician and so forth), there has to be an operational as well as strategic way of allowing people to work together for the public good for a shared goal, such as delivering the best palliative care outcomes. As Siouta and colleagues (2016, p.13) have put it:

> As the integration of [person-centred care] requires bringing together specialists from different backgrounds and their well-orchestrated coordination, the development of protocols that quantify their collaboration is imperative for the successful implementation of [person-centred care].

This ethos of collaboration, on top of 'co-production' (where nobody is left behind), should arguably also extend to different ways of working together in education and training. Interprofessional education has been defined as an activity that occurs when members of two or more professions (or students) learn with, from and about one another to improve collaboration and the quality of care (Pelone et al., 2015).

—— Concluding remarks ——————————

It is hard to say whether dementia care requires an incremental 'one last heave' approach or a fundamentally radical and innovative one. There are genuine concerns about whether the care home business model is fundamentally 'bust'. As Graham Ruddick (2016) commented in *The Guardian*:

> The financial pressure on older people and their families when trying to pay for social care is growing, with the average cost of a room in a care home now more than £30,000 a year. The cost of a care home room has risen by 5.2% in the last year, more than 10 times the average increase in pensioners' income.

And David Brindle (2016) reported with reference to Des Kelly, outgoing director of the National Care Forum, also in *The Guardian*:

> [Des Kelly] is adamant that the best social care, whether residential or at home, is local. While this does not mean it cannot be delivered by big

operators, with suitably decentralised structures, emerging findings from Care Quality Commission (CQC) inspections suggest that smaller is often better. About 80% of smaller care homes and homecare agencies in England are getting 'good' or 'outstanding' ratings, according to unpublished CQC analysis, compared to 68% overall.

But there are still reasons to be cheerful, perhaps. Caring for people living with dementia in care homes requires training in best dementia care practice and person-centred care. Baker (2015) provided an overview of the Positively Enriching and Enhancing Residents' Lives (PEARL) programme, which has been found to reduce antipsychotic medication use, depression scores and pain, and improve patient wellbeing. Notwithstanding, the future of integrated care more than ever before involves listening to what persons with dementia and their closest want and need, and how this can be delivered within the current public finances and legislative framework.

Fear of the future can be crippling, and it can be terrifying for people newly diagnosed with dementia to plan for it. It is said jokingly these days in corporate strategy that executives have taken to using the military acronym VUCA – Volatility, Uncertainty, Complexity, Ambiguity – to describe the world in which they operate (Berinato, 2014). There will soon be initial results from the new models of care reconciling enhancing health in care homes, with a small yet quite costly sample size, but will this be enough to draw any firm conclusions? As Vul and colleagues (2014) have framed the issue, 'If people are making decisions based on samples – but as samples are costly – how many samples should people use to optimize their total expected or worst-case reward over a large number of decisions?' (p.599).

We certainly cannot take anything for granted, a sentiment echoed by people living with dementia and carers. We have come a long way since the then Prime Minister's Dementia Challenge, but the overriding objective now must be to maintain an initial momentum which began with the seeds of 'dementia awareness' to mitigate against stigma and prejudice.

But where now?

There are very strong forces moving policy in the direction of community rehabilitation and a right to enhanced health and wellbeing, with a human rights focus. Person-centred care appears alive and well. And finally, we may – or may not – have a cure by 2025.

—— Essential reading ——

Brooker D, Latham I. 2015. *Person-Centred Dementia Care (2nd Edition): Making Services Better with the VIPS Framework*, London: Jessica Kingsley Publishers.
May H, Edwards P, Brooker D. 2009. *Enriched Care Planning for People with Dementia*, London: Jessica Kingsley Publishers.

Human rights

Rahman S. 2015. *Living Better with Dementia*, London: Jessica Kingsley Publishers, pp.251–253, 258–293.

Personhood

Rahman S. 2014. *Living Well with Dementia*, London: CRC Press, pp.101–120.

Other useful books

Hughes JC. 2014. *How We Think about Dementia: Personhood, Rights, Ethics, the Arts and What They Mean for Care*, London: Jessica Kingsley Publishers.

Mitchell G. 2016. *Doll Therapy in Dementia Care: Evidence and Practice*, London: Jessica Kingsley Publishers.

Rohra H. 2016. *Dementia Activist: Fighting for Our Rights*, London: Jessica Kingsley Publishers.

—— References ——

Agli O, Bailly N, Ferrand I. 2015. Spirituality and religion in older adults with dementia: a systematic review. Int Psychogeriatr, 27(5), 715–725.

Albers G, Pasman HRW, Rurup ML, de Vet HCW, Onwuteaka-Philipsen BD. 2011. Analysis of the construct of dignity and content validity of the patient dignity inventory. Health Qual Life Outcomes, 9, 45.

Alderwick H, Robertson R, Appleby J, Dunn P, Maguire P. 2015. *Better Value in the NHS: The Role of Changes in Clinical Practice*, London: King's Fund.

Allen DA, Gillen E and Rixson LJ. 2009. Systematic review of the effectiveness of integrated care pathways: what works, for whom, in what circumstances? International Journal of Evidence-Based Healthcare, 7(2), 61–74.

Askham J. 2005. The role of professional education in promoting the dignity of older people. Quality and Ageing, 6, 10–16.

Baker CJ. 2015. The PEARL programme: caring for adults living with dementia. Nurs Stand, 30(5), 46–51.

Berinato S. 2014. *A Framework for Understanding VUCA*, Harvard Business Review blog, available at hbr.org/2014/09/a-framework-for-understanding-vuca (accessed 3 Oct 2016).

Black N. 2013. Time for a new approach to assessing the quality of hospitals in England. BMJ, 347, f4421.

Bradford Dementia Group. 2005. *DCM 8 User's Manual*. Bradford: University of Bradford.

Brindle D. 2016. Social Care Interview. Des Kelly: 'More people will be paying for care' (18 May), available at www.theguardian.com/society/2016/may/18/des-kelly-people-paying-for-care-national-care-forum, accessed 23 Sept 2016.

Brooker D. 2005. Dementia care mapping: a review of the research literature. Gerontologist, 45(1), 11–18.

Buchert AR, Butler GA. 2016. Clinical Pathways: Driving High-Reliability and High-Value Care. Pediatr Clin North Am, 63(2), 317–328.

Burstin H, Leatherman S, Goldmann D. 2016. The evolution of health care quality measurement in the United States. J Intern Med, 279(2), 154–159.

Centre for Policy on Ageing. 2014. *The Effectiveness of Care Pathways in Health and Social Care*, London: CPA.

Chan DK. 2015. The concept of human dignity in the ethics of genetic research. Bioethics, 29(4), 274–282.

Chochinov HM. 2007. Dignity and the essence of medicine: the A, B, C, and D of dignity conserving care. BMJ, 335(7612), 184–187.

Devlin N. 2010. *Getting the Most out of PROMS: Putting Health Outcomes at the Heart of NHS Decision-Making, London:* The King's Fund.

Fyson R, Cromby J. 2013. Human rights and intellectual disabilities in an era of 'choice'. J Intellect Disabil Res, 57(12), 1164–1172.

Gallagher A, Li S, Wainwright P, Jones IR, Lee D. 2008. Dignity in the care of older people: a review of the theoretical and empirical literature. BMC Nurs, 7, 7–11.

Gastmans C. 2013. Dignity-enhancing nursing care: a foundational ethical framework. Nursing Ethics, 20, 142–149.

Greaves F, Pappas Y, Bardsley M, Harris M, et al. 2013. Evaluation of complex integrated care programmes: the approach in North West London. Int J Integr Care, 13, e006.

Ham C, Curry N. 2011. *What Is It? Does It Work? What Does It Mean for the NHS?* London: King's Fund.

Heath H, Phair L. 2009. Shifting the focus: outcomes of care for older people. Int J Older People Nurs, 4(2), 142–153.

Hecht B. 2013. Collaboration Is the New Competition. Available at hbr.org/2013/01/collaboration-is-the-new-compe (accessed 23 Sept 2016).

Heggestad AK, Slettebø Å. 2015. How individuals with dementia in nursing homes maintain their dignity through life storytelling – a case study. J Clin Nurs, 24(15–16), 2323–2330.

Higgins P. 2010. Using dolls to enhance the wellbeing of people with dementia in residential care. Nurs Times, 106(39), 18–20.

Hindle D, Yazbeck AM. 2005. Clinical pathways in 17 European Union countries: a purposive survey. Australian Health Review, 29(1), 94–104.

Institute of Medicine. 2001. *Crossing the Quality Chasm: A New Health System for the 21st Century,* Washington, DC: National Academy Press.

Johnston B, Narayanasamy M. 2016. Exploring psychosocial interventions for people with dementia that enhance personhood and relate to legacy – an integrative review. BMC Geriatr, 16, 77.

Johnston B, Pringle J, Gaffney M, Narayanasamy M, McGuire M, Buchanan D. 2015. The dignified approach to care: a pilot study using the patient dignity question as an intervention to enhance dignity and person-centred care for people with palliative care needs in the acute hospital setting. BMC Palliat Care, 14, 9.

Kane RA, Kling KC, Bershadsky B, Kane RL, et al. 2003. Quality of life measures for nursing home residents. Journal of Gerontology: Medical Sciences, 58A, 240–248.

Kitwood T. 1997. *Dementia Reconsidered: The Person Comes First,* Buckingham: Open University Press.

Manthorpe J, Iliffe S, Samsi K, Cole L, et al. 2010. Dementia, dignity and quality of life: nursing practice and its dilemmas. Int J Older People Nurs, 5(3), 235–244.

May H, Edwards P, Brooker D. 2009. Enriched Care Planning for People with Dementia, London: Jessica Kingsley Publishers.

McKeown J, Clarke A, Repper J. 2006. Life story work in health and social care: systematic literature review. Journal of Advanced Nursing, 55, 237–247.

Moody HR. 1998. Why dignity in old age matters. Journal of Gerontological Social Work, 29.

Mountford J, Davie C. 2010. Towards an outcomes-based health care system: a view from the United Kingdom. JAMA, 304(21), 2407–2408.

Muir Gray JA. 2011. *How to Get Better Value Healthcare (2nd Edition),* Oxford: Offox Press for Better Value Healthcare Ltd.

National Collaboration for Integrated Care and Support. 2013. *Integrated Care and Support: Our Shared Commitment, available at* www.gov.uk/government/uploads/system/uploads/attachment_data/file/287815/DEFINITIVE_FINAL_VERSION_Integrated_Care_and_Support_-_Our_Shared_Commitment_2013-05-13.pdf (accessed 23 Sept 2016).

Nelson EC, Eftimovska E, Lind C, Hager A, Wasson JH, Lindblad S. 2015. Patient reported outcome measures in practice. BMJ, 350, g7818.

Oosterveld-Vlug MG, Pasman HR, van Gennip IE, de Vet HC, Onwuteaka-Philipsen BD. 2014. Assessing the validity and intra-observer agreement of the MIDAM-LTC: an instrument measuring factors that influence personal dignity in long-term care facilities. Health Qual Life Outcomes, 12, 17.

Passmore MJ. 2013. Neuropsychiatric symptoms of dementia: consent, quality of life, and dignity. Biomed Res Int, 2013, 230134.

Pelone F, Reeves S, Ioannides A, Emery C, et al. 2015. Interprofessional education in the care of people diagnosed with dementia: protocol for a systematic review. BMJ Open, 5(4), e007490.

Reid PP, Compton WD, Grossman JH, Fanjiang G. (eds) (2005) Building a better delivery system: a new engineering/health care partnership, Washington, DC: The National Academies Press.

Riley S. 2015. Human dignity and the rule of law. Utrecht Law Review, 11, 2.

Roman G, Enache A, Pârvu A, Gramma R, et al. 2013. Ethical issues in communication of diagnosis and end-of-life decision-making process in some of the Romanian Roma communities. Med Health Care Philos, 16(3), 483–497.

Røsstad T, Garåsen H, Steinsbekk A, Sletvold O, Grimsmo A. 2013. Development of a patient-centred care pathway across health care providers: a qualitative study. BMC Health Serv Res, 13, 121.

Rothhaar M. 2010. Human dignity and human rights in bioethics: the Kantian approach. Med Health Care Philos. 2010, 13(3), 251–257.

Rotter T, Kinsman L, James EL, Machotta A, et al. 2010. Clinical pathways: effects on professional practice, patient outcomes, length of stay and hospital costs. Cochrane Database of Systematic Reviews, 3, CD006632.

Ruddick G. 2016. Care Home Rooms Now Cost More than £30,000 a Year, available at www.theguardian.com/society/2016/aug/17/care-home-rooms-now-cost-more-than-30000-pounds-a-year (accessed 23 Sept 2016).

Ryan L. 2014. 'If You Can't Measure It, You Can't Manage It': Not True, available at www.forbes.com/sites/lizryan/2014/02/10/if-you-cant-measure-it-you-cant-manage-it-is-bs/#5131bed43fae (accessed 23 Sept 2016).

Shaw S, Rosen R, Rumbled B. 2011. An Overview of Integrated Care in the NHS: What is Integrated Care? Nuffield Trust report.

Siouta N, Van Beek K, van der Eerden ME, Preston N, et al. 2016. Integrated palliative care in Europe: a qualitative systematic literature review of empirically-tested models in cancer and chronic disease. BMC Palliat Care, 15, 56.

Sleeman KE, Koffman J, Bristowe K, Rumble C, et al. 2015. 'It doesn't do the care for you': a qualitative study of health care professionals' perceptions of the benefits and harms of integrated care pathways for end of life care. BMJ Open, 5(9), e008242.

Smith B, Caddick N. 2015. The impact of living in a care home on the health and wellbeing of spinal cord injured people. Int J Environ Res Public Health, 12(4), 4185–4202.

Smith C, Hough L, Cheung CC, Millington-Sanders C, et al. 2012. Coordinate My Care: a clinical service that coordinates care, giving patients choice and improving quality of life. BMJ Support Palliat Care, 2(4), 301–307.

Steinmann R. 2016. The core meaning of human dignity. PER/PELJ, 19.

Stevens M, Biggs S, Dixon J, Tinker A, Manthorpe J. 2013. Interactional perspectives on the mistreatment of older and vulnerable people in long-term care settings. Br J Sociol, 64(2), 267–286.

The Nuffield Council on Bioethics. 2009. *Dementia: Ethical Issues. Nuffield Council Reports (1st Edition)*. London: Nuffield Council on Bioethics.

Thompson GN, McArthur J, Doupe M. 2016. Identifying markers of dignity-conserving care in long-term care: a modified delphi study. PloS One, 11(6), e0156816.

Timmins N. 2015. *The Practice of System Leadership: Being Comfortable with Chaos, London:* The King's Fund.

Tranvåg O, Petersen KA, Nåden D. 2013. Dignity-preserving dementia care: a metasynthesis. Nurs Ethics, 20(8), 861–880.

Tsai DF. 2001. How should doctors approach patients? A Confucian reflection on personhood. J Med Ethics, 27(1), 44–50.

Vul E, Goodman N, Griffiths TL, Tenenbaum JB. 2014. One and done? Optimal decisions from very few samples. Cogn Sci, 38(4), 599–637.

Waldron J. 2013. Is Dignity the Foundation of Human Rights? New York University School of Law, Public law and legal theory research paper series, working paper no. 12–73, January.

West D. 2013. Exclusive: Competition Rules Hold Back Quality, Says Nicholson, 25 November, available at www.hsj.co.uk/sectors/commissioning/exclusive-competition-rules-hold-back-quality-says-nicholson/5063515.article (accessed 3 Oct 2016).

WHO. 2008. Technical Brief No. 1: Integrated Health Services – What and Why?

Woolley RJ, Young JB, Green JR, Brooker DJ. 2008. The feasibility of care mapping to improve care for physically ill older people in hospital. Age Ageing, 37(4), 390–395.

AFTERWORD
Lucy Frost

First, I would like to congratulate Dr Rahman on this third book. As a nurse, specialising in the care of people living with dementia, and those who care for and support them, this will be a 'go to' text – for reference and for revisiting important topics relating to practice.

What seems to have been achieved in this book is a systematic analysis of the dementia care landscape. Throughout, this analysis aligns to the simple idea that dementia care should be about the person living with the dementia, and their families, friends and carers. Yes, this is a simple idea, yet the policy, variation in services geographically and a finite set of resources mean that dementia care is complicated. To produce a contemporary and definitive analysis of what care for people with dementia looks like today is a huge accomplishment.

Throughout this book, policy and the 'frameworks' that inform dementia care are considered and explained with clarity. The gaps that exist currently mean that people may not get the support they need, and it is very important they are not ignored.

Living with a dementia is without doubt complex, and will mean something different to each individual. Since 2000, I have had the privilege of working with people and families at different phases and stages of their experience of a dementia. Every person and family member feels something different; has a different question, a different worry, a different joy.

What they all have in common is a need for health and social care professionals to come into their lives with understanding, and a recognition of the need for the diseases that cause dementia symptoms to be understood, so that the person or their carer never feels they are being led blindly through our health and social care systems. They don't need us all to be experts in the scientific constructs of dementia, but they need us to know enough to respond sensitively and with confidence.

A better understanding of what person-centred care is, in the context of dementia, is what will help us to achieve this. I am hopeful that this book will appeal to specialists and non-specialists alike, and that it will inform and influence professionals who support people living with a dementia.

I believe that there is still a huge amount we don't know about dementia, why people experience different things and what 'excellent dementia care' really looks like in every setting. What we do know for sure is that, when we recognise unmet need, we can only respond well if we know who can help, where to find that help, and which part of the health and social care system is right for someone at any given time.

This book is an important milestone in the dementia care literature as it provides information to help us answer the difficult questions we face as professionals helping to support people and families. The different types of dementia all have in common that they cause a person to have needs around changing health and wellbeing. The discussion flowing through this book points to where the answers are in improving how we meet those needs.

Lucy Frost

SUBJECT INDEX

AUTHOR INDEX